Concepts of Epidemiology

An integrated introduction to the ideas, theories, principles and methods of epidemiology

Raj S. Bhopal

Alexander Bruce and John Usher Professor of Public Health
and
Head, Department of Community Health Sciences
University of Edinburgh, Scotland
formerly
Professor of Epidemiology and Public Health
University of Newcastle Upon Tyne

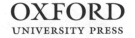
OXFORD
UNIVERSITY PRESS

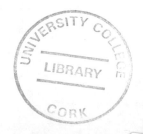

OXFORD
UNIVERSITY PRESS

Great Clarendon Street, Oxford OX2 6DP

Oxford University Press is a department of the University of Oxford.
It furthers the University's objective of excellence in research, scholarship,
and education by publishing worldwide in

Oxford New York

Auckland Cape Town Dar es Salaam Hong Kong Karachi
Kuala Lumpur Madrid Melbourne Mexico City Nairobi
New Delhi Shanghai Taipei Toronto

With offices in

Argentina Austria Brazil Chile Czech Republic France Greece
Guatemala Hungary Italy Japan Poland Portugal Singapore
South Korea Switzerland Thailand Turkey Ukraine Vietnam

Oxford is a registered trade mark of Oxford University Press
in the UK and in certain other countries

Published in the United States
by Oxford University Press Inc., New York

© R. S. Bhopal, 2002

British Library Cataloguing in Publication Data

Data available

Library of Congress Cataloging in Publication Data

Bhopal, Raj S.
Concepts of epidemiology : an integrated introduction to the ideas, theories,
principles, and methods of epidemiology / by Raj S. Bhopal.
Includes bibliographical references.
1. Epidemiology. I. Title.
[DNLM: 1. Epidemiology. WA 105 B575c 2002]
RA650 .B48 2002   614.4—dc21   2001052327

Typeset in 10\12 Minion
by Newgen Imaging Systems (P) Ltd, Chennai, India.
Printed in Great Britain
on acid-free paper by
Biddles Ltd, King's Lynn, Norfolk

ISBN 0 19 263155 1 (Pbk.)   978 0 19 263155 8

10 9 8

Foreword

When I was learning epidemiology in the late 1950s, I was inspired by the first edition of Jerry Morris's now classic little monograph, *Uses of Epidemiology*, but there were hardly any comprehensive current textbooks to guide me. The few available books were either unreadable, unhelpful, or failed to orient my thoughts along the directions my ideas were taking. How times have changed! Now there are so many good books that it is difficult for the uninitiated to select the most suitable one to meet their needs. In 1997, Raj Bhopal reviewed twenty-five textbooks of epidemiology, discussing their approach to the subject, and their strengths and weaknesses, in a critical commentary that is helpful to teachers and learners alike. Now, from the University of Edinburgh (where I spent five happy years in the 1960s), Raj Bhopal, who holds the Usher chair of public health, has written his own introductory textbook for graduate students who are embarking upon the detailed study of epidemiology.

This is an excellent introduction. Raj Bhopal's approach is conceptual—he describes and explains the underlying concepts and methods of epidemiology with clarity and with apt examples, and simple, elegant illustrations. Frequently throughout the text he asks penetrating questions that will test the limits of his readers' intellectual capacity— an admirable feature that other authors could copy with benefit to themselves and their readers. All the essentials are here: the person-population dyad, variation, error, bias, confounding, causality, the spectrum of disease, the 'iceberg' concept, risk and its relationship to disease frequency, study design, the ethical framework within which we practise epidemiology and conduct research, the relationship of epidemiology to other scholarly pursuits, and finally, some thoughts about the way the discipline has evolved and is likely to continue to evolve in the lifetime of those now entering upon careers in this field.

If I may speak directly to students starting the study of epidemiology: you can be grateful that there is a book like this to guide you along the fascinating pathway that leads to epidemiological enlightenment and understanding. This book will enable you to comprehend the connections between individual and population health, the natural history of disease, the methods of epidemiology, the interventions that work and don't work, and the role of epidemiology as the fundamental public health science. This is a book for you to buy, to read, to study, and to enjoy.

John M. Last
Emeritus Professor of Epidemiology,
University of Ottawa

I dedicate this book to my mother Bhagwanti Kaur Bhopal for impressing on me (and my siblings) the importance of education, and encouraging us to make up for her own lack of schooling and formal education; and to my father Jhanda Singh Bhopal for setting an example of how to work hard, shoulder responsibility, and strive for self-improvement.

Preface

The purpose of this book is to explain and illustrate the key concepts which underpin the science of epidemiology and its applications to research, policy making, health service planning and health promotion. The book emphasizes theory, ideas, and epidemiological axioms. In doing this I hope to counter the mounting criticism that epidemiology is an atheoretical discipline.

A concept is an idea, but the word is usually reserved for complex, or interrelated, ideas. A concept is the idea behind the word or phrase we use to describe something. This book, then, aims to explain the ideas underlying the language, principles, and basic methods in epidemiology. For example, the attributable risk and odds ratios are not considered merely as arithmetical equations or tools, but also in terms of the ideas underlying their calculation, applications, strengths, and limitations.

This book is primarily written for postgraduates beginning courses on epidemiology anywhere in the world, for the concepts are the same everywhere. Only the examples will differ. The book may be of interest to public health and other epidemiological practitioners interested in revisiting the fundamental ideas of their discipline. Undergraduates who are keen on epidemiology may find it helpful in deepening their understanding generally, or while studying some topics in a little depth. Health professionals (including busy doctors) may find this material an interesting adjunct to their use of epidemiological techniques or data. Finally, health service managers and policy makers may find this book a source of insights into the world of epidemiology.

There are 10 chapters. Many introductory courses are designed around 10–15 or so sessions. I envisage that the core of this book could be grasped in 10 days of committed study, preferably in the context of a taught course, but also independently.

The book is written in plain language but a basic understanding of biology is needed, as is some familiarity with illness and disease. However, medical terminology is explained and defined in a glossary. The learning objectives are expressed in terms of the reader acquiring understanding. I believe that achieving understanding is the highest form of learning; from that may flow a lasting and usable knowledge base, change of attitude, and the achievement of skills. There are exercises to help readers to deepen their understanding. Each chapter ends in a summary.

The motivation to write this book came from two directions, one in academia, the other in public health practice. As an examiner of both undergraduate and postgraduate students I was surprised, and crestfallen, to see how many students could not clearly explain basic ideas such as the difference between a case-control and cohort study, sometimes even after a year of study. In my duties in the health service I participated in many discussions on why service demands exceeded supply even after new investments were made. Not once did anyone invoke the crucial concept of the iceberg of disease and symptoms to explain this phenomenon, and clearly even those who knew of it did not make the leap from the classroom to the boardroom. This book is deliberately discursive, not simply descriptive, to help readers to achieve a deeper understanding and to help bridge the world of theory to that of practice.

Students rapidly grasp the importance and worth of studying concepts, and demand more. The depth of understanding of concepts gained from most books and courses is insufficient to permit students to apply what they have learned to the problems they are to solve. The acid test of this book is whether readers find themselves using epidemiological concepts in their everyday work, not seeing them merely as theoretical constructs for the classroom and examination hall.

The conceptual frameworks within which the practice of epidemiology operates take a slightly different perspective from those of the science of epidemiology. The nature of research questions, the relative value of the various methods, and the approach to data analysis, presentation, and interpretation differ. This book demonstrates these differences and makes the implications explicit.

The book places heavy emphasis on integrating the ideas of epidemiology. The interdependence of epidemiological studies and their essential unity is an important theme of this book. It is, therefore, designed to be read as a whole, either as a foundation text or as a refresher. Each chapter, however, can be read independently if necessary, with cross-references to other chapters for required definitions.

This book differs in many ways from alternatives, for example:

◆ The concepts of epidemiology are discussed in detail, and in an integrated way.

◆ The concepts are dominant whereas in other books the methods dominate.

◆ The epidemiological idea of population is explicitly the foundation of the whole book. In most other books the population idea is implicit and in some it is neglected.

◆ The practical applications of each concept are considered, and illustrated with examples drawn from contemporary research and public health practice, including healthcare policy and planning. The idea is that the reader will acquire the depth of knowledge to use the concepts and not merely be aware of them.

◆ The work is rooted in the basic ideas of the science of epidemiology, which are wholly applicable worldwide, not just in Europe or North America.

◆ The emphasis is on gaining understanding, and not on calculations, except where this is essential to understanding.

◆ Most of the exercises require reflection not calculation.

In short this textbook focuses on a theme which is the most important in any science, is too often overlooked, and which students demand more of: concepts.

R.S.B

Acknowledgements

My foremost debt is to the innumerable people who have taught me, whether in the classroom, seminar, and conference, or by their writings. One absorbs ideas and facts from others and over time synthesizes them with one's own thoughts and experiences. Eventually, it is impossible to distinguish one's own ideas from those of others. If my readers recognize their own ideas, and think they are incompletely acknowledged, then please accept my thanks and let me know.

Needless to say, I am responsible for all remaining errors of fact or interpretation—readers would do me a great favour by alerting me to any they discover (E-mail raj.bhopal@ed.ac.uk).

Many people have helped me by giving encouragement, information, constructive criticism, and by helping to prepare the manuscript. I can list only a few here; the others are not forgotten.

Marcus Steiner, an MSc (Epidemiology) student and graduate at Edinburgh University, was my postgraduate reader-critic and helper. His advice and help, particularly with the technical preparation and development of the figures, was immensely useful. His comment after reading an early draft, 'I wish I knew all this before', was highly motivating to me at times of difficulty.

Dr Sonja Hunt stimulated me to think about figure 10.1. Dr Colin Fischbacher helped me proof-read the manuscript and made several thoughtful observations. Professor John Last enthusiastically agreed to write the foreword.

Others who provided academic advice on one or more specific chapters include: Professor Carl Shy, Dr David Chappel, Dr Eileen Kaner, and four anonymous referees who commented on the book proposal and chapter outlines.

I thank Dr Mike Lavender for permission to use extracts from our joint unpublished paper on the role of epidemiology in priority setting, and co-authors on various publications that I have drawn on (these are referenced). I have drawn heavily on my publications to prepare Chapter 10 and acknowledgements are given below.

Helen Liepman, Commissioning Editor at Oxford University Press, deserves thanks for her enthusiasm, expert support, and patience.

I conceived this book while in my post as Professor of Epidemiology and Public Health at the University of Newcastle upon Tyne, England. The embryonic and fetal growth stages of the idea were nourished during my sabbatical at the Department of Epidemiology of the School of Public Health at the University of North Carolina at Chapel Hill, and on my return to Newcastle. The birthplace of the book, however, was in Edinburgh, during my tenure as Alexander Bruce and John Usher Professor of Public Health in the Section of Public Health, Department of Community Health

Sciences, Edinburgh University. I thank these departments and institutions, and my colleagues within them.

Secretarial support was provided chiefly by Lorna Hutchison, Carole Frazer (both Newcastle University), Betsy Seagroves (University of North Carolina), Janet Logan, and Hazel King (both Edinburgh University). Hazel bore the dual challenge of making sense of the styles of many other secretaries, and finishing the job.

It is customary to thank one's family, for many sacrifices including forsaking the dining room which is taken over by the author as a writing den. In my case I offer grateful thanks to my wife Roma for encouraging me to finish the project, for accepting the sleep disruption caused by early morning shuffling as I slipped out of bed and into the study, and for my lack of enthusiasm for late night revelries. She also allowed me to use the dining room as the second study in the last month of the project! I have four sons, Sunil, Vijay, Anand, and Rajan, and I ask their forgiveness for sometimes being too busy and distracted to give them and their passions the attention they deserved.

R.S.B.

Permissions

Permission to use material published elsewhere and due acknowledgements

I have drawn upon *A Dictionary of Epidemiology (4th Ed)* by J. Last throughout the book and, especially, the glossary (with the permission of the author). Direct quotations are attributed but readers will recognize the general debt I owe.

Chapter 2

Figure 2.2 is adapted from Figure 2 in G. Rose (1985) *International Journal of Epidemiology, 14*, 32–38 (with permission).

Chapter 3

Figures 3.1, 3.2, 3.3, and Table 3.4 are based on the concepts in R. Bhopal (1991) *Journal of Public Health Medicine, 13*, 281–9 (published with permission).

The artwork for Figs 3.4–3.7 was originally done by the Newcastle Medical School's Medical Illustration Unit under my direction.

Figure 3.7 and Tables 3.5 and 3.6 were first published in R. Bhopal *et al.* (1992) *British Medical Journal, 304*, 1022–7 (Figure 1 and Tables 2 and 3). They are published here with permission.

Figure 3.8 was first published in Bhopal *et al.* (1991)*British Medical Journal, 302*, 378–83, and Table 3.7 is an extract from the same paper (Table 2). They are published here with permission.

Chapter 4

The abstract in Box 4.6 is similar to the one published in Bhopal *et al.* (1998) *Occupational and Environmental Medicine, 55*, 812–22 (published with permission from the BMJ Publishing Group).

The data in Table 4.2 were first published by the Health Education Authority, a body that no longer exists. The source is acknowledged.

Chapter 5

The statistics for Table 5.1 are extracts from I. Semmelweiss's book *The etiology, concept, and prophylaxis of childbed fever*, republished in C. Buck *et al.* (1988) *The challenge of epidemiology*. PAHO, Washington.

The drawings of the triangle (Fig. 5.4) and wheel of causation (Fig. 5.7), now in widespread use, were inspired by those published in Mausner and Bahn (1985) *Epidemiology*, 2nd edn. Saunders, Philadelphia.

The model of the component causes (Fig. 5.11) is based on the ideas and diagrams in K. Rothman and S. Greenland (1998) *Modern Epidemiology*. Lippincott, Philadelphia.

Chapter 6

Figure 6.8 is based on figure 9.6 in Mausner and Bahn (1985) *Epidemiology*, 2nd edn. Saunders, Philadelphia. It is published with permission. Mausner and Bahn, in turn, based it on data from T. J. Vecchio (1966) *New England Journal of Medicine*, 274, 1171 (with permission).

Table 6.2 is prepared from text published in W. Holland and S. Stewart (1990) *Screening in health care*, pp. 12–13. Nuffield Provincial Hospitals Trust with permission.

Figure 6.10 is from Raffle, A.E. (2000) Honesty about screening programmes is best policy. *British Medical Journal*, **320**, 872 (with permission from the BMJ Publishing Group).

Chapter 7

Figure 7.3 is from unpublished work by R. Williams and based on data reported in an abstract (Bodansky, H. J., Airey, C. M., Chell, S. M., Unwin, N., & Williams, D.R.R. (1997) The incidence of lower limb amputation in Leeds, UK: setting a baseline for St Vincent. International Diabetes Federation Meeting. *Diabetologia*, A1850). The figure is published here with permission of the senior authors D.R.R. Williams and N. Unwin.

The bath model (Fig. 7.6) develops a diagram given to me by Ms Denise Howel: thanks are recorded.

The codes in Table 7.6 are extracted, with acknowledgement, from WHO's ICD-10 (International statistical classification of diseases and related health problems. World Health Organisation, Geneva, 1992).

Chapter 8

Table 8.1 is a small extract from a large table published in M. Marmot *et al.* (1984) *Immigrant mortality in England and Wales*. HMSO, London. The source is acknowledged.

Table 8.2 is a small extract of a table published in T. Pless-Mulloli *et al.* (1998) *Environmental Health Perspectives, 106*, 189–96. The source is acknowledged.

Table 8.12 extracts data from R. Doll and A. Bradford Hill (1956) *BMJ*, 2, 1071–81 as summarized by Mausner and Bahn in *Epidemiology*, table 7.4. Table 8.12 adapts this table (with permission of Saunders Co. and the BMJ).

Table 8.14 is based on that published on p. 29 in J. Mackintosh *et al.* (1998) *Step by step guide to epidemiological health needs assessment*. Newcastle University, Newcastle upon Tyne (there is no copyright, and R. Bhopal is the second author).

Table 8.15 is based on that published in *BMJ* (1994) *309*, 327–30 and is published here with permission.

Tables 8.17, 8.18, and 8.19 are based on work reported in Lee (1998) *International Journal of Epidemiology, 27*, 1053–6 (with permission of the author and the editor).

Chapter 9

The data in Table 9.3 are extracted from a large table in R. Bhopal *et al.* (1998) *Occupational and Environmental Medicine, 55*, 812–22 (with permission).

Chapter 10

Table 10.1 was first published by R. Bhopal in: S. Rawaf, V. Bahl (ed.) (1998) *Health needs assessment in ethnic minority groups.* Royal College of Physicians, London (used with permission).

Table 10.2 is adapted from a joint unpublished work with M. Lavender (published with permission of the co-author).

The text in Chapter 10 combines new and edited published writings. The edited material is as follows:

Discussion on paradigms, e.g. some of 10.1 and 10.5 draws on Bhopal, R. S. (1999) Paradigms in epidemiology textbooks: In the footsteps of Thomas Kuhn. *American Journal of Public Health, 89*, 1162–5. Copyright 1999 by the American Public Health Association (with permission).

Section 10.3 draws on an unpublished paper with M. Lavender (with permission of the co-author).

Discussion on the US and UK context, e.g. Section 10.8 draws on Bhopal, R. S. (1998) The context and role of the American School of Public Health: Implications for the UK. *Journal of Public Health Medicine, 20*, 144–8 (with permission).

Sections 10.10.1 and 10.11 on tobacco draw on Edwards, R., Bhopal, R. (1999) The covert influence of the tobacco industry on research and publication: a call to arms. *Journal of Epidemiology and Community Health, 53*, 261–2 (with permission from the BMJ Publishing Group).

Section 10.10.2 draws on Bhopal, R. S., Rankin, J., McColl, E., Thomas, L., Kaner, E., Stacy, R., Pearson, P., Vernon, B., & Rodgers, H. (1997) The vexed question of authorship: views of researchers in a British medical faculty. *British Medical Journal, 314*, 1009–12, and other work with these colleagues. This help is acknowledged.

Section 10.10.3 and other discussions on race, ethnicity, and health draw upon Bhopal, R. (1997) Is research into ethnicity and health racist, unsound, or important science? *British Medical Journal, 314*, 1751–6 (with permission from the BMJ Publishing Group).

Sections 10.14 and 10.15 draw on Bhopal, R. (2001) *Generating health from the pattern of disease.* Royal College of Physicians, London **31**, 293–8 (with permission).

The Section 10.12 draws heavily on P. Skrabanek and J. McCormick's book *Follies and fallacies in medicine* (with permission of the second author and the publisher).

Contents

Glossary

Acute An adjective commonly applied to diseases that have a short time course.

Adenocarcinoma A cancer of musosal cells.

AIDS Acquired immune deficiency syndrome is the serious multisystem disease resulting from infection by the human immodeficiency virus (HIV).

Allele See gene.

Anorexia Impaired appetite for food which can lead to serious illness; when caused by psychological factors it is called anorexia nervosa.

Angina See Rose angina.

Aristotle Greek philosopher, scientist and general scholar living 384–322 BC.

Arrhythmia An abnormal rhythm—usually applied to the heart, e.g. atrial fibrillation.

Association A link, connection, or relationship, between risk factors, diseases, and most usually between risk factors and diseases.

Asthma A respiratory disease characterized by difficulty in breathing caused by narrowing of the airways (which is reversible).

Atrial fibrillation An irregular heart beat resulting from very rapid and irregular contractions of the atrium (one of the chambers of the heart).

Autosomal A genetic disorder relating to any chromosome except the sex chromosomes.

Blood pressure Usually refers to the pressure in the systemic arteries (not veins and pulmonary arteries), as measured by sphygmomanometer (see below).

Bradford Hill (Austin) Statistician, 1897–1991, renowned for his work on smoking and cancer, and clinical trials, and on enunciating causal criteria.

Brucellosis An infection caused by Brucella microorganisms, characterized by recurrent fevers.

Capture–recapture methods A technique whereby two or more incomplete data sets are used to estimate the true size of the population of interest. Usually, the method is applied to elusive populations, e.g. the homeless.

Carcinogen(ic) A substance that increases the risk of developing a cancer (an adjective describing such a substance).

Case A person with the disease or problem under investigation.

Caseous An adjective applied to cheese-like lesions produced in response to inflammation, e.g. in tuberculosis.

Cataract An opacity in the lens of the eye.

Cause Something which has an effect, in the case of epidemiology, this effect being (primarily) a change in the frequency of risk factors or adverse health outcomes in populations.

Cholesterol A lipid (fatty substance) that is essential to many bodily functions that is transported in the blood via lipoproteins. Cholesterol and other lipids carried by low density lipoproteins (LDL/VLDL) are a risk factor for coronary heart disease (and like vascular diseases), while those carried by high density lipoproteins (HDL) seem to be protective.

Chromosome See gene.

Chronic An adjective commonly applied to diseases that have a long-lasting time course, and usually applied to non-toxic and non-infectious diseases.

Chronic bronchitis A lung disease characterized by production of excess sputum, wheezing, shortness of breath and eventual respiratory failure.

Circadian A rhythm with a cycle lasting about 24 hours, corresponding to each day.

Competing causes A concept where alternative causes of disease, or more usually causes of death, are in competition with each other; for example, in Afro-Caribbean populations one explanation of the comparatively low CHD rates is that the atherosclerotic process kills people from stroke. If stroke were to be controlled, it may be that CHD would become more common.

Confidence interval The interval, with a given probability, within which the true value of a summary measure such as a mean, or odds ratio, is contained.

Confounding The distortion of an association by other (confounding) factors that influence both the outcome and risk factor under study.

Contagion The infectious diseases that may be transmitted from person to person.

Congenital A health problem present at birth.

Cooling tower A term that describes a structure (sometimes including evaporative condensers, designed to extract heat from a liquid (usually water) before its re-circulation).

Coronary heart disease A group of diseases resulting from reduced blood supply to the heart, most often caused by narrowing or blockage of the coronary arteries that provide the blood supply to the heart.

Cot death A synonym for the sudden infant death syndrome, which is unexplained death in infancy (full definition in text).

Crohn's disease A disorder usually of the lower part of the small intestine, characterized by inflammation.

Cutaneous Associated with the skin.

Davey Smith (George) Epidemiologist, 1959–, working primarily in life-course epidemiology and inequalities in health.

Deep vein thrombosis Clotting of blood in the deep veins usually of the calves, thigh, and pelvis. The clots may lead to a pulmonary embolus.

Degenerative An adjective applied to disease thought to be resulting from deterioration of tissues over time, i.e. with age.

Demography The scientific study of population, particularly the factors that determine its size and shape, including birth and death. A cousin of epidemiology.

Diabetes (mellitus) A disease characterized by high levels of glucose in the blood caused by either lack or ineffectiveness of the hormone insulin.

Diethylstilboestrol A medication containing the hormone oestrogen.

Differential diagnosis A preliminary list of the most likely diseases in a patient, to be confirmed by further investigation.

Disease A bodily dysfunction, usually one that can be described by a diagnostic label. (For simplicity, this book concentrates on discussing diseases and uses this word when other words describing other health problems would also be appropriate, e.g. death, disability, illness, sickness, etc.)

Distribution The frequency with which each value (or category) occurs in the study population. The distribution of many variables takes on a characteristic shape. (See normal distribution.)

Down's syndrome A congenital genetic disorder, leading to mental retardation and a characteristic face caused by the presence of three chromosomes instead of two at the site of the 21st chromosome.

Durkheim (Emile) 1858–1917, French social theorist and eminent sociologist.

Einstein (Albert) Physicist, 1879–1955, most famous for the theory of relativity.

Elective In health care, a procedure done at a time chosen for its convenience, as opposed to being dictated by an emergency, e.g elective surgery.

Electrocardiogram (ECG) A recording of the electrical activity of the heart made by an instrument called an electrocardiograph.

Emphysema When applied to the lungs (pulmonary emphysema) a condition caused by destruction of lung tissue with gaseous distension.

Environment A broad concept in epidemiology, sometimes meaning everything except genetic and biological factors, and sometimes more qualified and narrow, e.g. physical environment.

Epidemiology See Chapter 1, but in short it is the science and craft that studies the pattern of diseases (and health, though usually indirectly) in populations to help understand both their causes and the burden they impose. This information is applied to prevent, control or manage the problems under study.

Evans (Alfred) Epidemiologist, 1917–1996, who developed criteria for causality, based on the Henle–Koch postulates.

Exposure A general term to indicate contact with the postulated causal factors (or agents of disease) used in a way similar to risk factor.

Fetal origins of disease hypothesis The phrase encapsulating the idea that early life circumstances, particularly in utero, have an important and lasting effect in determining health and disease in later life.

Gene The discrete basic unit (made of DNA or deoxyribonucleic acid) of the chromosome, which itself consists of numerous genes and other DNA material. Genes carry information coding for specific functions, e.g. making proteins. There are two copies of each gene, one on each of the pair of chromosomes. The two copies of the gene at a particular location on the pair of chromosomes are called alleles. There are 23 pairs of chromosomes in each cell in human beings (46 in total), and the number of genes is variously estimated as 25–50,000.

Genetic drift Genetic evolution, characteristically observable in small populations, arising from random variations in gene frequency.

Gestational diabetes High levels of blood glucose in association with pregnancy (see diabetes).

HDL See cholesterol.

Heaf test A skin test similar to the Mantoux test (see below).

Health A desired ideal, which includes being alive and free of disease, disability, and infirmity, characterized by well-being and efficient functioning in society.

Helicobacter pylori A bacterium that lives in the human stomach, and in some circumstances causes gastritis, ulcers, and stomach cancer.

Herd immunity The resistance of an entire community to spread of infection arising from immunity to the infection in a high proportion of the population preventing easy spread of disease.

Herpes Infection with the herpes simplex virus, characterized by small blisters, usually in and around the mouth (type I virus) and on and around the genitals (type II virus).

Histology The examination of tissues microscopically (and the results thereof).

Human papillomavirus (HPV) A viral micro-organism that causes, among other problems, cervical cancer.

Hume (David) Scottish philosopher and historian living 1711–1776.

Hypersensitivity reaction An abnormally powerful reaction by the immune system to exposure to some substances (allergens) such as peanuts, fur or pollen.

Hypertension A condition of having blood pressure above an arbitrarily defined level (presently 140/90). Hypertension is associated with many adverse outcomes, particularly atherosclerotic diseases.

Hypertrophy Unnatural enlargement of the tissues or structures.

Hypothesis A proposition that is amenable to test by scientific methods. (See null hypothesis.)

Illness The state of being unwell, usually due to disease.

Kaposi's sarcoma A cancer of cells (called reticuloendothelial cells) that is characterized by brown/purple patches on the skin.

Kuhn (Thomas) Science philosopher, 1922–1996, who is renowned for his work on the nature of scientific revolutions.

LDL/VLDL See cholesterol.

Lead-time The extra time gained by earlier than usual detection of disease, as in screening.

Legionnaires' disease A pneumonia usually caused by the bacterium *Legionella pneumophila* (so-called because of the major outbreak among the US Legionnaires attending a convention in Philadelphia in 1976).

Leprosy A multisystem infection caused by the bacterium *Mycobacterium leprae.*

Leukaemia A group of cancers of blood cells, with various types, e.g., chronic myeloid leukaemia, acute leukaemia, etc.

Life-grid approach A technique of data collection from the past where the information of interest, say, smoking habits, is linked to key life events, e.g. date of marriage, change of job, etc.

Logistic regression See multiple regression.

Lyme disease An infection caused by the microorganism Borrelia burgdorferi, characterized by skin rash and arthritis.

Lymph glands or nodes The fluid from the spaces between cells drains into the lymphatic system, a network of tubes. The lymph glands/nodes are lymphatic organs connecting into the lymphatic system, and are important in the immune system.

Mantoux test A skin test to assess the level of immune response to tuberculosis, using a protein derived from the tubercle bacillus.

Mean A statistical measure of the average, where the values for all the members of a group are added up, and the total is divided by the number of members.

Median A statistical measure of the average; the value that divides a group into two equal parts, those below and those above the median.

Melanoma A skin cancer of the pigment producing cells of the skin or eye.

Meningitis/meningococcal meningitis An inflammation of the lining around the brain (meninges), as, for example, caused by infection by the meningococcus bacterium.

Miasma An impurity in air capable of causing diseases, the impurity arising from a number of sources including decaying matter and from cases of disease. Cholera was long thought to be caused by miasma.

Micro-organism A term to refer to unicellular organisms including viruses, bacteria, protozoa, and algae.

Mm Hg Pressure recorded as millimetres of mercury (Hg) because traditionally mercury has been used in the sphygmomanometer.

Mode A statistical measure of the average; simply the most commonly occurring value.

Multiple (logistic) regression In regression analysis a mathematical model is constructed to describe the relation between one variable X (say, height), and another Y (say weight). The method then predicts Y, knowing X (the independent variable). Multiple regression permits the simultaneous assessment of the relation between several variables (X1, X2, etc.) and Y. The multiple logistic model is a variant where the predicted variable (Y) is the probability of an event and hence is of particular interest in epidemiology.

Natural history of disease The course of disease from inception to resolution (or death).

Neoplasm/neoplastic A new growth, usually applied to a cancer/an adjective usually used to describe something that is cancerous.

Normal distribution A distribution that describes well a great many biological variables. The mean, median and mode values are identical, the distribution is symmetrical around this value, and one standard deviation encapsulates 68 per cent of the population.

Null hypothesis A testable hypothesis stated in a way that implies that there is no difference between comparisons, other than that which could occur by chance alone.

Osteoporosis Loss of bone density caused by loss of calcium and phosphorous from bone.

Participant The word that is replacing subject, as in study participant.

Pathogen An organism (usually reserved for micro-organisms) that causes disease.

Pathogenesis The mechanisms and processes by which disease occurs.

Pellagra A nutritional deficiency disease caused by lack of the vitamin niacin with problems including dermatitis and neurological disorders.

Person-to-person spread Direct transmission of disease, usually infections, resulting from close proximity of persons.

Phenylketonuria A genetic disorder in which the amino acid phenylalanine cannot be metabolized properly, leading to mental deficiency.

Placebo An inactive substance or procedure used as a therapeutic intervention for psychological effect; and commonly used in the control group in a trial.

Popper (Karl) Philosopher, 1902–1994, who contributed to science by promoting the key idea of falsifying rather than proving hypotheses.

Population A complex concept with multitude meanings in epidemiology, but crucially, the group of people in whom the problem under study occurs, and in whom the results of the research are to be applied. The concept is discussed extensively in the text.

Prognosis Forecast of the outcome of a disease or other health problem with appropriate management (cf. natural history, which is without such management).

Proportional mortality (or morbidity) ratio (PMR) A summary measure of the proportion of deaths/disease due to a specific cause in the study population compared to either all causes or another cause.

Prostate A gland at the base of the male bladder.

Public health (medicine) An activity to which many contribute, most usually defined as the science and art of prolonging life, preventing disease and promoting health through the organized efforts of society.

Public health medicine is one of the many names given to the specialty of medical doctors who focus on public health.

Pulmonary Associated with the lungs.

Pulmonary embolus A blood clot lodged in the artery structure of the lungs.

Ramanujan (Srinivasan) Mathematician, 1887–1920, renowned for his intuition that led him to enunciate complex formulae that are still being proved.

Regression See Multiple regression.

Risk factor A factor associated with an increased probability of an adverse outcome, but not necessarily a causal factor.

Rose angina Angina is the characteristic chest pain arising from a shortage of oxygen to the heart muscle. Rose angina is the measure of whether chest pain is angina using the Rose angina questionnaire (also known as the London School of Hygiene and Tropical Medicine questionnaire).

Rothman (Kenneth) Epidemiologist, 1945 to 19–, known for conceptual and technical advances, and for his text *Modern Epidemiology*. (See References.)

Rubella syndrome A complex set of congenital malformations caused by infection of the mother by German measles (rubella) and transmitted to the fetus.

Sarcoidosis A disease of unknown cause, where the histology resembles tuberculosis. Most commonly affects the lungs, liver, eyes and skin.

Scurvy A disease caused by vitamin C deficiency, characterized by symptoms/signs including bruising and bleeding readily.

Senile dementia Brain disease characterized by loss of intellect, usually irreversible and caused by degenerative processes associated with old age.

Sexually transmitted diseases (STDs) The group of diseases mainly transmitted during sexual behaviour, e.g. syphilis. Some STDs may be transmitted in other ways too, e.g. AIDS.

Sickle cell disease/anaemia A genetic disorder, whereby the haemoglobin, the oxygen-carrying molecule in red blood cells, crystallizes and distorts the blood cell into a sickle shape when oxygen in the cell is low.

Sickness The state of being unwell or dysfunctional, usually as a result of disease.

Significance Usually shorthand for the phrase statistical significance, as given by the *P*-value (see Significance test).

Significance test A shorthand for tests of statistical significance whereby *P*-value is the probability that the observed difference could have been obtained by chance alone.

Skrabanek (Petr) Epidemiologist living 1940–1994, known for his capacity for critical appraisal.

Smallpox A severe viral disease, now extinct, characterized by skin blistering.

Sphygmomanometer A device for measuring arterial blood pressure using an inflatable cuff (usually applied to the upper arm). The cuff is inflated until blood flow stops, then deflated until blood flow begins (systolic blood pressure) and then occurs freely (diastolic blood pressure).

Standard deviation A measure of variation around the mean, measured as the square root of the variance (see below).

Standardized mortality (or morbidity) ratio (SMR) A summary measure of the rate of death/disease in a population adjusted for one or more confounding factors (usually age or sex or both) using the indirect method. The ratio is of deaths observed/deaths expected if the rates in the standard population had applied in the study population.

Statistical significance See significance.

Stratified sample The people selected for (or participating in) a study where the sampling frame is organized by subgroups, e.g. men and women, or age groups. Then random samples are chosen within each subgroup.

Streptococcus/cocci One of a number of species of bacteria, some of which cause serious human diseases.

Subject A person who is studied, i.e. a member of the population under study (see participant).

Target population The population about which inferences or generalizations are to be made or interventions designed for.

Tesh (Sylvia) Public health scholar (1937–) and author of a wide ranging and controversial book on public health—*Hidden Arguments*.

Theory A system of ideas offered to explain and connect observed factors or conjectures. A statement of general principles or laws underlying a subject.

Trisomy 21 See Down's syndrome.

Tuberculosis A multisystem infection caused by the bacteria *Mycobacterium tuberculosis*.

Variance A measure of the variation in a set of observations, defined as the sum of the square of the deviation of each value from the mean (in other words, each value is subtracted from the mean value and squared (always a positive number)), divided by the degrees of freedom (often the number of observations minus 1).

Zoonoses Diseases transmitted from animals to humans.

Chapter 1

What is epidemiology?
The nature and scope of a biological, social, and ecological science and of epidemiological variables and outcomes

Objectives

After reading this chapter you should understand:

- that the prime focus of epidemiology is on the pattern of disease and ill-health in the population;
- that epidemiology combines elements of clinical, biological, social and ecological sciences;
- that epidemiology is dependent on clinical practice and the clinical sciences to make a diagnosis, the starting point of epidemiological work;
- that the central goal of epidemiology as a science is to understand the causes of disease variation and use this knowledge to better the health of populations and individuals;
- that the central goal of epidemiology as a practice is preventing and controlling disease in populations, guiding health and healthcare policy and planning, and improving health care in individuals;
- that good epidemiological variables should meet the purposes of epidemiology;
- that epidemiology is based on theories though these may not be made explicit.

1.1 The individual and the population

Humans cherish the fact that they are unique, not only in their physique but also in their character, personality and behaviour (though identical twins may be excepted here). The health history of an individual is also unique, and only the facts of birth and death are universally shared experiences.

Some people who smoke heavily develop lung cancer and others do not. Some people drink alcohol and become aggressive, while others become passive. These outcomes are not easily predictable at the individual level. It is self-evident, nonetheless, that the characteristics and behaviours of individuals play a part in causing their diseases, and this has been recorded since the time of Hippocrates but was no doubt known much earlier. According to Hippocrates, whoever would study medicine should consider the health of the inhabitants of a place, for example, 'are they heavy drinkers and eaters and consequently unable to stand fatigue or, being fond of work and exercise, eat wisely but drink sparely?' Hippocrates also wrote at length about the role of the environment on disease, particularly the seasons, the winds and water (see Chadwick and Mann 1950).

It is less intuitive, but true, that population groups have unique and distinctive patterns of disease. This pattern is a result of variations in the exposure of the individuals in the population to the causes of disease that are mainly behavioural and environmental. If different populations were exposed equally to the same causes they would have more or less the same patterns of disease. Some variation would remain due to genetic differences, which are extremely small between populations (but these too are ultimately due to environmental pressures).

The population pattern of disease is not solely dependent on the characteristics of individuals but also on the interaction between individuals with each other and the environment in which they live. Distinctive population patterns of diseases arise from difference in the interaction of individuals in a social setting. For example, sexually transmitted diseases arise only when having more than one sexual partner is common practice in society. If a non-diseased man had multiple sexual partners in a society where a single sexual partner was the norm for others, his own behaviour would not raise his own risk of sexually transmitted disease (nor that of others in the society). The protection given to children who are not immunized against measles by the immunization of other children in the society, a phenomenon known as herd immunity, is another example. Forms of social interaction and organization lead to stresses which cause mental disorders such as anxiety, depression and eating disorders such as anorexia nervosa. The population has a pattern of disease arising from its intrinsic social characteristics. If society or the environment changed, the individual's risk of disease would also change, even when the individual resists change personally – as reflected in the examples of sexually transmitted disease and immunization against measles. Patterns of diseases in populations, therefore, result from the characteristics of individuals, societies and environment (as discussed in detail in Chapter 2). The science and practice of epidemiology seeks to describe, understand and utilize these patterns to improve health.

1.2 Definition of epidemiology and statement of its central paradigm

The identity of the person who coined the term epidemiology is unknown but it is derived from the Greek words meaning study upon populations (epi = upon, demos = people, ology = study). This derivation does not convey what is studied or the nature of that study and is effectively the same as demography which is the study of the characteristics of populations, such as size, growth, density, distribution, and vital statistics. Epidemiology is concerned primarily with disease, and how disease detracts from health. A more descriptive word would be epidemiopathology (pathos is the Greek word for suffering and disease) but it is too clumsy to recommend.

The word epidemic was used by Hippocrates, but his writings were mainly compilations of the case histories of affected people and not a study of the causes or descriptions of the pattern of the epidemic in the population. The early applications of epidemiology were in the study of infectious disease epidemics, environmental hazards and nutritional problems. The examination of social inequalities in mortality patterns was also an early focus of epidemiology. Most epidemiology is on human populations but veterinary epidemiology is important both in its own right and in the interaction of humans and animals, causing the diseases known as the zoonoses.

Last's (2001) dictionary gives a detailed definition of epidemiology that includes these words 'The study of the distribution and determinants of health-related states or events in specified populations, and the application of this study to control of health problems'.

Based on what it has done in the last 150 years, epidemiology is the science and practice which describes and explains disease patterns in populations, and puts this knowledge to use to prevent and control disease and improve health. Thomas Kuhn's (1996) influential concept of scientific paradigms is helpful (and is discussed in more detail in Chapter 10). Kuhn's concept of a paradigm is the matrix of examples, theories, applications, and instrumentation which underpins a tradition of scientific research. The central paradigm of epidemiology is that patterns of disease in populations may be analysed systematically to provide understanding of the causes and control of disease. The key strategy, then, of epidemiology is to seek out the differences and similarities ('compare and contrast') in the disease patterns of populations to gain new knowledge. Most epidemiologists are interested in health but study it indirectly through disease partly because of the difficulty of measuring health. Nearly all the examples used in textbooks and in collections of great epidemiological papers are based on this paradigm. Epidemiology is, however, evolving new paradigms as discussed in the next section and again in Chapter 10.

The valid measurement of the frequency of disease and factors which may influence disease, which are therefore potential explanations for the observed patterns, is crucial to the epidemiological goal (Chapters 3, 4, 7, 8). Measurement, however, is a means to an end. Excellence in measurement will not, in itself, yield excellence in epidemiology. The quality of epidemiology must be judged by its contributions to its goals. The same applies to the design of epidemiological studies (Chapter 9). A technically well-designed study may reach the wrong conclusions, and a technically poor one the right ones.

1.3 Directions in epidemiology and its uses

A great expansion in the scope of epidemiology is underway; the ideas which have proven themselves in the study of disease are used increasingly to study health, and health care. Epidemiology has also been useful in the laboratory, both in contributing to the provision of ideas to help us to understand biological processes and in pragmatic ways such as defining standards and ranges for the normal values of biological and social measures. Normal values are usually derived by demonstrating the distribution of the values in populations or, better, by demonstrating the adverse health effects associated with particular values. Epidemiology is becoming a key tool in the practice of clinical medicine, and though its uses have been insufficiently demonstrated, its potential for the professions allied to medicine, such as nursing and physiotherapy is promising.

The standard definitions of epidemiology such as the science of the distribution and determinants of disease, or the occurrence of disease in populations, do not capture the essence or potential of applied epidemiology in healthcare settings, though they do describe well the tradition of the science. Morris's (1964) classic book, *The Uses of Epidemiology*, fully recognized the huge contribution of epidemiology to health care, opening the chapter on community diagnosis with these words, 'Epidemiology provides "intelligence" for the health services' (1964, 2nd edition). Modern epidemiology is becoming more than a science; it is becoming a craft, vocation and profession; a partner of public health, not just a science of public health. Currently epidemiology is seen as useful in:

+ yielding understanding of what causes or sustains disease in populations;

+ preventing and controlling disease in populations;

+ guiding health and healthcare policy and planning;

+ assisting in the management and care of health and disease in individuals.

1.4 **Epidemiology as a science, practice, and craft**

Nearly all definitions of epidemiology say it is a science, and there is a claim for it to be the underlying science of public health (Chapter 10). Some critics have claimed epidemiology is not a science but a tool kit of methods for other sciences and professions to use. An understanding of whether epidemiology is a science is important in this era when the label 'science' is vital to the credibility of research. Try the exercise in Box 1.1 before reading on.

Box 1.1 **The nature of science in relation to epidemiology**

+ What are the characteristics of a science?

+ Name some disciplines which are sciences.

+ Name some which are not. Compare the disciplines which are sciences to those which are not.

+ Is public health a science?

+ Is epidemiology a science?

+ Is there some aspect of a science which epidemiology does not fulfil?

Science is about knowledge, for the word is derived from the Latin *scientia* meaning knowledge and the French *scíre*, to know. Dictionary definitions of science tend to be complex such as:

1 the observation, identification, description, experimental investigation, and theoretical explanation of phenomena

2 such activities restricted to a class of natural phenomena

3 any branch of knowledge based on systematic observations of facts and seeking to formulate general explanatory laws and hypotheses that could be verified empirically.

There is a wide range of other meanings where the word is used to indicate a systematic way of doing anything. Clearly, not all systematic study is science; for example, literature, art, philosophy, and religion are not sciences, though they may be rigorous and systematic, and even emulate the methods and measurement techniques of science. I think of science as the systematic study of natural phenomena. Furthermore, science is not just about the methods and techniques, which can be applied in many non-scientific circumstances, for example political polling, but the mode of thought. The mode of thought is the quest for new knowledge based on, and extending, theory and verified by direct research-based observation. Scientists are engaged in extending or consolidating the knowledge base, sometimes through deliberate repetition of research. Science is a creative endeavour and relies as much on questioning, imagination and exploration as art, but the difference is that science tests out its ideas by seeking empirical evidence rooted in the natural world. The idea to be tested is often stated as a study question and if it is expressed in a way which lends itself to systematic test, it is called a hypothesis. Reflect on the importance of the testable question in science as emphasized in Box 1.2.

The idea, the question, the testable hypothesis, the research test, and the interpretation of the research data to advance understanding of natural phenomena, together, comprise science. Epidemiology studies the nature of diseases, and their causes, and it uses systematic methods of measurement to test ideas, questions and hypotheses, and hence it is a bio-science, serving medicine and public health just as medical sciences such as pathology and microbiology do.

Box 1.2 **The question as the basis of science**

♦ That is the essence of science: ask an impertinent question, and you are on the way to a pertinent answer.

Jacob Bronowski (1908–74), British scientist, author of (1973) *The ascent of man*, ch. 4.

Epidemiology has come to be perceived as particularly relevant to medicine rather than laboratory science, but the increasing collaboration between geneticists and epidemiologists is changing the balance, once again. Epidemiology is, however, primarily concerned with disease and health hazards in populations and not individuals. Human populations live in societies, where behaviour and attitudes are shaped by interaction among people, which in turn are governed by the conventions and laws of the society. In short, epidemiology studies disease within a cultural context, and is particularly concerned with social organization. Epidemiology is, therefore, not only a bio-science but also a social science. Populations exist in a physical environment which is a dominant force in determining health. The study of life in relation to the environment is ecology (the word derives from the Greek for house), so epidemiology is, in addition, the science of the ecology of disease.

The science of epidemiology, therefore, combines elements of biology, social sciences, and ecology: a bio-social-environmental science focusing on disease in populations. By its nature, epidemiology is multidisciplinary. The closest partner of the epidemiologist is the statistician, for reasons that will become apparent.

Epidemiological science is applicable to practical purposes. Understanding the causes of diseases, more than any other information, transforms the practice of clinical care and public health. For example, the observations that infants put to sleep on their front are at higher risk of sudden infant death than those placed on their back, or that smokers have a much higher risk of a multiplicity of diseases than non-smokers. Epidemiological data has also demonstrated its value for actions such as creating a health policy for the nation or providing data essential for a plan to meet the needs for health care of patients with cancer.

While many epidemiologists are simultaneously engaged in both theoretical and practical applications, usually in public health but sometimes in clinical and laboratory medicine, some are wholly occupied in applying available knowledge. This applied work is not science, though it draws upon science. In this regard, epidemiology is no different to, for example, geology and chemistry, where there are scientists and practitioners, and often the two roles are combined. Scientific research and practice in epidemiology are symbiotic, but not synonymous, activities. Recent criticisms of epidemiology may partly arise from a failure to separate the roles of epidemiology as a science and as a craft or practice. Analogously, there are criticisms of physics for discoveries which have underpinned poor energy policy (disasters in nuclear energy power plants, for example) and criticisms of biology for unethical and erroneous interpretation of data on intelligence (for example, the Immigration Bill of 1924 in the USA kept Jews from migrating to America on the basis of their supposedly low intelligence). The paradigms within which the practice of epidemiology operates are somewhat different from those of the science of epidemiology. The research questions, the value of the various methods, data analysis, presentation, and interpretation may differ; a matter which needs to be appreciated. These differences and their implications will be emphasized throughout the text.

1.5 **The nature of epidemiological variables**

The word variable is in common use in epidemiology, but its meaning in an epidemiological context is seldom defined. A variable is anything which varies and has different values. Clearly, this applies to most phenomena, but only a few are chosen for epidemiological analysis. Variation in disease pattern is the foundation of epidemiology, but in epidemiology the word variable is less often applied to diseases, which may be referred to as outcome variables or simply outcomes, but to factors which help to describe and understand disease pattern. These are also called exposure variables.

Epidemiological variables aid in the depiction, analysis, and interpretation of difference in disease patterns within and between populations. Analysis of disease by age, sex, economic status, social class, occupation, country of residence, country of birth, region of residence, and racial or ethnic classification are all powerful ways of showing variations in a broad range of diseases and health states. Most variables used in epidemiology are markers for complex, underlying phenomena of interest which cannot be measured easily, if at all. For example, social class is an indirect indicator of various differences between populations in factors such as occupation, income, education and styles of consumption. Sex may act as a proxy for genetic, hormonal, psychological, or social status in different studies. It is important, therefore, that we can disentangle and study separately the component influences of the epidemiological variable.

Before reading on do the exercise in Box 1.3.

Box 1.3 **The epidemiological exposure variable**

◆ What qualities should an exposure variable have to make it worth pursuing in epidemiology?

◆ How do the purposes and uses of epidemiology help to assess the potential value of a variable?

A good epidemiological variable should:

◆ have an impact on health in individuals and populations;

◆ be measurable accurately;

◆ differentiate populations in their experience of disease or health;

◆ differentiate populations in some underlying characteristic relevant to health e.g. income, childhood circumstance, hormonal status, genetic inheritance, or behaviour relevant to health;

◆ generate testable aetiological hypotheses, and/or

  • help to develop health policy, and/or

  • help to plan and deliver health care, and/or

  • help to prevent and control disease.

These criteria, which are closely tied in to the purposes of epidemiology, can help to evaluate an exposure variable. In Chapter 10, and other parts of the book, they will be used to illustrate the points more deeply, particularly in the context of the controversial and difficult variables of race and ethnicity (10.10.3).

Table 1.1 summarizes the concepts here in the context of age, the most influential and important of all epidemiological variables. Before reading on, however, try the exercise in Box 1.4.

Box 1.4 **Thinking about age as an epidemiological variable**

◆ Is age easily and accurately measured?

◆ Is age good at showing population differences in disease experience?

◆ What underlying differences between people does age reflect?

◆ How can these differences be used to advance understanding of disease causation, or health policy or healthcare planning?

Biological changes related to ageing profoundly influence susceptibility to many diseases. For example, disorders of growth and development occur in the young;

Table 1.1 Age as an epidemiological variable

Criteria for a good epidemiological variable	Criteria in relation to age
Impact on health in individuals and population	Age is a powerful influence on health
Be measurable accurately	In most populations age is measurable to the day, but in some it has to be guessed
Differentiate populations in their experience of disease or health	Huge differences by age are seen for virtually every disease, health problem, and for factors which cause health problems
Differentiate populations in some underlying characteristic relevant to health e.g. income, childhood circumstance, hormonal status, genetic inheritance, or behaviour relevant to health	Differences in disease patterns in different age groups reflect a rich mix of environmental factors and may also reflect population changes in genetic factors, particularly in populations where migration has been high
Generate testable aetiological hypotheses, and/or	It is hard to test hypotheses because there are so many underlying differences between populations of different age
help in developing health policy, and/or	Age differences in disease patterns profoundly affect health policy
help to plan and deliver health care and/or	Knowing the age structure of a population is critical to good decision making
help to prevent and control disease	By understanding the age at which diseases start, preventive and control programmes can be targeted at appropriate age groups

degenerative diseases such as osteoporosis or senile dementia mostly in the old. The occurrence of specific disease, however, is a result of the interaction of biological, social, and environmental factors—and age is relevant to all three, as discussed below.

In most populations age is easily and accurately measured by asking subjects their date of birth. Alternatively, the age can be obtained or checked using birth registration data. In some populations, mainly in developing countries, where the system of registration at birth is not operative or effective, the age may not be known or may be approximated. In some societies, for social reasons, there is a tendency to exaggerate age on self-report, in others to underestimate it.

Age is superb at illuminating and sharpening the picture of variations in most diseases (see Table 8.17, Chapter 8). Variations by age seldom yield easy explanation, for the causes underlying the variations are a complex mix of social, environmental, and biological factors. Causal hypotheses constructed around the age variable are not easily tested. As a generalization, the more complex the concept captured by the variable, the harder it is to both explore and to understand the underlying reason for the associated variation in disease experience. This is why it is imperative to understand the underlying concept behind the variable, for in causal studies additional data will be needed and this will be dependent on such understanding. The epidemiological concept of ageing is a mix of a biological and environmental component; that is, as one grows older the biology changes, but at the same time the body absorbs a barrage of environmental insults, the combined effects leading to differences in disease patterns in different age groups and in different generations. Furthermore, the social circumstances, and particularly social support networks, of people change greatly at different ages and these affect health. The differences in disease experience at different ages, giving a different pattern of health in places where the population is older than average, are profoundly important to making sound health policy and to effective healthcare planning.

The epidemiological concept of sex is also largely biological though differences in the lifestyle of men and women and their social circumstances means that the concept is also a mix of biological and social. Try the exercise in Box 1.5 before reading on.

Box 1.5 **Categorizing the differences between sexes**

List the differences between women and men which could explain their different patterns of disease. (You may wish to focus your thinking using heart disease which is more common in men than women.) Can you put them into categories?

To begin to understand the well-known variation by sex in the occurrence of coronary heart disease, the investigator needs to know what differences there are between men and women in the context of the population studied. Table 1.2 categorizes some

Table 1.2 Categorizing and analysing the factors which may underlie an epidemiological variable: the example of male/female differences in heart disease

Category of underlying difference	Example of possible specific differences by sex	Implications for science of epidemiology
Biological	Hormonal, e.g. oestrogen levels	Collect biological data
Co-existing diseases	Women may have less of the other diseases which raise the risk of heart disease e.g. diabetes	Collect clinical data
Behavioural	Women eat more fruits, vegetables, and salads than men, and generally smoke less	Collect data on behaviours relating to health
Social	Women spend more time with friends and family	Collect psychosocial data as potential explanations
Occupational	The pattern of working, including likelihood of employment, the hours worked and the type of occupation is substantially different	Collect data on employment histories
Economic	Women earn less than men	Collect data on differences and their effect on lifestyles and stress
Health care	Women with heart disease are treated differently from men by health care professionals	Collect data on level and timing of interventions

of the differences as biological, co-existing disease (or co-morbidity), behavioural, social, occupational, economic, and health care. There are complex differences between men and women so using this variation to explain the different patterns of heart disease is an immensely difficult exercise. To ascribe differences solely to genetic factors would be a serious though tempting error. By contrast, differences between men and women in the risk of breast cancer are likely to be biological and for cervical cancer are, of course, wholly biological because men don't have a cervix. The depth of the analysis will, therefore, be disease and context specific. Differences in health care between men and women, as explanations for disease variations, arouse great controversy, because inequitable health care is unethical.

Scientific understanding of the reason for the variation by sex is extremely helpful in shaping rational interventions, but in its absence the information can be used to set priorities and target resources. For the science of epidemiology, concerned to advance causal knowledge, variables which highlight variations between and within populations in diseases of unknown aetiology are *potentially* of great value. If disease variation has not previously been demonstrated using other variables it is of particular value. The repetitious demonstration of variations is, however, seldom of scientific value.

For example, huge variations between countries in the incidence of cancer have been demonstrated, and these conclusively demonstrate that population variation in cancer is largely determined by environmental factors. New observations on cancer variations by country would be of scientific value only if they advanced (or refuted) rather than confirmed this interpretation. A great deal of effort is presently underway to show racial and ethnic variations in cancer. These mainly reconfirm the insights from international studies. Unless some new perspective can be achieved, their additional value in aetiological research needs to be questioned. In an analysis of the role of epidemiology as a science Skrabanek (1994) argued that epidemiologists must advance understanding of the underlying basis of the associations between epidemiological variables and disease patterns that they describe. He cited a review of 35 case-control studies of coffee drinking and bladder cancer, which failed to provide important information on whether coffee causes bladder cancer. He likened such repeated work to repetitively punching a soft pillow. A dimple forms and refills rapidly. The totality of the repeated blows is no more than the first alone. He called this 'black-box' epidemiology, and another epidemiologist, Kuller (1999), has criticized a similar phenomenon that he called circular epidemiology.

1.6 A disease and health problem: an illustration of the interdependence of clinical medicine and epidemiology

Investigating the causes and understanding the means to control the problem is, in essence, the science of epidemiology and taking the steps to prevent and control the problem, including providing the appropriate health services is, in essence, public health. The craft of epidemiology is presenting the scientific evidence in ways which lead to effective public health action. Epidemiology cannot begin its work until some basic clinical and pathological issues have been resolved, for example, on the definition of the disease. The science of epidemiology, therefore, functions in close partnership with clinical medicine and pathology. Read Box 1.6 and try the questions before reading on.

Box 1.6 A puzzle for medicine and a challenge for epidemiology: sickness X

A sickness of unknown type, which appears as outbreaks, sometimes affecting whole communities, is spreading across a large part of continental Europe. Years later it will emerge in the USA. It will be shown to be present in many countries, though it may remain unrecognized in normal medical practice, for it may occur as solitary cases or in small numbers and not outbreaks. Sick people have a wide range of symptoms and signs on examination. Their many symptoms include simply feeling unwell, with loss of appetite and abdominal pain, disturbances of the gastrointestinal tract including diarrhoea, a skin rash on parts of the body exposed to the sun, and mental disturbances.

Box 1.6 (*continued*)

It leads to progressive physical and mental deterioration. People who contract the sickness are likely to die, with the mortality rate as high as 60 per cent in some outbreaks. If a sufferer recovers the sickness can recur.

The sickness clusters in families, and it affects the poor living in rural areas more than any other group. Sharecropping and growing of corn are common in areas where the disease occurs. The problem is greatest in spring, though the early symptoms occur in winter. The sickness is common in prisoners and patients in asylums. It does not affect staff in the institutions.

Physicians cannot agree on the cause of the sickness and the many 'cures' tried by physicians and quacks give variable results.

Questions

- Can you form a definition of this sickness X? If not, how would physicians make a diagnosis? How could the number of cases of the sickness be counted?

- If you can define it how would you do it? What would be the components of your definition?

Sickness X (Box 1.6) illustrates why epidemiology requires clinical collaboration. Since the cause is unknown the disease must be defined on the clinical picture, or laboratory tests. If a definition cannot be agreed or the definition is inaccurate, cases cannot be diagnosed and epidemiology is paralysed, or led to error. The first question for the epidemiologist, in any investigation, is the nature and validity of the definition of the disease or other problem under investigation. Clinicians need to study cases and agree on a definition which will permit the classification of sick people into one of two groups: probably suffering from the disease or probably not. Diagnoses are no more than statements of probability, and their accuracy will depend on the clarity of the definition of the disease. A definition of sickness X which accepted only patients with a rash as cases would miss those without a rash. To accept cases of disease without a rash means that more people suffering from other disorders will be wrongly diagnosed with sickness X.

Pragmatic choices will need to be made. For the purposes of scientific investigation, a definition which includes people with a high probability of disease is likely to be better than one which includes many people without. For public health action the same definition may be inadequate, for it underestimates the size of the problem and misses the people most likely to benefit: those with early symptoms. A possible definition would be that a case of sickness X is, for the purpose of epidemiological research,

- an illness diagnosed by a physician;
- one of a cluster or outbreak of cases;

- one that occurs in an ill person who has at least two out of these three problems:
  - gastrointestinal disturbance
  - skin rash
  - mental disturbance
- one with no other clear diagnosis.

Using this pragmatic definition physicians can be asked to inform the researchers of the occurrence of cases, which can be counted and studied. The effect of error in the definition on the estimated frequency of the disease may be huge and comparison of different populations is likely to be misleading as will be discussed in Chapter 3, but an approximate definition is still essential.

Consider, for comparison, the definition used by Fraser and colleagues (1977) in their investigation of the 1976 Legionnaires' disease outbreak in Philadelphia: a case had a *fever of at least 102 degrees and a cough, or a fever allied to chest X-ray evidence of pneumonia, plus some association with the Legion convention.* The definition was designed to separate those who were probably linked to the outbreak from those who were not. Later, when the importance of the Bellevue Hotel in Philadelphia as the source of exposure became clearer, the definition was revised to include only people who were American Legion conventioneers or who had entered the Bellevue Stratford Hotel after 1 July 1976. The change in definition caused confusion in the minds of the public and the media, and changed the numbers of cases involved and dead. Similarly, a change in the definition of AIDS some years ago led to changes in the numbers of cases. Changes in case definition are common, reflecting the fact that diagnosis is often pragmatic.

Even at this stage some possibilities in the underlying disease processes and causation of sickness X can be ruled out on the basis of general clinical and pathological principles about the nature of disease. Try the exercise in Box 1.7.

Box 1.7 **The nature and possible causes of sickness X**

- What thoughts come into your mind about the nature of the sickness? What kind of sickness/disease is it?
- What kind of sickness/disease is it not?
- What sort of factors could cause a sickness such as this?

Table 1.3 summarizes some reasoning on the nature of sickness X. This disease is not a chromosomal or gene defect, congenital, an immune disorder, a result of injury, a degeneration of age, or a result of uncontrolled cell division (cancer). It may be a result of infection, exposure to toxins, or a deficiency of some essential substance. This basic reasoning is based on epidemiology, which draws upon the other relevant sciences.

Table 1.3 Types of disease and some preliminary reasoning on sickness/disease X

Type of disease	Reasoning for and against sickness X being this kind of disease
Genetic	Genetic diseases do not vary in their frequency over short periods of time, and do not selectively avoid certain populations e.g. staff in institutions
Congenital	Congenital problems tend to affect the young and are not usually epidemic
Degenerative	As above. They do not tend to affect the young
Cancers	As above. They do not exhibit marked seasonal variation
Injuries	The cause of injuries is usually apparent
Infections	The picture fits, though the reason for some populations being immune is a puzzle
Toxins	The picture fits
Nutritional deficiency	The picture fits
Immune disorders	These do not present as epidemics

Information on causation based on population studies may be used by the clinician in managing the individual patient. Therapeutic ideas may be sparked by understanding of causation and tested on populations of patients. The results derived from populations will then be applied to individuals.

1.7 Seeking the theoretical foundations of epidemiology

A theory is a statement which provides an explanation or coherent account of a group of ideas, facts, or observed phenomena, like the theory of evolution. Epidemiology has been criticized as an atheoretical discipline, comprising a mixed bag of tools, useful for solving particular problems but neither adding up to a science, nor providing a theoretical basis to the study of health and disease. Epidemiology, however, both draws upon and contributes to theories of health and disease. It may be that epidemiologists spend little time reflecting on the theories underpinning their work, but the same criticism would probably apply to other sciences. In most disciplines theories are at the core of thinking and practice. Priscilla Alderson has argued that it is not possible to think about health care without theory even though it may be implicit rather than explicit. Before reading on do the exercise in Box 1.8.

Box 1.8 Spotting theories and principles underlying epidemiology

Can you discern any theories which have guided this chapter so far? What general principles follow from these theories?

The main epidemiological theories and principles that have guided this chapter include these:

- Disease in populations is more than the sum of the disease in individuals.
- Populations differ in their disease experience.
- Disease experiences within populations differ in subgroups of the population.
- Disease variations can be described and their causes explored by assessing whether exposure variables are associated with disease patterns.
- Knowledge about health and disease in human populations can be applied to individuals and vice versa.
- Health policies and plans, and clinical care can be enriched by understanding of disease patterns in populations.

Methods and techniques in epidemiology are designed to achieve the promise inherent in these theories, but in turn, their development and use leads to new or refined theoretical understanding. Epidemiology's contribution to the theory of health and disease will be a recurrent theme of the book, and will be summarized and developed in Chapter 10 (Section 10.1).

Summary

Populations, as with individuals, have unique patterns of disease. Populations' disease patterns derive from differences in the type of individuals they comprise, in the mode of interaction of individuals, and in the environment in which the population lives. The science of epidemiology, which straddles biology, clinical medicine, social sciences, and ecology, seeks to describe, understand, and utilize these patterns to improve health. As a science, epidemiology's central paradigm is that analysis of population patterns of disease provides understanding of the causes of disease. Epidemiology is useful in other ways, too, including preventing and controlling disease in populations and guiding health and healthcare policy and planning. Causal understanding is not always essential in these latter applications. Epidemiology also helps to manage the health care of individuals.

A good epidemiological exposure variable reflects the purposes of epidemiology and is measurable accurately, differentiates populations in their experience of disease or health, and generates testable aetiological hypotheses, or helps in developing health policy and healthcare plans or to prevent and control disease. For advancing causal knowledge, variables which highlight differences between and within populations in diseases of unknown aetiology are *potentially* of great value. The more complex the concept captured by the variable the harder it is to understand the reasons for the associated variation in disease experience. For health policy and planning, variables which show variations in diseases for which effective interventions are possible are particularly valuable.

Understanding the epidemiology of the disease demands clinical collaboration. Clinicians need to agree on a definition which will permit screening or diagnosis. The first question for the epidemiologist, in any investigation, is the nature and validity of the definition of the disease or other problem under investigation. Then follow decisions on which populations are to be studied and the methods for making accurate measurement of the frequency and pattern of disease and the postulated risk factors. In turn, epidemiological knowledge is used by clinicians to help make diagnoses in individuals, to prescribe effective treatments, and to offer patients information on the natural history and prognosis of disease.

Epidemiology is both founded on, and contributes to, theories of health and disease, though these are seldom made explicit.

Chapter 2

The epidemiological concept of population

Objectives

On completion of your reading you should understand:

◆ the meaning and applications of the idea that epidemiology is a population science;

◆ the profound influence of the characteristics of a population on its disease patterns;

◆ the potential and limitations of epidemiology in the absence of demographic population data;

◆ the expansion of possibilities in epidemiology which occurs when demographic population data are available;

◆ the impact of change in population size and characteristics on health.

2.1 The individual and the population

Epidemiology is invariably defined as a population science. It is primarily concerned with reaching an understanding of disease through the comparison of the pattern of disease in populations over time, between places and in different types of people as symbolized in Fig. 2.1.

Populations do, of course, comprise unique individuals. Humans, however, are social animals who thrive in families, groups, and communities and it is extremely rare for people to live in isolation. (Solitary confinement is one of the severest penalties in society.) The family is the basic unit of the group or community but nearly all humans live in and relate to much larger populations. The interaction of humans in societies is, without doubt, the keystone of epidemiology as a medical science. No epidemiological study can be done on one person, but other medical sciences such as pathology and physiology may gain much from the detailed study of one person, or even parts of a person. Even therapeutic trials can be designed for one individual thus advancing clinical knowledge.

To compare and contrast disease status and disease pattern, the basis of epidemiology, you need at least two individuals. While epidemiology may be on very large groups—sometimes millions of people but nearly always hundreds or thousands—it can be done on very small groups. The classic experiment of Lind in 1747 was on

- Populations comprise individuals, families, groups and communities
- Epidemiology seeks variation in disease pattern over time, between subgroups and between places
- Understanding such variation yields knowledge on causation and prevention of disease

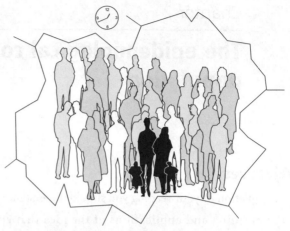

Fig. 2.1 The individual and population: the triad of time, place, and person.

Box 2.1 **The triad of epidemiological questions**

- How does the pattern of this disease vary over time in this population?
- How does the place in which the population lives affect the disease pattern?
- How do the personal characteristics of the people in the population affect the disease pattern?

12 persons, divided into six pairs of two, with each pair receiving a different nutritional supplement to try to prevent scurvy (Lind 1988). A definitive study of adenocarcinoma of the vagina by Herbst and colleagues (1971) was based on eight cases and 32 people without disease as controls.

Epidemiology aggregates the health experiences of individuals and tries to generalize the findings to the population from which the individuals have come. These aggregate experiences are analysed in terms of the questions summarized in Box 2.1 to seek patterns over time, between places and between sub-populations with different characteristics; this is known as the triad of time, place, and person. Time, place, and person can be thought of as exposure variables. We are, then, examining how time, place, and personal characteristics are associated with disease pattern. The strategy of epidemiology is to discover the causes of these patterns, and ultimately the causes of disease. (A theme developed in later chapters, particularly Chapter 5.)

Answer the questions in Box 2.2 in relation to disease X described in Chapter 1, Box 1.6, before reading the answers in Table 2.1.

As the analysis in Table 2.1 shows, epidemiological data can help us to understand causes of disease in populations and also to forecast the probability (risk) of disease and its outcome in individuals, albeit poorly. For example, we can reassure staff in institutions where disease X is present that their chance of developing disease is low. In

Box 2.2 **Exercise: Application of the triad to disease X**

Apply the questions in Box 2.1 to disease X.

◆ Now, does this information help you to understand the causes of the disease?

◆ How might you use this information to begin more detailed scientific investigation and to plan the control or prevention of disease?

Table 2.1 The epidemiological triad of questions applied to disease X (Box 1.6) and contribution to causal understanding

The epidemiological questions	The questions applied to sickness X
How does the pattern of disease vary over time?	The sickness is a new, emergent problem It sometimes occurs as outbreaks It is seasonal It follows times of economic hardship
How does the place in which the population lives affect the disease pattern?	It is worst in people living in low lying areas It affects people in institutions more, but only the inmates, not staff
How do the personal characteristics of the people in the population affect the disease pattern?	Living in poverty and sharecropping increase risk Being related to a person with the disease increases the risk It affects all ages, and both men and women

Moving from triad to causes

Now, does this information help you understand the causes of the disease? How might you use this information to begin more detailed scientific investigation and to plan the control or prevention of the disease? With the great variation in disease over time, between places, and by personal characteristics the evidence points to an environmental rather than a genetic cause. The various associations e.g. emergence in the spring, the link to poverty, the effect on those living in institutions, etc. permit hypotheses to be developed and tested. Also they point to populations for study e.g. those living in institutions. At this stage no specific control or preventive actions are compelling but the disease seems to be preventable.

studies to pinpoint the cause of the disease we will be looking for particular types of environmental exposures.

Epidemiological conclusions are directly applicable to the groups studied, but only indirectly to individuals, and then only to those who are reasonably typical of the population which has been studied. For example, for populations, the causal link between smoking and lung cancer is solid and can be accurately quantified but for an individual it may not apply, for there may be environmental or genetic reasons why that person is not susceptible to the carcinogenic effect of tobacco. The risk of a disease outcome for an individual can seldom be estimated accurately, except in unusual circumstances. This contrasts with some other fields of life. For example, school examination grades can be predicted fairly accurately for an individual from previous examination achievements. Individuals can also assess the risk of being struck by a car while crossing the road, based on their own experiences. The difference is that most diseases are rare so few individuals get them; many diseases only occur once; and for disease you either have it or you do not; while school grades are estimated many times and crossing the road is a daily event. Predicting the individual's risk of developing the common cold over, say, a five year period is more feasible than predicting whether an individual will develop, say, stroke or lung cancer.

While the knowledge gained by the study of groups is not directly applicable to any one individual it still benefits individuals. Surprisingly, information gained from groups may sometimes be more helpful to individuals than information from the individuals themselves. Physicians from the time of Hippocrates have devoted much effort to prognosis, the prediction of outcome once a disease has occurred, which is essential to both the practice and the science of medicine. A great deal of attention has been paid to symptoms, signs, and tests which would indicate the prognosis of an individual, but prognosis at the individual level remains an erroneous art. Before reading on reflect on the questions in Box 2.3.

Box 2.3 **Thought exercise on prognosis**

+ How would you assess the prognosis for a patient with a terminal illness who asks, how long have I got to live?
+ How would you advise a parent of a 5-year old son with asthma who asks, will my child have asthma for the rest of his life?

Even in the dying, the outcome is nearly impossible to predict accurately. In a study in Chicago hospices of the terminally ill, experienced physicians overestimated survival by a factor of 5.3. The likelihood of an individual child with asthma continuing to have it in adulthood cannot be predicted from the signs and symptoms or characteristics of the individual. Prognosis can, however, be expressed as a probability derived from population studies. This probability only informs the individual what happens on average, although the physician may use the individual's data to try to refine the prediction. Imperfect and unsatisfactory as this extrapolation from the population to the individual is, the approach has been widely adopted within medicine as the best available pending the development of accurate measures of prognosis based on the characteristics of individuals (this is a massive challenge for future clinical research which will be greatly assisted by advances in genetics).

Where a disease or manifestation of a disease occurs repeatedly in the same person, individual-based prediction becomes possible, and is likely to be superior to predictions based on population averages and distributions. For example, the experience of a child who has an asthma attack once or twice a week, mostly at nights, can be used to predict the occurrence, timing, and outcome of the next attack. By contrast the likely occurrence and outcome of meningococcal meningitis, which is rare, is only predictable from population studies.

Information about the demographic and socio-economic characteristics of a population tells us a great deal about the likely health state and disease risk of individuals within that population. For example, knowing that a population on average is a rich one leads us to predict a pattern of death for most individuals in the population that is dominated by heart disease, stroke, cancer and not by infections and nutritional deficiency disorders. This generalization will, of course, be subject to individual exceptions but will apply at the population level. The reason these generalizations are possible is that population characteristics influence individual risk of disease, as discussed next.

2.2 Harnessing heterogeneity in individual and group level disease and risk factor patterns

Epidemiology is interested in understanding the underlying factors that cause recognizable patterns of disease as in the example of disease X in Box 1.6. These factors are usually complex interactions between individuals, their physical environment, and their society. To understand the pattern, therefore, needs detailed understanding of the circumstances in which the population under study lives.

Epidemiological study of disease patterns should be based, therefore, on populations defined in terms of location, size, age and sex structure, and a wide range of data on the life and environmental circumstances of the people. The idea is to define and utilize the inherent heterogeneity of the population, and measure characteristics that are potential explanations for disease variation. In studying variation in a disease such as chronic bronchitis, for example, we would need to know whether the population studied is exposed to air pollution, tobacco, poverty or poor housing. This is the central message in the famous quotation from Hippocrates (Chapter 1, p. 2), and the idea captured in most definitions of epidemiology. Do the exercise in Box 2.4 before reading on.

Box 2.4 Heterogeneity of exposure to potential causes of disease in epidemiology

- How would epidemiology study the link between tobacco and lung cancer in a society where every adult smoked 20 cigarettes per day?
- How would one investigate epidemiologically the effect of the gas nitrogen on human health? What about oxygen?
- Neutrinos are interstellar particles which bombard the Earth penetrating deep into the Earth. How would we investigate, epidemiologically, their impact on health?

In a society where everyone smoked cigarettes, say 20 per day, epidemiology would be virtually powerless to assess the effect, for while lung cancer would be common, the exposure to what we know to be the major cause would be uniform. The key strategy of comparing and contrasting the disease pattern in people with and without the postulated cause (exposure) is not possible here. The solution would be to persuade some of the population to decrease or stop smoking, in other words, to do an experiment. Experiments usually need to be closely justified by data supporting a plausible hypothesis; in the circumstances described this would be difficult.

While experimentation might be possible in humans in the case of tobacco, it could not be accomplished easily with respect to oxygen, nitrogen, and neutrinos, for experimentally stopping, or even substantially reducing, exposure to these substances would not be feasible except for very short periods of time. The effects of these gases and particles on long-term human health are not amenable to rigorous epidemiological study. Nonetheless, useful information might accrue from studies on animals or cell cultures.

Paradoxically, the heterogeneity so vital to epidemiological investigation of disease poses challenges in interpreting and applying research. While tobacco and alcohol, for example, are damaging to health in populations, there are people and groups for whom these substances are harmless and perhaps even beneficial in some respects. For example, tobacco use is clearly linked to fewer problems with ulcerative colitis, and it suppresses the appetite and prevents weight gain. Alcohol in small amounts is widely agreed to reduce the risk of atherosclerotic heart disease and possibly stroke too. Whether, for a particular individual, tobacco or alcohol consumption is advisable or not is beyond the limits of epidemiology, which permits judgements at the population level. The health damage caused by tobacco in all populations far outweighs the health benefits. The position in regard to alcohol consumption is less clear, but the harm and damage at a population level is more in balance than that for tobacco.

The next section will discuss why the disease and risk factor patterns in populations are more than the sum of measures in the individuals comprising the population.

2.3 Disease patterns as a manifestation of individuals living in changing social groups

Diseases are expressed biologically in individuals. It is tempting, therefore, to assume that the causes of disease and the solutions to their control and prevention are also biological and lie at the individual level. Many diseases, however, are caused only by the interaction of individuals within and between populations, and most are profoundly influenced by such interactions. In other words the causes of disease are often social.

Individuals shape society, and in turn society exerts a powerful influence on individuals, which manifests itself in attitudes, behaviour, and diseases.

Do the exercise in Box 2.5 before reading on.

Box 2.5 **Impact of social organization and disease**

Imagine a world in the future where humans lived an isolated lifestyle, avoiding others whenever possible, using technologies to communicate, and using physical barriers to reduce contact, when this was inevitable. Children would be raised by one parent, perhaps. Imagine that the physical environment remained similar to that we experience now; that is, people lived in housing of similar quality and used similar cars etc.

◆ What would be the effect on disease patterns?

◆ Which diseases would be more common and which less so?

◆ What would the influences be on lifestyles?

Chapter 1 introduced the idea that disease patterns were influenced by the interaction of social, environmental, and individual level factors. The examples emphasized then were of infections. This central concept applies to a wide range of diseases. Suicide is a particularly clear-cut example. While suicide and parasuicide are linked to psychotic disorders, particularly depression, they are behaviours which are hugely influenced by convention. Durkheim, a French sociologist working in the 19th century, held that common values are the bonds of social order, and that the loss of such values leads to social and individual instability and suicide. Durkheim's studies on suicide (1951) showed huge variations which he believed to be an attribute of the society, or social reality, which in turn determined the suicide-related behaviour of individuals. This principle has now been demonstrated in wider circumstances, and most recently in the context of inequalities in health.

Mortality rates, generally, and for some specific causes of death are associated with increasing inequality of wealth in society. For a given level of wealth, societies that distribute the wealth more equally have higher life expectancy (and other health outcomes are better) than those that distribute wealth less equally. Economically unequal societies also have poorer mental and physical health than expected. Such societies show an excess of both overtly social problems such as murder and accidents, and other apparently biological problems such as cardiovascular diseases. The explanations for these observations are complex and controversial. The main hypothesis under examination is that unequal societies are less likely to invest in activities that improve health, and/or that they undermine social cohesion and increase stress. There is some evidence that the adverse effects of income inequality are greatest in the poorer and middle income groups and least in the wealthiest groups. In short, being relatively poor in society is associated with poor health, and being poor in an economically unequal society adds a further burden on health. Many industrialized countries, including the UK and US, have become both wealthier and more unequal in the late twentieth century, so these observations have particular relevance to public health.

The effects of society even have an impact on genetic diseases. Down's syndrome, a genetic disorder called trisomy 21, provides a specific example of how social expectations and behaviours alter disease patterns. Societies that encourage birth at older ages will have a higher rate of Down's syndrome than those that encourage childbirth in the late teens and twenties because the genetic abnormality becomes more common as the mother ages. Prenatal screening is available for this disorder, and the choice of abortion of the fetus is possible. So, the amount of Down's syndrome depends on age of the mother at conception, availability and uptake of screening and acceptability of abortion—all socially determined issues.

The pattern of disease depends, therefore, on the way society is organized and it is the role of epidemiology to understand this. Individuals and their societies live in a physical environment which is the prime determinant of health and illness (an argument developed in Chapter 4 on causal thinking). Epidemiology must, therefore, analyse the pattern of disease using variables that characterize individuals, society, and the environment.

In the imaginary future world alluded to in Box 2.5, which will soon be feasible, diseases which are transmitted from person to person would occur rarely. The causes of such diseases would not be able to propagate and would become extinct. So, an isolated individual or small group would not develop diseases such as tuberculosis, leprosy, influenza, the common cold, measles, mumps, AIDS, and sexually transmitted diseases. Smallpox would not have been the genocidal scourge it was. Some of the micro-organisms causing these diseases are exclusively human pathogens (e.g. the leprosy bacillus, mumps virus, measles virus) so they would not survive, and would rapidly become extinct. Assuming that in the world of Box 2.5 humans also isolated themselves from animals, the zoonoses (diseases transmitted from animals to humans), including Lyme disease and brucellosis, would not occur. The human/animal cycle necessary for the propagation of parasitic diseases would be broken. The effect would not just be on the highly contagious diseases. Ulcers associated with infection by *Helicobacter pylori* would be less common. Cancers linked to infection would not occur or their incidence would be profoundly reduced; for example, cervical cancer, which is primarily caused by human papillomavirus transmitted sexually, and gastric cancer, assuming the hypothesis that it is a consequence of chronic gastritis from *Helicobacter pylori* infection. The health problems linked to passive smoking would be avoided.

The pattern of mental health problems would be profoundly different; the stresses of living in complex societies would be replaced by problems associated with isolation and loneliness. The influence on common diseases such as cancer and heart disease would also be huge, either directly from changes in the nature of human interactions or indirectly from the changes in behaviours which are themselves an outcome of societal and peer pressures; for example, smoking, alcohol drinking, and the amount and content of diet. Even our concept of the desired body shape is determined by the society we live in. In the world of isolated beings the pattern of behaviour would change hugely, causing massive (but unpredictable) alterations in the pattern of disease.

The thought exercise in Box 2.5 is not theoretical. For most of their history humans have lived as small groups of hunter-gatherers and not in large settled communities. There are small groups of humans who are effectively isolated. Influenza and measles are killing disorders in populations previously unexposed to them and therefore lacking in immunity. Smallpox, a scourge for any society, was near genocidal in isolated populations exposed to it. Over the last few hundred years isolated groups have been rapidly exposed to populations of strangers with devastating consequences for their health. The Tasmanian aborigines were made extinct by their interaction with European settlers and North American Indians were decimated by the new patterns of disease arising from both the interaction with Europeans, and later the new social expectations and roles imposed upon them. As a form of germ warfare, European settlers gave American Indians 'presents' of blankets that had been contaminated with material from smallpox patients. In more modern times, in 1857 the British colonized the Andaman Islands (east of India, west of Thailand) where the tribe Great Andamanese comprised 5000 people. In 1988, 28 were left. Measles and influenza took their toll. The Jarawa tribe remains isolated on the Andaman Islands. They are now making contact with the outside world. The result is predictable.

The swift move to urbanization following the industrial revolution, still continuing in the industrialized nations and accelerating in the developing ones, has exposed billions of people to new environments, disease agents, and different forms of human interaction. Migration and population mixing has a profound effect on the disease patterns of society. As a generalization, over some generations, the migrant population takes on the pattern of disease prevailing in the country to which migration takes place. The process of change is usually slow, with intermediate patterns occurring. Emigrants from India to wealthy industrialized countries develop chronic diseases such as heart disease and diabetes at a level far higher than predictable from the rate of disease in India and from the pattern of established causal factors. The explanations for this exceptionally rapid change are under study. Migration also changes disease on a local scale. For example, the strongest explanation for the observed high rates of childhood leukaemia around nuclear power stations currently is that the disease is linked to the pattern of childhood infections. There was substantial population mixing because of the inward migration of workers into relatively isolated communities during and following the building and commissioning of power stations. If the hypothesis is correct, local migration changing the pattern of childhood infection, and not radiation, is the fundamental cause of the excess of leukaemia in these areas (see Kinlen *et al.* 1995).

The twenty-first century may see a reversal, at least in wealthy industrialized countries, of the process of population mixing which has been so profoundly important to the industrial revolution. Firstly, easier transport and new communications technology are offering people the chance of enjoying the benefits of the city while mostly living in isolation, either in the countryside or within fenced and guarded compounds in the city. Computer links at home, work that can be done solo, environmental concerns and an increase in costs of office space in cities are likely to accelerate these trends.

Secondly, with increasing inequality in income the wealthiest people have both the resources and incentives to isolate themselves geographically from their societies, thereby avoiding the health and social consequences of living in proximity to the poor.

The population, then, has patterns of health and disease which are caused by the interactions of individuals living in complex, organized society. Some diseases would not arise at all in isolated individuals and small groups. For nearly all diseases the pattern would be greatly different if the social organization differed. Disease patterns are generated in, and by, populations and need to be described, explained, and predicted in a population setting. While all individuals must sicken and die it is the nature of the population they live in which has a profound effect on which sicknesses they develop, when they develop them, and at what age they are likely to die within the range determined by biological processes. The close link of epidemiology to public health, the science and art of prolonging life, preventing disease, and promoting health through the organized efforts of society, is clear in this context. This sets the stage for considering the late Geoffrey Rose's idea of the sick population.

2.4 Sick populations and sick individuals

Rose proposed a radical and still controversial vision of health in his book, *The Strategy of Preventive Medicine* (Rose 1994). His central proposition was that people with overt diseases and health problems—people with hypertension, alcohol problems or obesity – were simply at one end of the spectrum, or distribution; that is, they are not deviant, merely an integral part of the whole. To prevent such problems required changes in the population as a whole, or a shifting of the whole distribution. For example, on Rose's argument, prevention of alcoholism requires that the entire distribution of alcohol consumption shifts, so the average and total consumption declines. To quote Rose, 'the supposedly "normal" majority needs to accept responsibility for its deviant minority—however loth it may be to do so'.

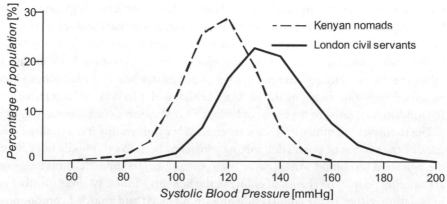

Fig. 2.2 Distribution of systolic blood pressures in middle-aged men in two populations (Source: Rose *Int J Epidemiol* 1985; **14**, 32–8, see Permissions).

Rose developed the idea of sick and healthy populations, distinct from sick or healthy individuals, by reflecting on questions arising from international studies of high blood pressure and cardiovascular disease, and the exercise that follows is based on that. Currently a systolic blood pressure of 140 mmHg or more is considered a matter of concern and one of 160 mmHg would cause some alarm. In the exercise consider a value of 140 mm as *indicative* of hypertension. Before reading on, reflect carefully, but broadly, on Fig. 2.2 using the questions in Box 2.6. Figure 2.2 is a graph showing the systolic blood pressure on the *x*-axis and the percentage of the population with that level of pressure in each of two populations.

Box 2.6 **Reflection on the distribution of blood pressure values in Kenyan nomads and London civil servants**

Examine Fig. 2.2 and reflect on these questions:

◆ In what ways do the shapes of the distributions differ in the two populations?

◆ Roughly, what percentage of Kenyans and London civil servants have hypertension?

◆ Is there any suggestion from Fig. 2.2 that the cause of high blood pressure in an individual Kenyan nomad and a London civil servant is likely to differ?

◆ What is the cause of the different distribution of blood pressure in the two populations?

◆ Are the causes of sickness in the population different from the sickness in the individual?

Figure 2.2 shows that the shape of the two distributions of blood pressure is similar, and of the shape that is described as a normal (or Gaussion) distribution as shown in Fig. 2.3 (normal distributions are symmetric, the mean, median and mode are the same, and 68 per cent of the population lies within one standard deviation of the mean value, and 95 per cent within two standard deviations, see glossary). The distribution in London civil servants is far to the right of that of Kenyan nomads. One simple indication of the impact of this on the amount of disease is the percentage of the population with hypertension. Based on the cut-off of 140 mmHg, a large percentage of civil servants have hypertension (about 40 per cent) and a small number of nomads do (about 10 per cent). Based on a cut-off of 160 mmHg substantial numbers of civil servants have hypertension (about 15 per cent) while such values are rare indeed in nomads. Rose and Day showed that the population mean (average) predicts the number of people with the health problem. For systolic blood pressure their data predicted a 10 per cent increase in the percentage of the population with hypertension for every 10 mmHg increase in mean systolic blood pressure.

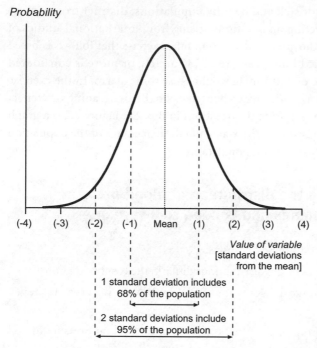

Fig. 2.3 The normal distribution.

The cause of high blood pressure in individuals is usually not pinpointed and is named essential hypertension. In about 10 per cent of cases a specific cause (such as a kidney problem) is found. While Fig. 2.2 does not inform us about the causes of hypertension in individuals the similarity in the shape of the distribution, and the range of difference between the two extremes, suggest similarities in the forces that shape the distribution. Rose surmises that the specific causes of hypertension in nomads may be the same genetic, environmental, and behavioural factor as those operating on civil servants. Certainly, renal failure will cause hypertension in a Kenyan and a Londoner alike.

The stark difference in the location, as opposed to the shape, of the blood pressure distributions indicates that powerful forces are operating. It is likely that the nomads are closer to the normal pattern and the Londoners' distribution has shifted rightwards. The question of what causes this is a different one from what causes hypertension in an individual. We can speculate that the causes of the rightward shift are dietary factors (including high fat, high salt, high calories), obesity, insufficient exercise, stress, and relationships between these and genetic factors. These and other factors are acting on the entire population. The question of causes, therefore, needs to be studied in relation to the whole population and not just individuals. The causes of sickness in the population—for example, London civil servants comprise a group with an abnormal blood pressure distribution—are conceptually different from the causes of sickness in the individual, and need to be studied differently too. Rose emphasizes that information on the population distribution of the risk factors, and the shape of the risk factor-disease outcome relationship is vital to the population approach to preventive medicine.

Similar analysis could be done for many other health problems such as alcoholism, obesity, and diabetes. While the cause of alcoholic liver cirrhosis is alcohol (by circularity of argument in the definition) its incidence varies hugely among populations and indeed within subgroups of the population. What is the cause of this population variation? Plainly there are differences in the population distributions in the consumption or metabolism of alcohol. Why are there such differences? Again the causes of differences in the population are likely to be different from the causes in the individual. The individual may be an alcoholic as a response to anxiety, depression, unemployment, or simply a fondness for alcoholic beverages that led to addiction. Populations, however, have high and low consumption for different reasons including religion, tradition, customs of hospitality, availability, income, and taxes.

Understanding causes of phenomena in the population is the primary responsibility of population scientists, and in regard to health and disease of epidemiologists. Rose referred to the causes of population variations as the causes of the causes. The major cause of lung cancer is tobacco. What causes people to take up smoking even when they are knowledgeable about its harm? Why does the amount of smoking vary so much between populations? The causes of the causes tend to be social and environmental, not biological.

The idea that the causes in individuals may differ from causes in populations, leads to a radically different population-based strategy for disease control based on both the causes, and the causes of the causes, and a goal of changing the distribution of risk factors in populations as opposed to individuals. Figure 2.4 illustrates the strategic difference between the so-called high risk and population-based approaches. A distribution of alcohol consumption is shown in part (a), with the level at which health risk increases (say risk of alcoholic liver damage). Part (b) of the figure shades the high risk group. The high risk approach concentrates on this group. If the strategy is successful, the end result would be as shown in (c), a highly artificial result. The population approach concedes that a distribution like (c) is not feasible. To achieve a similar result in terms of reducing risk, the aim is to shift the entire distribution leftwards. Such shifts require social action whereby the acceptable or average levels of consumption are based on reducing the harm, not merely in the individuals, but the population as a whole. This matter is discussed again in Section 2.8. Do the exercise in Box 2.7 on whether sickness X is a disease of individuals or of populations, before reading the material in Table 2.2. (You may wish to re-read the material in Box 1.6.)

Box 2.7 **Sickness X: individual and population perspective**

◆ Was sickness X (Box 1.6) a disease of sick individuals or of a sick population?

◆ What might have been the causes of the causes in sickness X?

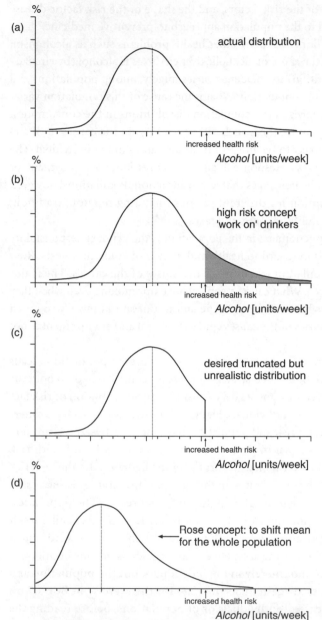

Fig. 2.4 The actual, high risk, truncated, and shifted distributions.

Isolated cases of sickness X did occur independent of outbreaks usually in the mentally deranged or in people with addictions such as alcohol. More usually it occurred in outbreak or epidemic form in whole communities. Knowledge of the specific 'causal' agent did not achieve control of the disease at the population level though it did cure the individual treated.

Table 2.2 Some observations on disease X as a sickness of populations

Sickness X

Never occurred in humans free to choose their own way of life

Occurred after populations were thrown into poverty

Did not decline even after its specific cause was well understood in biological terms

Continued to occur, in hundreds of thousands of people every year, in some extremely rich countries that would not accept that the cause had been discovered even though other countries virtually eliminated the problem by acting upon available knowledge

Declined when a war led to a change in the mode of life in the USA

Declined when economic disaster led to a marked change in the mode of living and working in rural areas

Was virtually defeated by government action

Sickness X is pellagra, a disease caused by deficiency of a vitamin, niacin. The investigation of the causes of pellagra by Joseph Goldberger is a compelling, classic tale. The biology of the disease is now clear. But, to say the cause of pellagra is niacin deficiency, or even a nutritional deficiency is a simplification, particularly as it does not provide a course of action for controlling the disease in the population. The characteristics of the disease in a population context, some of which are identified in Table 2.2, give clues to the wider causes of the specific cause (niacin deficiency): poverty, loss of freedom of populations and individuals to choose their diet, and eating too narrow a range of foods. The causes of the disease are, therefore, nutritional deficiency of niacin, lack of milk and meat in the diet, lack of variation of foods in the diet, poverty, farming practices inappropriate to the needs of the population, and loss of the freedom to farm according to one's own judgement.

The effective actions to bring the disease under control have included: treatment of individuals with niacin, free distribution of yeast which is rich in niacin to supplement niacin intake, increasing the range of foods offered to captive populations, phasing out sharecropping, flour enrichment, reduced unemployment, military service, and food rationing. In the USA flour enrichment started in1941 and was made compulsory by a war order in 1943, and this action virtually wiped out pellagra. Pellagra outbreaks continue to occur, but thankfully are now rare. A pellagra outbreak with 908 cases between July 1999 and February 2000 occurred in Kuito, Angola, mostly in war refugees. Diseases with socially based causes of causes, require socially based remedies.

2.5 **Individual and population level epidemiological variables**

Information collected at the individual level may not portray, in a valid way, the true state of the society or population. Equally, information on a population or the environment may not have meaning at an individual level. Before reading on reflect on the questions in Box 2.8.

Box 2.8 **Individual and population measures**

Under what circumstances might individual measures be meaningfully applied to populations and vice versa? Reflect on such measures as age, sex, blood pressure, household size, population density, and gross national product.

Individual attributes such as age, age at death, blood pressure, and serum cholesterol can usually be aggregated meaningfully and described in the population as a whole. To provide a meaningful picture the data must be from either the whole population or a characteristic (representative) sample. If this is not the case the measure of the population's health status may be grossly inaccurate, even though the individual measures are accurate.

Imagine a study to determine the distribution and mean value of cholesterol in a population aged 18–64 where state-of-the-art methods were applied to ensure accurate measurement. If the investigators called for volunteers to participate, their measures may lead to erroneous conclusions because the people studied are untypical. For this reason epidemiology is generally based on studies of the entire population of interest and, when this is too large, on samples selected using methods to achieve representative samples (e.g. random sampling, stratified sampling, etc.). In other words the investigator exerts control of who is in the study. These are known as probability methods of sampling. As representativeness is a key requirement in epidemiology, small studies on representative samples tend to be of greater value than large ones on unrepresentative samples. Typically the response rate would be 60–70 per cent of those called to participate. Participation is usually least in young poor men living in the inner city. Even with excellent measures and best practice in terms of sample selection, therefore, the end result may be inaccurate as a population measure.

The attributes of a population need to be described by both the frequency distribution and summary measures of the distribution such as the mean and standard deviation (see Fig. 2.3). The population distribution of most biological measures follows a normal or Gaussian distribution as shown in Fig. 2.3. When this is the case the mean, median and mode value is the same; one standard deviation includes about 68 per cent of the population, and two standard deviations include 95 per cent of the population. In epidemiological studies the population distribution must be examined to assess whether it follows the normal distribution. If it does, then the mean and standard deviation provide an accurate picture of the distribution. If not, the distribution should be shown because summary statistics do not permit the reader to envision it accurately. The distribution and the summary statistics of measures made on representative samples of individuals often do provide meaningful information on the whole population. Sometimes individual measures have no value when aggregated. Table 2.3(a) lists fingerprint patterns and personality as examples of such measures. Societies do not have a personality or a fingerprint pattern and applying individual data to groups is purposeless quantification. Measures of the

Table 2.3(a) Some individual measures which, conceptually, have no meaningful interpretation when aggregated into populations

Fingerprint patterns
Personality
Eye colour
Loneliness

Table 2.3(b) Some population and environmental variables which, conceptually, have no direct and meaningful individual counterpart

Population variables	Environmental variables
Population density	Air quality measure such as particulate matter or sulphur dioxide
Income and wealth inequality index	Road traffic density
% of population unemployed	Ambient temperature
Indexes of socio-economic deprivation	
Gross national product	Land use

population or the environment also may be meaningless when applied to the individual. Epidemiological findings based on variables that have no meaningful individual counterpart may be applicable only at the population level. Some population and environment level variables of this kind are listed in Table 2.3(b). It is a paradox that some data collected from individuals (e.g. the number of people who live in the household), when used in aggregate (e.g. as population density of an area), cease to be meaningful at the individual level. While social variables are usually measured in individuals, environmental variables are usually not so measured. Contemporary challenges in epidemiology include the accurate measurement of environmental exposures in individuals, and the measurement of social characteristics in aggregate. Social characteristics including cohesion in society, teamwork, and the state of economic transition, are likely to have profound effects on health and yet be incompletely captured and described through individualized approaches to measurement. Advances in epidemiology are being driven by critical re-analysis of the concept of population (see also Chapter 9). The next section examines the interdependence of demography and epidemiology.

2.6 Epidemiology and demography: interdependent population sciences

Demography is the study of population, including the impact of birth, death, fertility, marriage, migration, and other social factors on population structure and trends.

Box 2.9 **The importance of demography to epidemiology**

- Imagine a country or region where there was no demographic data, so the number of people and the age and sex composition of the population were unknown.
- Imagine also that an epidemic (of pneumonia, food poisoning, depression or attempted suicide) is suspected.
- You are asked to develop a plan to prevent and control the epidemic in the area.
- You are also asked to advise on the future needs for medical personnel in the area.

There is an obvious overlap in the disciplines of epidemiology and demography. Epidemiology is hugely dependent on demography and is difficult to do well when demographic data are not available or are erroneous. To understand the importance of demography in epidemiology try the exercise in Box 2.9 before reading on.

It is hard to imagine a place without demographic data, for in modern society we are bombarded with population statistics. A census of population is fundamental to modern life. The US census has taken place every ten years since 1790 and the UK one since 1801. Indeed, our first public health action on encountering a society without a population count would probably be to fill the gap by undertaking a survey of population size (census). Accurate population counts are hardest to obtain in fast changing societies and in countries where people do not live in wood, stone or brick-built homes on land they own or rent.

Even in the industrialized world there may be a lack of reliable population size data in the inner city, in economically deprived areas, in holiday towns where there is a flux of population, holiday theme parks (although these may operate turnstile counts), war zones, refugee camps, or at major public gatherings such as pop festivals. In most developing countries census data are usually available but are probably less reliable, particularly for small localities.

Lebanon is an advanced middle-income country in the Middle East. It is unusual in not having had a census since the 1930s. The reason for this is political. Population size and structure is, nonetheless, estimated in various ways. With the recent civil war, the continuing border battles and the large number of refugees and soldiers, an accurate population count is not possible. Furthermore, registration of deaths takes place at the locality of family origin as registered in the last census and not at the place of residence or death. A medical diagnosis is not a requirement for a death certificate. Without such base information, describing disease patterns on a national scale and monitoring trends is difficult. The circumstances of a refugee camp, though extreme, illustrate the principles well.

Imagine that the epidemic referred to in Box 2.9 occurs in a refugee camp, where the population size is variable and where there has been a large intake in recent days (the

- Count of cases possible
- Limited health care planning possible on case count
- Trends in case counts useful if population is stable
- Changes in case count cannot be interpreted easily if population is unstable

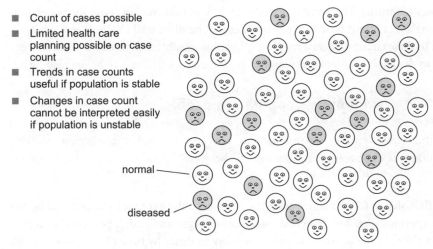

normal

diseased

Fig. 2.5 Potential and limits of undefined populations

camp population is represented in Fig. 2.5 with each circle being a person and cases of sickness/disease are shaded). An outbreak of pneumonia is suspected. What can the epidemiologist do?

The epidemiologist can count the number of cases, and relate this information to the date of disease onset, date of diagnosis, and the age and sex of the patients. This information is useful to assess the level of need for care. For example, if there are 20 cases who become sick today perhaps we can assume there will be a similar number tomorrow. So, facilities can be organized and supplies can be ordered. What if the number of cases per day declines or rises? The daily trend can be described and used to make a prediction and the facilities and supply order adjusted. Using information on the age, sex or other characteristics of cases, appropriate refinements can be made to the plan of needs. So, if 90 per cent of the cases are children, the need for antibiotics can be adjusted, because they need small doses and possibly different drugs. This is a useful and practical application of epidemiology, and arguably simple epidemiology such as this should be applied more widely. Nonetheless, the information is sorely limited.

Without a knowledge of population size and composition, we cannot estimate the number of cases that are to be expected in normal circumstances, so we cannot say with certainty whether there are more than expected, and hence whether an epidemic is underway. Changes in daily numbers may simply be reflecting changes in population size. We cannot assess whether the disease is affecting some groups, such as men more than women, or whether it is commoner in some parts of the camp than others. The number of cases over time gives some, but not definitive, insight into whether the disease is controlled or not, for a rise may occur if the population is increasing even in the face of successful control. Only if the population size is stable can changes in the number of cases reflect change in disease incidence. Epidemiological investigations into the reasons why outbreaks (here pneumonia) occur usually focus on comparing cases with non-cases (controls). This work is impeded by lack of information about the population of potential cases and potential controls, as will be discussed in Chapter 9 on study design. In these circumstances a rational, epidemiologically based disease control strategy is hard to design, implement and monitor. Try the exercise in Box 2.10 before reading on.

Box 2.10 **Developing a population profile**

Imagine that accurate information on the age and sex composition of the inhabitants is to be collected. How will this be done?

The first step is to set some boundaries of which the geographical one will be the most important (Fig. 2.6). Where does the camp begin and end? The second step is to define a time for the census. The count is likely to differ by time of year, day of week and probably time of day. The third step is to define who is to be included. It is likely that some people are visitors, others are helpers, some are staff, and some refugees will move in and out of the camp. The fourth step is to decide what information is to be collected and how. Once these decisions are made, the number, age, and sex of the inhabitants can be ascertained. Now that we have done a census the case numbers can be expressed as a proportion of the population from which they arose. The number of cases per unit of population can be calculated either overall or separately by the characteristics of the people in the camp (e.g. by age, sex, type of resident etc.).

- Set a boundary
- Decision about those on the boundary
- Define a time
- Count the population
- Describe the population
- Count migrations, births and deaths
- Link population counts to health data to calculate birth and death rates, and disease specific rates
- Surveillance by time, place and person
- Monitoring
- Design of studies to understand the burden and causes of disease

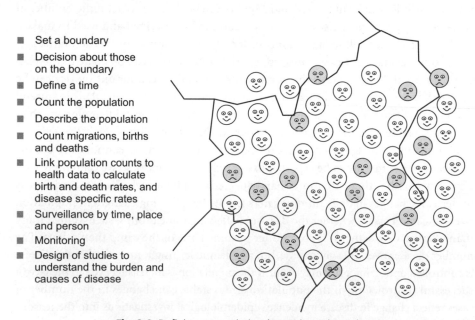

Fig. 2.6 Defining a population by setting a boundary.

Box 2.11 **A public health and epidemiological framework for solving the problem of the epidemic in the camp**

Imagine yourself as the health officer of this camp responsible for controlling the epidemic.

◆ Which questions do you need to answer to bring to bear a rational control strategy and to declare the problem controlled?

◆ Which epidemiological data do you need, in general terms, to answer the questions?

◆ How does the census help you?

If there is a change in the number of cases over time, there are two main explanations: either the number of people has changed or the rate of disease has changed. Since the population is unlikely to remain stable for long in a refugee camp, it is likely that the number of cases will change due to population size fluctuations. The obvious answer is to recount the population regularly, perhaps weekly, but this will be impractical in a camp and in most real life circumstances. In practice, the occasional census needs to be combined with a means of keeping track of population change, which requires recording deaths, births and migration. This system of recording 'vital' statistics permits the census data to be updated routinely.

The collection of vital statistics is an incomplete and error prone exercise, so population counts become out of date, particularly in small geographical areas, and the census needs to be repeated. In the setting of a camp this need may arise monthly. Most nations repeat the census every 5–10 years or so. Cities generally need counts between census years. Reflect on the questions in the exercise in Box 2.11 before reading on.

The questions the health officer needs to ask and answers are summarized in Table 2.4. With the population count by age and sex, basic but important epidemiological questions of whether the disease frequency has altered, and is altering in the face of control measures, can be answered (see part (a) of Table 2.4). For understanding of cause (part (b) of Table 2.4) the level of information needed is greater. For designing, implementing, and evaluating effective strategies for the prevention and control of disease, knowledge of the culture and politics of the refugee camp and the society it is in, will need to be integrated with the epidemiology.

The work of demographers and health statisticians who work to develop disease rates clearly overlaps with that of epidemiologists and yet differs from it in one important goal: epidemiology needs to understand, explain and use, and not just describe, the patterns of disease and that means understanding enough about the population to generate and test causal hypotheses. The epidemiological population, as with a demographic one, is usually defined using geographical boundaries (Fig. 2.6). The epidemiological population may also be defined by the characteristics of the population such as age and sex, or

Table 2.4 Answering public health and epidemiological questions using data

The public health and epidemiological questions	Data needs
(a) Frequency and pattern	
How common is this problem?	Case numbers sufficient for rare diseases and when the population is stable, otherwise population counts are essential
Is the problem increasing, decreasing, or about the same?	Accurate numbers and population counts are essential
Where does it occur most?	Case numbers and population counts by area are essential
Who is affected most?	Case numbers and population counts by population characteristics such as age, sex, economic, and ethnic group are essential
(b) Understanding cause	
What are the causes of the problem?	Detailed information on the population and its social and environmental context is essential. The data need to be collected to test hypotheses on causation
(c) Control	
What strategy is needed to prevent or control the problem?	Understanding of the causal chain of the disease and outbreak and of the resources available, together with understanding of the refugee camp in its social context
Are control measures working?	Case numbers and population data are usually essential for monitoring effectiveness of control measures; together with understanding of other changes occurring in the population and environment

consist of, say, people with diabetes, children attending a particular school, or the homeless. The epidemiological population also needs to be bounded by time limits. In addition to a population size estimate in a defined place and time, epidemiology needs an understanding of the social and environmental circumstances of the people under study.

The idea of generalization (applicability elsewhere) is crucial to many scholarly disciplines and sciences. Ideally, epidemiological conclusions should be applicable not just to the people actually studied but also to others similar to them elsewhere. In practice, as human populations are highly variable in biological, environmental, and social ways, generalization is fraught with difficulty. Figure 2.1 has deliberately depicted human figures, for it is too easy to forget the complexity of a human when using symbols (of which numbers are the prime example), but for simplicity the many figures in this book use ovals to represent human beings. A clear and detailed description of the population, in its environmental and social context, is essential to assess the potential for generalization. Unfortunately, it is common for investigators to ignore this cardinal rule, to generalize too readily and to err. When generalization is not appropriate, epidemiological data can still be used for local assessment of the health state of the people actually studied.

2.7 The dynamic nature of human population

In natural living communities the size and composition of populations is constantly changing owing to deaths, births and migrations. However, even when the population size remains fixed, the population is still changing. Obviously, within any fixed group the individuals are getting older so the average age increases, and that will have a profound effect on the pattern of disease. In a more subtle way, the same trend can occur in whole societies. In the industrialized world we have witnessed the phenomenon of increasing lifespan arising from better socio-economic conditions, nutrition, environment, and health care. The average lifespan has increased by several decades in the last two hundred years or so (and continues to rise). Simultaneously, such societies typically have moved to having smaller families, in some countries too small to replace those dying. This phenomenon has led to societies where the population is, on average, older than it was. This is labelled the demographic transition.

Imagine, however, a place where the number of people is fixed, and whenever an individual dies, or leaves, he/she is replaced by another. Imagine that over time the age, sex and ethnic composition of the group stays the same. A place of this kind might be a jail or a long-stay institution such as a nursing home. Even then, the population's health patterns are not fixed because human behaviours are constantly evolving and their environments changing. The jail environment in the UK has changed by, for example, the introduction of television, alteration in diet, and the development of a drug-taking culture. The wider social trends in behaviour, including smoking, influence these enclosed populations. In short, for epidemiological purposes there is no fixed human population, only dynamic ones, always in transition. Epidemiology is of necessity the study of the pattern of disease in changing populations.

While all human populations are dynamic, the concept of a fixed population is helpful in shaping epidemiological thinking about the measurement of disease occurrence. Cohort studies (discussed in Chapter 9) are an attempt to create a defined or 'closed' population, while studies on vital statistics are on natural living or 'open' populations. In closed populations people who are dying and migrating are not replaced. In open populations there are gains as well as losses, as people are born and migrate into the population. The change in size of the closed population can be predicted if we know the death rates and emigration rates. The prediction of the size of the natural living population is much more difficult and requires, in addition to the above, estimates of immigration and fertility patterns. Predicting the size and composition of open populations is a key component of demography. If the number of people entering a population is balanced by the number exiting, the population is in a steady, but not unchanging, state.

Changes in the environment and behaviour over time lead to time-period influences on disease patterns. For example, 30–40 year old women were less likely to be smokers in the decade 1920–1930 than 30–40 year old women in 1950–1960. In an examination of the close and positive relationship between age group and lung cancer, say in 2001, the investigator would need to consider both the direct effect of ageing, and the period effect (cohort effect) of changing exposures to the causes of lung cancer over time.

The combination of the demographic transition and the effects of wider influences on health (environment, behaviour, etc.), leads to a profound change in the pattern of disease, with the dominance of chronic disease. In many countries we have witnessed increasing wealth and the dominance of diseases of affluent lifestyle and older age groups. This phenomenon is labelled the epidemiological transition and is emerging rapidly in middle-income countries such as Mauritius, Chile and urban India. For epidemiology as a science these transitions are a boon, because they have led to greater variation in disease patterns and exposures to causes, and provide the fuel for the epidemiological endeavour.

Most epidemiologists live and work in relatively wealthy and stable countries. In these countries improvements in most established quantitative indices of health have been both dramatic and inexorable. This must not lead to complacency. In the face of economic, political, and social disturbance, health gains can be rapidly reversed. The decline in life expectancy in Russia and other East European countries in recent decades is a perfect example of the epidemiological transition in reverse. The extremely high infant mortality (in excess of 100) in Iraq, in comparison with adjoining countries of similar economic standing and social circumstances, is almost certainly directly related to the trade blockade imposed on the country following the Gulf War.

2.8 Applications of the population concept

The concept of population, as outlined above, has a huge influence on every aspect of health care, but it is often implicit. Health policy is nearly always based on the concept of population. Policy is usually directed either at the whole population or at subgroups identified by some important characteristic, such as geographical location (a nation, a city, or economically deprived area), the age group or gender, or some other characteristic such as ethnic or racial group.

Traditionally, healthcare systems have been designed around those who voice their need by consulting a doctor or other healer. Increasingly, healthcare systems are broadening their scope and focusing on their goals of improving the health of the whole population by using the concept of population in a number of ways. Firstly, they are planning services based on the pattern of health problems in the population as a whole, taking into account variations in the health of subgroups within the population, and not just of users of the service. Secondly, they are delivering modified services to sub-subgroups of the population who differ in their needs and are not making effective use of existing services, for example the homeless, those in rural areas, or those who speak a foreign language. Thirdly, by using knowledge of population trends in health status they are anticipating the need for future services.

The theory of health promotion is based on the population idea. Indeed, the social sciences and psychology, which underpin health promotion theory, emphasize how peer influences dominate the actions of individuals. The population concepts of epidemiology, particularly as interpreted by Rose, may lead to a radical shift in practice. The concepts shift attention away from the individual-orientated programmes to the population as a whole. The concept requires a radical idea: the targeting of interventions at people in the middle of the distribution (the average person) and not the extremes of the distribution (the deviants as described by Rose).

Clinical practice based on the epidemiological concept of population is potentially transformed. The clinician is presented with new challenges, a means of increasing the impact of medical science, personal responsibility to the wider society, and acute ethical dilemmas. Clearly, the purpose of the health professions is greater than just the alleviation of the pain and illnesses of individuals. Their purpose includes the acquisition of knowledge (research) and organization of care for the benefit of people who access the service, the people who need the service but do not access it, and the generations to come.

For the individual clinician the people to be served are primarily those who have elected to consult, whether in the 'walk-in' manner of the American healthcare system or by registration with the general practitioner and referral as in the British NHS. Clinicians have or develop a list of people for whom they are responsible. For clinicians, collectively, the list comprises all the people in the society within which they live and work. This population philosophy provides the foundation for clinical epidemiology and evidence-based health care. The example of diabetes care illustrates the need for and power of this approach.

Diabetes is a chronic disabling disease with a prolonged progression (natural history, which is discussed in Chapter 6) which may not be diagnosed until after the damaging effects have occurred. Only about half of all people with diabetes are actually diagnosed at any time. This poses a huge problem for clinicians managing diabetes. The traditional form of clinical care would involve awaiting the development of symptoms and problems severe enough to lead the person with diabetes to present for clinical care, for example infections, fatigue, organ failure, or even coma. The population approach is to take advantage of our epidemiological knowledge to promote the early diagnosis of disease and the prevention of complications. At present, early diagnosis is through widespread awareness rather than through screening tests. Diabetes physicians are among the early adopters of the population perspective and are increasingly assessing their effectiveness in terms of how well diabetes is detected, diagnosed, prevented, and controlled in the population and not just in individual patients.

This requires them to identify all people with diabetes and to have means of indirectly influencing them through other healthcare providers. Practising population-based medicine requires diabeticians to study health and disease in the community setting, to understand the epidemiology of the disease and to have access to information on the impact of their work in the population setting. The key tool for achieving all this is a population register of patients with diabetes. In future, such registers may also include people with impaired glucose tolerance, which is at least for some a precursor of diabetes.

Despite Hippocrates' exhortation to doctors to understand diseases by studying the airs, waters and places affecting their patients, medical sciences concerned themselves with understanding how body systems worked and disease process occurred in individuals presenting themselves for medical care. In the nineteenth century epidemiology established its credentials as a mode of enquiry which could overturn causal ideas derived from these sciences and now it is considered as an essential part of clinical research and practice.

Biomedical scientists can also use and apply the population concepts in epidemiology. Firstly, they can use hypotheses generated by epidemiological observations in populations for their own studies whether on cells, organs, animals, or individual human beings. Secondly, they can test out their own hypotheses based on their research by seeing whether disease patterns in populations are in line with their predictions. Thirdly, they can ground their own work in a defined sample of population and not rely on cells, organs, and other specimens from volunteers, or from selected patients.

2.9 **Conclusion**

Thinking about populations drives epidemiology and its applications. Population thinking emphasizes that disease patterns are the outcome of the interaction between groups of individuals and their environment. It emphasizes that effective understanding of the causes and control of disease needs to be based on these interactions and not on an analysis of individuals in isolation. If applied by all the health professions the population approach promises to enhance the impact and effectiveness of their endeavour, not least by providing a broader scientific rationale to practice. The concept underlies the discipline of health and healthcare needs assessment. No policy document or healthcare plan is complete without a population view, and health promotion and health education work also thrive within the population perspective. Clinical practice is embracing the idea. Medical science has always had the ambition of being generalizable to the whole population and is increasingly moving from the study of the individual and the organs, to studying these in the context of representative samples of the population.

The underlying theories that underpin this chapter are that disease patterns in individuals and societies are profoundly influenced by the mode of interaction of individuals with each other, animals, and the wider environment; and that the pattern of disease in society is more than the sum of disease in individuals. The central principle that can be drawn from this chapter is that the causes of disease lie in populations and their societies as much as in individuals and their biology.

Summary

Epidemiology is a population science in several senses. Firstly, it studies disease patterns, which are hugely influenced by the interaction of individuals living in communities. Secondly, it depends heavily upon demographic population data to achieve its goals. Thirdly, its findings are drawn from, and applied to, groups (or populations) of people. Conclusions and recommendations from epidemiological data may be applied to individuals with caution (in a probabilistic way), and with open acknowledgement of individual variation.

Epidemiology without demographic data is limited in its scope, for then disease patterns can only be studied in populations which are stable in size and composition. Without accurate demographic data, interpretation of comparisons between population groups is possible only when there are stark differences. Epidemiological studies do not work well without an understanding of the composition of the population under study and important errors in interpretation of data may arise from the use of erroneous demographic statistics.

A prime purpose of epidemiology is the application of findings in health promotion, health care, and health policy to improve the health of populations. The focus on population is the defining feature of epidemiology, which distinguishes it from clinical research and the other medical sciences, which primarily study the individual, the organ, and the cell.

Chapter 3

Variation in disease by time, place, and person
A framework for analysis

Objectives

On completion of this chapter you should understand:

- that virtually all diseases vary in their incidence and prevalence over time, across geographical areas and between population subgroups;

- that apparent disease variations can be artefacts of errors or changes in data collection systems;

- that variations must be analysed systematically to check that they are real, and not illusory;

- that real variations are driven by environmental and social change over the short term, with a genetic contribution in the long term;

- that real variations, which are nature's experiments, provide a potentially powerful means of understanding the causal pathways of disease;

- that study of clusters and outbreaks, which reflect abrupt changes in disease frequency, may yield both causal knowledge, and information to control the public health problem;

- that real variations help to develop and target health policy and health care;

- that variations generate observations of associations, which in turn spark causal hypotheses.

3.1 Introduction

Diseases wax and wane in their population frequency over time and the pattern varies between populations. This simple but profoundly important observation, which holds virtually without exception, is one of the axioms of epidemiology. Medical and public health practice are often given credit for bringing about a decline in disease when it is due to natural causes (but medicine and public health practice rarely take the blame for rising disease rates). Diseases which have undergone massive change in incidence within the last 50 to 100 years, largely uninfluenced by deliberate human interventions, include peptic ulcer, stroke, gastric cancer, AIDS, and infections including tuberculosis.

This chapter introduces a systematic mode of analysis of disease variations, particularly to ensure that observations of variation are real, and not illusory products of data errors and artefacts.

The framework for the analysis of changes in disease frequency presented in this chapter applies to all measures of disease frequency. For reasons discussed in Chapter 7 (Sections 7.2 and 7.3, Table 7.2), for aetiologically orientated investigations, the soundest measure is the incidence rate, a measure based on new cases. The likelihood of artefact being the explanation for changes in disease frequency is greater with prevalence measures (these are measures of existing disease) than with incidence rates.

3.2 Reasons for analysing disease variations

Consider the questions in Box 3.1 before reading further.

Box 3.1 Benefits of studying variations

- What potential benefits are there from investigation of changes in disease frequency?
- Is a decline in disease as worthy of investigation as a rise?

There are three principal reasons for investigating a change in disease frequency. Firstly, to help control an abrupt rise in disease incidence, especially of a suspected cluster or outbreak (the commonest public health emergency) of an infectious or environmental disease.

Secondly, for understanding the factors which influence disease frequency, and hence to gain insight into the causes of disease. Thirdly, and an increasingly important goal, to use the time trend in disease, and its causes, to develop health policy and healthcare plans and to predict and alter its future course.

The investigation of a decline in disease frequency is, for understanding causes, as worthy of investigation as an increase. In practice, a rise in disease incidence is a problem for society, while a decline is the resolution of a problem, and so is given lesser priority.

The key strategy in epidemiology is to seek out and quantify disease variation, and then develop and test hypotheses to understand the causal mechanisms which led to it. The variation is analysed by asking the question: why does the disease vary over time, between places, and between populations with different characteristics? As already discussed briefly in Chapter 1 and Chapter 2 (Section 2.1, Box 2.1) this strategy and question is one of the keystones of epidemiology. In the first analysis, as discussed in Chapter 5, causes are distinguished as genetic and environmental, the latter being used broadly to mean everything that is not genetic.

Before reading on, do the exercise in Box 3.2.

Box 3.2 **Reasons for variation**

- Why, in general terms, do diseases vary over time, between places, and between subgroups of the populations?
- What is the relative importance of genetic and environmental influences in bringing about population differences in disease?

Variation in disease occurs over time in populations because the characteristics of the people or of their environment alter. Some of these characteristics influence disease frequency. As such changes are not geographically uniform, this generates different patterns of disease in different places. In addition, within apparently homogeneous populations the disease experience of subgroups usually varies too because of differences in their characteristics, including genetic inheritance, behaviour, and local environment. Even if the social and physical environment were constant, however, some changes in population patterns of disease over time would still occur albeit much more slowly, for genetic changes are inevitable and will influence disease.

All humans belong to one species, with mating and reproduction occurring between all human populations in natural circumstances, so genetic variation between populations is small in scale. Genetic change arises from a number of processes including genetic drift and genetic mutation, which cause random variation in gene frequency from generation to generation. In small populations genetic drift can lead to important genetically driven disease differences.

In large populations, however, genetic make-up is relatively stable. Changes in disease frequency in large populations occurring over short periods of time, meaning years or a few decades, are almost wholly due to environmental factors. There must, of course, be the genetic potential to develop a disease for it to occur. For example, hypertension is extremely common in urban-living Africans, especially those living in wealthy, industrialized countries, but not in rural Africans. Diabetes is common in urbanized Australian Aborigines but not in those living traditional lifestyles. The increase in disease prevalence in urban settings is due to changes in environmental factors in populations with a genetic potential to develop these diseases. Most diseases result from an interaction of environmental and genetic factors. Though changes over longer time periods, meaning several hundreds or thousands of years or more, may be due to genetic factors, even they are also much more likely to be due to environmental ones. The varying genetic potential for disease in different populations is acquired (and lost) over evolutionary timescales.

To take an analogy from theatre, in shaping the pattern of disease in large populations, the environment is the leading player and genetics the stage. This is not to deny the importance of genetic and hence biological factors in disease occurrence. The main cause of lung cancer is the growth and consumption by inhalation of tobacco. If humans were not biologically susceptible to the carcinogens in tobacco, then tobacco would not cause lung cancer in populations. In shaping the risks of disease in individuals as opposed to populations, genetic make-up is profoundly important, for genetic variation between individuals is great. This can be stated as one of the public health paradoxes: for populations the environment is the dominant influence on the pattern of disease, for individuals genetic inheritance may be equally or more important. This paradox underlies the argument between those who emphasize the environment and those who favour genetics as the dominant cause of disease. Disease is, of course, caused by the interaction of the genome and the environment. Nonetheless, the control of disease does not usually involve influencing the interaction, but in choosing between genetic or environmental manipulation, the latter usually being easier than the former.

In the last few hundred years change in the environment has been rapid and has profoundly changed disease patterns, particularly in populations which have industrialized and become wealthy. A decline in birth rates and death rates leads to a shift in the age distribution of the population, with the average age increasing (the demographic transition). Industrialization, wealth creation, ageing of the population, and the other profound changes alter the pattern of diseases (the epidemiological transition). In a few decades or a century or so, infectious disease can decline dramatically as a cause of death and serious disease, and chronic diseases such as coronary heart disease, stroke, diabetes and cancers of the lung, breast, and colon, can become dominant. This transition is reversible, for when poverty strikes either as a result of economic or political turmoil or in war, infectious diseases return. These massive shifts in disease patterns invariably overshadow the impact of both medical care and public health efforts, at least in terms of the population, if not the individual.

International differences in disease patterns mainly, though not wholly, reflect the fact that the populations are at different stages in the demographic and epidemiological transitions. Some of the differences, however, are due to local environmental factors (e.g. climate) and some to genetic factors. For these reasons international variations will be much reduced, though not eliminated, as the demographic and epidemiological transitions progress. Similarly, the disease patterns of migrant populations converge towards those of the population that they join. The same conclusion and underlying principles apply to differences in disease patterns in subgroups within a geographically defined population. Disease differences between social classes or ethnic groups, for example, largely reflect differences in the environment and not in genetic composition. These differences, too, can be conceptualized as a result of sub-populations being at different stages of the demographic and epidemiological transition.

3.3 Variations and associations: real or artefact?

When changes in disease frequency are natural, or real, and not a result of the way diseases are diagnosed or counted (illusory, apparent, or artefactual), the underlying reasons as discussed above are often exceedingly difficult to pinpoint. Changes in disease pattern can be considered as an experiment of nature, posing a challenge to science.

For causal understanding of disease variation, the first step is to exclude artefact as the explanation, the second is to develop a hypothesis stated as an association, the third is to design a test of the hypothesis, and the fourth is to assess the results in relation to frameworks for causal thinking. Much of this chapter and Chapter 4 concern the process by which artefactual (or illusory, spurious, or apparent) variations and associations are identified and excluded. The process in epidemiology for assessing the causal basis of such hypotheses is considered in Chapter 5.

Demonstrating variation in disease is the first step towards establishing an epidemiological association which, in turn, may generate explanatory hypotheses. The association is a postulate that there is a link (or relationship) between a disease and another factor (called risk factor, see Chapter 7 for discussion), whether this factor is another disease, or a characteristic of the person or population under study. For example, in the UK, coronary heart disease (CHD) mortality rates rose steadily in the twentieth century until the 1970s when they declined, a rise and fall similar to that seen in many industrialized countries. First, we measure and demonstrate the association of disease rates and time periods. We attempt to explain the time trend by developing our understanding of social, environmental, and lifestyle changes over these time periods. Then, we develop and test specific hypotheses; one might be that the rise and fall reflect the changing levels of factors that are known to cause CHD, for example exercise patterns, consumption of dietary fats and fruits and vegetables, and levels of blood pressure and its control in the community. Further studies are then done to confirm or refute such hypotheses. The solution will be quantitative; how much of the decline in CHD can be explained by the changing pattern in these factors? The epidemiological association, thus, fuels a process of analysis and research which either strengthens causal understanding or raises new questions by failing to confirm the hypotheses. In this example, the decline in CHD is too rapid to be a result, solely, of change in the factors mentioned. Better treatment of established CHD reducing or delaying death from this disease has contributed and there are other unexplained factors.

The epidemiological association can be based on theory alone or observations only on one or a few persons. For example, a doctor may observe a few cases of renal failure in patients taking a particular drug, as happened for phenacetin and other anti-inflammatory drugs used for arthritis. The epidemiological association implies that disease and an associated factor may be causally connected. The epidemiological challenge is to demonstrate what the factor is (when it is unknown), to quantify the association, to assess whether the association is causal, and, if so, to explain how. Ultimately, the challenge is to understand the mechanisms by which the risk factor affects disease. Understanding of mechanisms invariably requires collaboration with other sciences.

The first and crucial question is this: is the variation in disease an artefact or real? If it is an illusion, then there is no epidemiological association to explain. Before reading on, do the exercise in Box 3.3.

Box 3.3 **Why variations and resulting associations may be illusory**

Consider the possible reasons why a variation in disease pattern might be an arte-fact rather than real. (You may find 7–10 reasons.) Can you group them into three or four categories of explanation?

Most often disease variations are an illusion arising from the following:

* Chance. The numbers of cases are randomly fluctuating over time.

* Errors of observation. Biased techniques are the most common reason for making erroneous observations, and this is discussed in detail in Chapter 4.

* Changes in the size and structure of the population from which the cases arose. This was discussed in the previous chapter (Section 2.6).

* The likelihood of people seeking health care and hence being diagnosed and eventu-ally counted in statistics. This varies with their level of knowledge, expectations and the accessibility and acceptability of health care.

* The likelihood of the correct diagnosis being reached, which is dependent on avail-ability and use of medical care, the level of skill of the doctor, and the quality of the diagnostic facilities available (Chapters 6 and 7).

* Changes in the clinical approach to diagnosis, which are dependent on changing med-ical trends, for example whether wheezing is to be called wheezy bronchitis or asthma.

* Changes in data collection methods; for example, when computerization of medical records takes place with structured methods of entering a diagnosis and automatic data extraction, the numbers of cases is likely to rise.

* Changes in the way diseases are diagnostically coded, which is influenced by both the versions of disease codes used and the interpretation of the disease data by the coder (Chapter 7).

* Changes in the way data are analysed and presented; for example, merely altering the 'standard' population used in adjusting disease rates for differences in age and sex (discussed in Chapter 8) can spuriously alter disease incidence.

These 'illusory' explanations, summarized in Table 3.1, can be categorized as: chance; measurement error in counts of cases or populations; diagnostic variation; data pro-cessing and presentation. The role of chance is assessed using statistical probability methods (the reader will need to consult a statistics textbook), and measurement and data processing errors by quality assurance methods (see Chapter 4). Errors in popula-tion counts may be difficult to find and correct, so the key is a high level of awareness. Diagnostic activity can usually be assessed indirectly by observing changes in staffing

Table 3.1 Summary of illusory, apparent, or artefactual explanations of disease variations and associations

Chance
Error
Change in size and structure of underlying population
Healthcare seeking behaviour
Diagnostic accuracy
Diagnostic fashion
Data collection
Coding
Analysis
Presentation

and facilities, or directly by counting the number of tests done. Where specialists in a particular disease are employed, the number of tests done for the disease of interest will rise, and the disease frequency will appear to rise. For example, the north-east of England has an extremely high prevalence and incidence of primary biliary cirrhosis, and the prevalence has risen dramatically over the last 20 years. One possible explanation for this is that the number of gastroenterologists interested in this disease has increased. This was indeed the case. Diagnostic activity measured by the number of tests can be related to the number of cases diagnosed to test a hypothesis that a high number of cases in a locality or time period reflects excessive diagnostic activity. If this were the case, we would predict that a large number of tests would be done for each case diagnosed (test to case ratio would be high). If, however, there was a high incidence of disease, and no excessive testing then the test to case ratio would be low. Figure 3.1 illustrates this in relation to a study of Legionnaires' disease.

Geographical variations are particularly likely to be artefactual, because the mode of clinical practice varies greatly between places. One real, yet potentially misleading cause of geographical variation is short-term fluctuation in disease incidence. Figure 3.2 illustrates the point. Over the three year period the disease incidence in places A and B was identical. A study done in any one year, however, would have concluded that the incidence of disease varied. This is an example of medium-term changes in disease incidence masquerading as geographical variation, when in the long term there is none.

If such artefactual explanations are incorrect, the variations in disease may be real. Before reading on try the exercise in Box 3.4.

There are numerous explanations for disease variations; for example, human beings may change their behaviour, their mode of social interaction, or their reproductive patterns. The causes of disease might change; for example, a micro-organism might

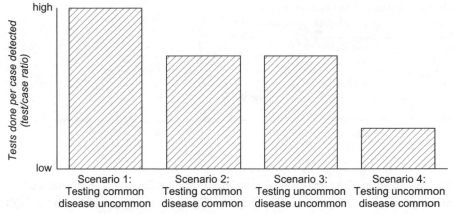

Fig. 3.1 Assessing the effect of diagnostic activity on disease frequency (Adapted, Bhopal, *J Pub Hlth Med* 1991; **13**, 281–9, see Permissions).

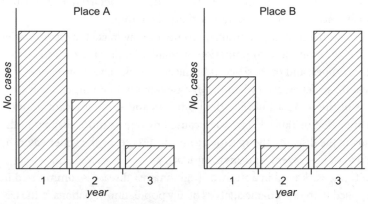

Fig. 3.2 Variations in time masquerading as variations in place (source, Bhopal, *J Pub Hlth Med* 1991; **13**, 281–9, see Permissions).

Box 3.4 **Explanations for real changes in disease frequency**

◆ What explanations can you think of for a real change in disease frequency?

◆ Can you group these into three or four categories of explanation?

mutate so that it becomes less or more virulent (as happens with influenza) or crosses the species barrier (as has probably happened with HIV infection and new variant Creutzfeldt-Jakob disease). The virulence of the causes of disease (agent factors) changes over time; for example, the lowered incidence of rheumatic fever is at least partly due to lesser virulence of the causal organism, the streptococcus.

Table 3.2 Summary of real explanations of disease variation and examples: the causal triad

Host	Genetics
	Behaviour
Agent	Virulence
	Introduction of a new agent
Environment	Housing
	Weather

The composition of the cause of a disease might change; for example, the reduced tar content of modern cigarettes reduces the risk of lung cancer compared with the high tar, unfiltered cigarettes of the past.

The susceptibility of people to acquiring disease may change for many reasons including genetic, nutritional, social, and medical. For example, successful measles immunization programmes in childhood led to this disease occurring rarely, but increasingly in adolescence and adulthood rather than in children.

Changes in the social, chemical, or physical environment may make the disease easier or harder to contract. For example, a combination of smaller family size, the move from extended to nuclear families, and more space at home and work, have reduced the incidence of tuberculosis in societies, even when the disease remains endemic and common in some subgroups of the population (e.g. the homeless and some migrant populations). If so, as summarized in Table 3.2, they are caused by one or more changes in the host (person acquiring the disease), the specific agents of disease, or the wider environment (the causal triad of host, agent, and environment).

The real-artefact framework used in a study of Legionnaires' disease is summarized in Fig. 3.3. It can be applied to the systematic analysis of any population variations in the frequency of disease. Section 3.4 provides the opportunity for you to apply the framework.

3.4 **Applying the real-artefact framework**

Imagine you are the epidemiologist responsible for surveillance of infectious diseases in a city of about 1 million people. You are examining the statistics on the numbers of cases of Legionnaires' disease, which is an environmentally acquired bacterial pneumonia with no person-to-person spread. This pneumonia is rare, with a reported incidence rate of about 3 cases per million population in the USA and England and of about 8 cases per million in your country.

The main sources of the causative micro-organisms, the 'Legionellacae' or, for short, the legionellas, are complex water systems, particularly cooling towers and hot water systems, which are usually found in large buildings or as part of industrial machinery. The incidence rate varies geographically (between localities, cities, and nations) and over time (seasons and years).

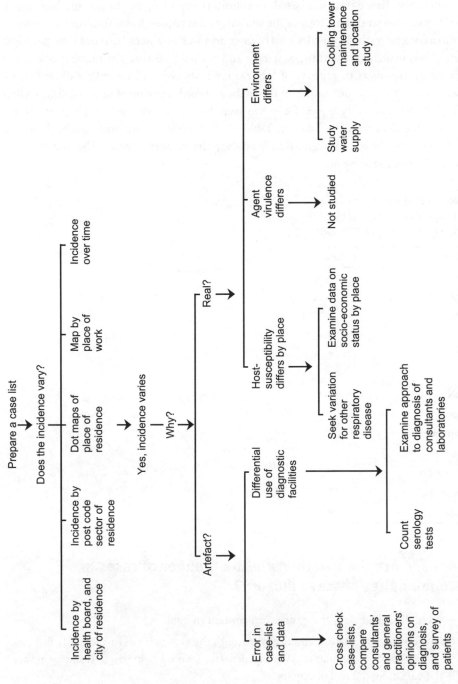

Fig. 3.3 Plan of studie of Legionnaires' disease: framework for geographical variation (source, Bhopal, *J Pub Hlth Med* 1991; **13**, 281–9, see Permissions).

Your surveillance system is based on voluntary reporting by clinical and laboratory colleagues who send you a copy of the laboratory test request form. Your data are entered onto a computer which provides a list of cases on a week-by-week basis but your statistical analysis is usually on monthly, quarterly, and annual statistics. The number of cases is based on numbers of reports of laboratory tests compatible with a diagnosis of Legionnaires' disease per month. Your database records the date of onset of illness when this is on the laboratory request form. You keep the original request forms in paper files.

Examine the surveillance data in Table 3.3 and use the framework and background information above to systematically analyse the pattern. Answer the questions in Box 3.5 before reading on.

Table 3.3 The number of cases of Legionnaires' disease by month in the City of X in 1984

Month	Cases
January	0
February	2
March	3
April	0
May	1
June	26
July	4
August	4
September	6
October	7
November	7
December	12
Total	72

Box 3.5 **Are the variations in the number of cases of Legionnaires' disease illusory?**

◆ First, describe briefly the nature and content of Table 3.3.

◆ Now, work your way systematically through the factors listed in Table 3.1, and discussed above, for guidance. What information would help you to decide whether the variations are real or apparent?

◆ Now, make a judgement on whether the findings represent an outbreak of Legionnaires' disease.

Table 3.3 shows the number of cases of disease in 1984 per month, and shows a month-by-month fluctuation in the number of cases with an abrupt rise in June. At 72 cases per million population the incidence rate in this city is exceedingly high, in relation to national rates (8 per million), and cannot be ignored. There is no automatic means of judging whether an outbreak has occurred and whether some action is required. Judgement has to be exercised. In this case, chance (random fluctuation) seems to be a remote possibility. Yet, an outbreak of 26 cases in one month is a major public health problem, with serious repercussions, so there is no room for misjudgements by declaring an outbreak when there isn't one. We first need to exclude explanations based on error.

Was there, for example, a problem in the techniques used to handle laboratory specimens leading to false positive results? The issue needs to be discussed with the laboratory staff and, if appropriate, the specimens need to be double checked. Two common and important types of errors are misdiagnosis and miscoding. On computerized databases the disease is usually given a code number. Could information on other diseases, say pneumococcal pneumonia or influenza, have been miscoded as Legionnaires' disease? A cross-check of the codes against the original report forms, which will have the full diagnosis, is required to rule out this possibility. These two simple checks will prevent the embarrassment of lengthy and inappropriate investigation arising from illusory changes in disease incidence which turns out to be a pseudo-outbreak.

Has there been a batch of reports in June, possibly arising from some doctor accumulating reports over some months or even years and submitting them together? Alternatively, someone may be re-testing positive specimens from previous years. This can happen in the context of research projects where large numbers of blood tests may be submitted as a batch. If the people on whom the tests have been done are currently sick then this is an unlikely explanation. The date of onset of disease will help to clarify this. If the date of onset varies greatly, say it spans years, then we are not looking at an outbreak. Examine the original laboratory request form, and for cases where the date of disease onset is not given ask the physician-in-charge. Ideally, surveillance systems should analyse cases by date of onset but unfortunately this information is often not available, leaving the epidemiologist to use the much less satisfactory date of receipt of the specimen or of the report.

Has the number of people at risk altered? Most of the analysis above is concerned with the number of cases, also known as the numerator. A change in the size of the population denominator from which the cases are drawn can change the number of cases, though the rate remains the same. This is important for popular tourist areas where the population can increase many-fold. If the reputation of the doctors, healthcare system, or laboratory becomes enhanced, patients can be referred from a wider catchment area. This is an unlikely explanation for the data in Table 3.3, the change having occurred so fast. However, one possibility worth considering for environmentally acquired disease is travel abroad. An increase in international travel can increase the number of cases. Information on the number of travellers is not readily available.

The rise in cases in June could reflect a travel-associated outbreak. It is possible that the cases could be returning from a package tour to a particular destination. This matter can be resolved by questioning the cases about their whereabouts. In fact the data in Table 3.3 are on locally infected cases only.

Has the likelihood of diagnosis increased, either because of greater vigilance by doctors or of people using the healthcare system? A common problem which causes pseudo-outbreaks is the new doctor who is unusually thorough in reporting certain diseases, either because of a diligent commitment to the concept of disease surveillance or because of a research interest in the frequency of these diseases. (It is worth noting that there may be, as in the UK, a fee attached to the notification to a health authority of certain diseases.) This diligence causes problems because the surveillance of disease is normally incomplete, due to a mixture of non-diagnosis and non-reporting. Effective surveillance relies more on stability in the levels of reporting, than on the absolute levels of reporting. Local knowledge of the doctors and their reporting habits helps to assess this possibility. Here, the recent appointment of a chest physician or infectious diseases specialist would increase the possibility both of pseudo-outbreaks and of detecting real ones. Research projects increase the likelihood of the correct diagnosis being reached both because of greater awareness of the diagnosis among the doctors involved and more resources and techniques being available to make the diagnosis. As research may be of a personal nature, and may not be recorded in research databases, it may be difficult to detect that this is the cause of an apparent outbreak. The investigator will be alerted to this possibility if there is a predominance of reports from one or a small group of doctors particularly when one of them is a newcomer to the area; or predominance of recovered rather than ill cases.

Have there been changes in diagnostic fashion or disease definition? Diagnosis is not a fixed or rigid entity but relies on medical knowledge, beliefs about how to manage patients, facilities to practice medicine, and case definitions. The cause of, and diagnostic methods for, Legionnaires' disease were discovered in 1977. Following such a discovery, the incidence of the new disease will inevitably appear to rise and that of the other similar diseases (here, other forms of pneumonia and viral infections such as influenza) will appear to fall. Abrupt changes such as those in the table are unlikely to arise merely from changes in diagnostic fashion.

Have there been changes in the completeness of the data collection methods? Any change in the process by which surveillance is organized will lead to a changed frequency of disease. For example, if following notification of a case of Legionnaires' disease a microbiologist contacts the reporting doctors to request more information and to discuss the case, the extra education and interest is likely to spur those doctors into notifying and diagnosing Legionnaires' disease in future. More obviously, during the investigation of a declared outbreak doctors are alerted by health officials of the need to report disease and to do the necessary tests for it. The greater likelihood of testing, diagnosing, and reporting is likely to last for a while. In the case of the data in Table 3.3, these explanations seem improbable for the 26 cases in June but are likely to be contributing to the cases after that.

Has there been a deliberate change in the way diseases are coded, analysed or data presented? Disease coding systems change. At that time, as there was no specific code in the International Classification of Diseases for Legionnaires' disease, the codes were probably created locally. In other cases, a new edition of the code book may change the coding rules or codes. For instance, the principal global source of codes, the International Classification of Disease (ICD), is revised every ten years or so (see WHO 1992). Major fluctuations in the apparent frequency of some diseases is the result in the transition period as new editions are adopted. Guidance is given with each revision on how to maximize comparability across different revisions of the ICD.

The decision on whether a change in disease frequency is real or apparent can usually be taken rapidly. The important thing is to consider the questions and to judge the likelihood of each possibility. In this example, once error is excluded, the date of onset of illness in the cases has been checked, and the symptoms and signs found to be of a pneumonic illness, the likelihood is that the rise in case numbers is real and there is an outbreak.

The challenge now is to develop a testable explanation, a hypothesis, to unveil the underlying reason for the rise in the disease. One obvious and crucial question is whether the cases were local or travel-acquired infections and this is easily resolved by questioning patients. The rise was in locally acquired cases and there was no excess in travel-associated cases. This simple observation, showing a degree of specificity in the rise of disease frequency, helps both to rule out some sources of artefact (e.g. a laboratory or coding error would not be confined to non-travel cases) and to refine the hypothesis. The same reasoning would be applied to other disorders; for example, is a rise in obstructive airways disease affecting both chronic bronchitis and emphysema and asthma? Is a rise in heart disease confined to coronary heart disease or also affecting, say, rheumatic heart disease? Specific changes are less likely than non-specific ones to arise from artefact.

The rise in locally acquired Legionnaires' disease can be analysed as follows using the host, agent, environment framework (Table 3.2), and the question in Box 3.6.

Box 3.6 **Changes in host, agent, and environment as explanations for the outbreak of Legionnaires' disease**

Do changing susceptibility of the local population, changing virulence of the causal micro-organism, or changes in the environment explain the occurrence of the outbreak? What might the nature of these changes be?

Susceptibility to disease is a result of both genetic and acquired characteristics. Genetic factors, immunization, past exposure to organisms, nutrition, general health status and other relevant risk factors determine the susceptibility of the population.

As the susceptibility of the population usually changes over long periods, and in the case of genetic factors over generations, this is not the explanation for the findings in Table 3.3. If the same data were for decades, not months, such factors might need to be considered.

The virulence of micro-organisms is very difficult to determine, and baseline data rarely exist. The virulence of many micro-organisms is constantly changing; the influenza virus, streptococcus, and staphylococcus are such organisms. Virulent legionellas may have colonized water systems in May or June 1984 and led to the abrupt rise in disease incidence. In this instance, and indeed in most circumstances, an interaction would be required between the agent and environment. In practice, change in virulence is unlikely to be demonstrable and such an explanation will be based on exclusion of other possibilities. While virulence is usually associated with microbes, the concept can be applied to some other causes too, for example, cigarettes and tar content.

A rise in the number of cases could reflect an increase in the level of exposure to the micro-organisms either because the environment has become more hazardous or the contact between the environment and the population has become closer. In our example, the following changes could have occurred:

- The weather changed leading to the switching on of water systems in air conditioning units that harboured virulent legionellas.
- The winds and humidity changed such that virulent organisms could be delivered to a susceptible population at the infective concentration.
- Protective mechanisms (such as the drift elimination mechanisms or chemical decontamination procedures in a cooling tower, or temperature control in a hot water system) broke down.

A large number of explanations of this type can be generated and tested, some quickly, some with difficulty. To re-emphasize, the key to a successful investigation is the systematic analysis and explicit statement of the possible explanations.

In reality a rise in cases will be a result of an interaction of factors. Indeed, both real and artefactual factors will be relevant. For example, the rise in Legionnaires' disease shown in Table 3.3 probably arose because of environmental changes which permitted a virulent organism to colonize a complex water system and which permitted the organisms to be dispersed so that many people were exposed, of whom a small proportion (maybe 1 per cent) were susceptible. Once the excess of cases was publicized and case search procedures started, cases were unearthed which normally would have remained undiagnosed (e.g. patients originally diagnosed as pneumonia or influenza being re-tested for antibody to legionellas, even after they have recovered). This enhanced surveillance will lead to a lasting excess of cases.

In practice, teasing out the different explanations is a complex task. In studies of the geographical epidemiology of Legionnaires' disease in Scotland, 1978–1986, I prepared a case-list of all 372 potential cases diagnosed over the period. The explanations for geographical variation are listed in column one of Table 3.4. The solutions generated to

Table 3.4 Summary of problems arising in the demonstration and interpretation of geographical variation in disease with solutions adopted in a study of Legionnaires' disease in Scotland

Explanations	Solutions adopted
Time variation	
Geographical variation results from varying incidence in time	A long time period was studied (1978–1986)
Artefact	
Differences in case-definition	Standard case-definition applied
Missing cases/incomplete surveillance	Cross-checked case-lists; used data from several sources
Errors in address data/postcodes (Zip codes)	Addresses checked against medical records; all postcodes confirmed using postcode directory; patients asked to check basic details
Differential hospital admission rates	Examined hospital admission rates for other diagnoses (effect would be non-specific); compared travel and non-travel-related Legionnaires' disease cases
Differential use of diagnostic tests	Ratios of serology tests to pneumonia and serology tests to Legionnaires' disease used as an indicator; consultants' and laboratories' approach to diagnosis surveyed
True variation	
Host susceptibility differs	Assessed whether geographical variation existed for other diseases which share risk factors; assessed whether populations differed in terms of socio-economic status
Agent virulence differs	Not studied
Environmental factors differ	Developed hypotheses on most likely source; collected new data on location and maintenance of cooling towers

Adapted from Bhopal, *J Pub Hlth Med* 1991; **13**, 281–9 (see Permissions).

provide evidence to choose between the explanations are in the second column. The chart showing the plan of the studies is in Fig. 3.3. The plan clarifies which hypotheses need exploring, the studies that are to be done, and indeed which explanations remain untested. Such an analysis and overview is necessary in all investigations of disease variations, both as a guide to the actions needed and as a means of data interpretation.

3.5 Disease clustering and clusters in epidemiology

According to the *Oxford English Dictionary* a cluster is a collection of things of the same kind, a bunch, a number of persons close together, a group or crowd. In epidemiology, according to *Last's Dictionary*, a disease cluster is an aggregation of relatively rare events or diseases in time or place, or both. The terms clusters and clustering are not used in the context of common diseases because clustering is inevitable due to chance alone, or for infectious diseases that spread from person-to-person for clustering is the norm. A disease cluster is a mini-epidemic or outbreak of a rare event; that is, occurrence of disease clearly in excess of that expected.

The disease cluster is a special instance of disease variation. Typical examples might be four cases of leukaemia in one street, or three cases of primary biliary cirrhosis in a single nursing home, or five cases of Legionnaires' disease in a factory. Once observed such a cluster presents a public health problem that cannot be ignored, and a difficult epidemiological puzzle. From a scientific perspective, if the factors that lead to the cluster can be identified then the cause of the disease might become clearer. The cluster can be considered as a potential causal goldmine. From a public health perspective the fear is that unless the cause of the cluster is discovered and action taken there may be further cases; that is, the cluster heralds a large outbreak or even widespread epidemic. Clusters of a few cases of a rare disease are an especially difficult problem in epidemiology, for the causes of the clustering are rarely discovered while the difficulties of judging the appropriate public health action remain.

Typically, clusters are identified by an observation by a member of the public or a local health professional of an excess of cases in a locality or over a short time period. For example, Alistair Gregg observed that in 1941 the number of cases of congenital cataract, an exceptionally rare problem, far exceeded the normal. He saw 13 cases of his own, and 7 of his colleagues. He hypothesized that this cluster was associated with a preceding outbreak of German measles (rubella). He was correct and rubella syndrome was discovered. It is less common, but quite possible, to identify a cluster on the basis of the personal characteristics of cases; for example, if all cases of a particular disease were in 6 year old children we might suspect that the problem arose in a classroom set-ting. Similarly, if cases were in bus drivers we might suspect the cause to be at the bus depot. Clusters may also be identified through examining routinely collected surveil-lance data, and this becomes easier if cases are mapped or plotted over time. The opportunities to seek clustering of disease are expanding with the development of automated ways of searching for clustering on large data sets. For example, geographi-cal information systems (GIS) make it easy to examine the space and time location of cases. The geographical analysis machine is an example of a software program (devel-oped at Newcastle upon Tyne, England, by Stan Openshaw (Openshaw and Blake 1995)), that searches a data set for clusters and plots these on a map. Clearly the key data requirements for seeking clusters are spatial co-ordinates usually obtained from postcode, time (usually date of onset of disease) and the personal characteristics of the case such as age, sex, occupation.

Identification of a cluster of cases is not the solution to any problem, rather it is the beginning of a problem. Leukaemia clusters have been observed for about 100 years, but explaining them has been extremely difficult. Clustering, however, points to an environ-mental basis to disease. Clustering of childhood leukaemia around nuclear power sta-tions occurs. Intuitively, the explanation would be expected to be exposure to low levels of radiation. The radiation hypothesis for such clustering has not held. The currently favoured hypothesis is that leukaemia is one rare outcome of a common childhood infec-tion, possibly deferred to a later time, and that leukaemia clusters are a consequence of a

Is this a cluster?

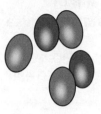

Perhaps. The challenge is
statistical and causal.

Fig. 3.4 Clusters I: are these
grapes in a cluster?

Box 3.7 **Do the five grapes make a cluster?**

Reflect on whether the five grapes in Fig. 3.4 make a cluster. What characteristics
make you think that they may be?

---

change in the pattern of such an infection resulting from the migration and population
mixing that occurs when a nuclear power plant is built and put into operation.

As clustering is merely a specialized variant of disease variation the analysis of clustering follows the principles discussed in Section 3.4. Clusters, as with all disease variations, may arise from data error, or chance. Clusters are, however, also easily missed in
clinical practice and even by routine surveillance systems, because of either incomplete
data (e.g. the date of onset of disease is missing), or the insensitivity of data presentation and analysis methods.

The concept of a cluster in epidemiology goes beyond that of merely a group of
cases, as shown in Fig. 3.4, using the analogy of grapes. Do the exercise in Box 3.7
before reading on.

The five grapes may or may not be part of a cluster but they certainly seem to be. They
look the same and are close together spatially. The fact that they look equally fresh sug-
gests that they share a common origin in time. If two of the grapes had been light in
colour, one was a plastic replica and one dried and shrivelled, we would not perceive
them as a cluster. So we would probably conclude that the grapes in Fig. 3.4 are part of a
cluster. The next step is to prove this. This analogy is directly applicable to a disease cluster. Imagine five cases of acute leukaemia are reported from a single street in a small
town. The first action is to verify this observation. If all five cases are indeed recent cases
of acute leukaemia we would be inclined to judge this as a cluster. If one turns out to be
a misdiagnosis (say anaemia), one occurred 15 years ago, one was chronic myeloid
leukaemia and only two were acute leukaemia in childhood, we would be disinclined to
treat them as a cluster. A mixed bag of diagnoses makes an unconvincing cluster,
as does a mixed bag of grapes. The epidemiological challenge is to discover how the
cluster came together. Do the exercise in Box 3.8 before reading on.

Box 3.8 **Assessing whether the cluster of grapes and of leukaemia is an artefact or whether there is a common cause**

Reflecting on both the cluster of grapes and five cases of childhood leukaemia, what evidence would you seek to help you to exclude artefact and to ascertain a common cause?

Is this a cluster?

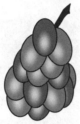

Yes, but, significance unclear i.e. how or why the grapes are together.
The challenge is causal.

Fig. 3.5 Clusters II: what is the significance of this cluster? How did it come about?

Evidence that the grapes are bound together by a common stalk would be compelling. Diseases, in contrast to grapes, have a background rate of occurrence. Five cases of leukaemia close together in time and place could occur by chance. Statistical tests are available to help to assess the role of chance. The close occurrence of leukaemia cases could be an artefact. Just as the grapes may have come from disparate bunches and have been placed together, so the cases of leukaemia may come from several localities; for example, a children's hospice opened in a particular locality may bring cases together. An even more mundane explanation would be a coding error in relation to postcode so that cases are wrongly being given the same but erroneous postcode. Figure 3.5 shows the grapes bound by a common stalk and part of a larger bunch, and leaves no doubt that the cluster is real. Similarly, if our investigation of leukaemia cases had shown that these and possible other cases were all bound by common factors such as type of leukaemia, age group, residence, time of disease onset, and exposures to causal factors we would be convinced the cluster is real. The next step is to explain mechanisms. This is easy in terms of grapes; we simply study the mechanisms by which grapes grow on vines (Fig. 3.6) and the biological and environmental processes that promote clusters of grapes. For diseases, the processes are far more difficult to study. Nonetheless, the guiding concepts are similar. In studying the cluster the investigator's job is incomplete unless these steps are achieved—and that is rare. The final step is to explain why the cluster arose both in terms of biology and in the wider environment. We now return to Legionnaires' disease.

Is this a cluster?

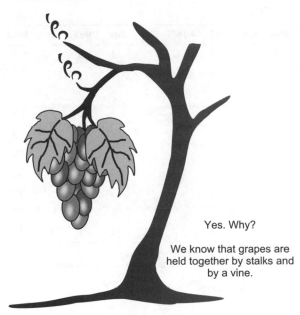

Yes. Why?

We know that grapes are
held together by stalks and
by a vine.

Fig. 3.6 Clusters III: explaining the
cluster: the vine.

Legionnaires' disease cases may occur in outbreaks, or in sporadic form. The cause of
outbreaks has often been tracked to cooling towers or complex hot water systems, as
the sources of infective aerosol. What of sporadic cases? By definition, these are solitary
cases, unconnected in space and time to others. The source of infection for such cases
is harder to study. I studied non-outbreak, non-travel Legionnaires' disease in and
around the City of Glasgow 1978–1986. The results are in Table 3.5.

Before reading on do the exercise in Box 3.9.

Box 3.9 **Defining and assessing clusters of Legionnaires' disease**

- On first principles, what would you expect the distribution of cases to be like in
  time? What possible clusters do you see in Table 3.5?
- What additional information would you like to assess these?

As these were apparently sporadic cases no clustering was expected, but there was.
Nine cases occurred in July–September 1979, six in November 1983, and 36 between
October 1984 and February 1985. The next step is to see whether there is clustering in
space too. Table 3.6 shows the suspected clustered cases by postcode, the number of
hospitals and the number of hospital consultant physicians in charge of each cluster,
and Fig. 3.7 shows similar data on a map.

Table 3.5 Number of non-travel, non-outbreak cases of Legionnaires' disease in Greater Glasgow Health Board by year and month

Year	Jan	Feb	Mar	Apr	May	Jun	Jul	Aug	Sep	Oct	Nov	Dec	Total
1978				1	1		1			1	3		7
1979					3		2	4	3		3		15*
1980	1							1	2		1		5
1981	1			1		1			1	1			5
1982						1	1			1			3
1983	2	2					1	1	3		6	1	16
1984		1	2			2	1	3	2	7	6	12	36
1985	4	7	1	2	1	1	1		1	3	4	4	29
1986										1	1		2
Total	8	10	3	4	5	5	7	9	12	14	24	17	118

* For one case neither the month of onset nor the date of serological testing was known.
Source: Bhopal *et al. British Medical Journal* (1992), **304**, pp. 1022–27, with permission from the BMJ Publishing Group.

Table 3.6 Clusters of apparently sporadic cases of Legionnaires' disease by area of residence, date of onset of disease and numbers of hospitals and consultants (hospital specialists) involved

Health Board and postcode sector of apparent cluster*	No of cases	Date of onset	Number of hospitals	Number of individual consultants in charge of each group
Greater Glasgow				
G5.0	3	Oct, Nov 1978	2	3
G21.1, G21.3	2	Nov 1983	2	2
G11.5, G12.8	2	Nov 1983	2	2
G4.0	2	Aug, Nov 1983	1	1
G33.5	2	Sep, Dec 1983	1	2
G4.0	5	Mar, Jun, Aug, (2 cases), Oct 1984	2	5
G31.4, G31.3, G31.1	6	Oct, Nov 1984; Jan, Feb, Apr, Nov 1985	2	4
G33.3	3	Jul, Oct, Nov 1984	2	3
G13.4, G13.3	2	Sep, Dec 1984	2	2
G72.8	3	Nov, Dec 1984	2	3
G5.8, G5.9	2	Feb 1985	2	2
G21.2, G22.6, G21.4	5	Jan, Feb, Oct 1985	3	6

* Postcodes in a row are contiguous areas.
Adapted from Bhopal *et al. British Medical Journal* (1992), **304**, pp. 1022–27, with permission from the BMJ Publishing Group.

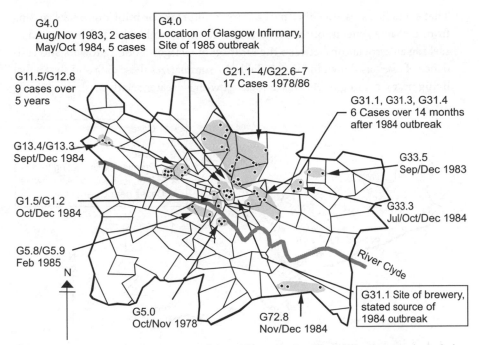

G4.0
Aug/Nov 1983, 2 cases
May/Oct 1984, 5 cases

G4.0
Location of Glasgow Infirmary,
Site of 1985 outbreak

G11.5/G12.8
9 cases over
5 years

G21.1–4/G22.6–7
17 Cases 1978/86

G31.1, G31.3, G31.4
6 Cases over 14 months
after 1984 outbreak

G13.4/G13.3
Sept/Dec 1984

G33.5
Sep/Dec 1983

G1.5/G1.2
Oct/Dec 1984

G33.3
Jul/Oct/Dec 1984

G5.8/G5.9
Feb 1985

N

River Clyde

G31.1 Site of brewery,
stated source of
1984 outbreak

G5.0
Oct/Nov 1978

G72.8
Nov/Dec 1984

Internal lines are simplified postcode sector boundaries

Fig. 3.7 Community acquired, non-travel, and apparently sporadic cases of Legionnaires' disease in Glasgow suspected to constitute a space–time cluster (Bhopal *et al. British Medical Journal* (1992), **304**, pp. 1022–27, with permission from the BMJ Publishing Group).

These data indicate that many of the sporadic cases were actually part of space-time clusters. Questions which arise include these: why were these clusters missed, and what is their cause? The findings showed that clusters can be easily missed in clinical practice, possibly because of the dispersion of small numbers of patients to several hospitals and physicians and because of incomplete data. For example, the six cases in postcode sectors G31.4, G31.3 and G31.1 in October 1984–November 1995 were spread over time, admitted to two hospitals and cared for by four hospital consultants. The routine surveillance system's data on postcode and date of onset were, in fact, incomplete. In these circumstances, identification of clustering on a routine basis is problematic. Effective surveillance requires proactively seeking, completing and analysing data to find patterns of disease. The final step of ascertaining cause requires us to develop and test hypotheses as to why there are apparently sporadic Legionnaires' disease clusters. Aside from artefacts the principal three hypotheses generated were these:

(a) People living in different parts of Glasgow are differentially susceptible to Legionnaires' disease. This seemed highly unlikely.

(b) The clusters reflect the intermittent virulence of Legionella. This hypothesis seems unlikely and is extremely difficult to test.

(c) That sporadic cases are either part of larger outbreaks or mini-outbreaks, arising from the same general sources of aerosol as for most outbreaks. This was tested by seeking an association between the location of Glasgow cooling towers and residence of cases, as shown in Fig. 3.8. Table 3.7 summarizes these data and shows that living near a cooling tower was associated with a greater relative risk of sporadic

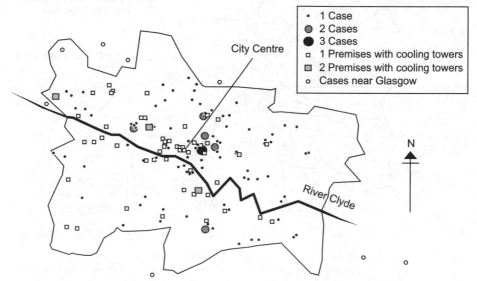

Fig. 3.8 Clusters: map of the location of cooling towers in the city of Glasgow and in relation to the residence of non-travel, community acquired, non-outbreak cases of Legionnaires' disease (Bhopal *et al. British Medical Journal* (1991), **320**, pp. 378–83, with permission from the BMJ Publishing Group).

Table 3.7 Relation between distance of patients' homes from cooling tower and risk of Legionnaires' disease

Study Group	Distance of home from nearest cooling tower (km)*	No. of cases observed (No. expected)	Relative risk of disease compared with group living >1.0 km from nearest cooling tower
Legionnaires' disease:	≤0.25	12 (4.4)	3.89
no history of travel	>0.25 to ≤0.5	28 (13.2)	3.00
abroad (*n* = 107)	>0.5 to ≤0.75	15 (17.9)	1.19
	>0.75 to ≤1.0	14 (17.9)	1.11
	>1.0	38 (53.7)	1.00

* The denominator population living within each distance category varied from year to year owing to the varying numbers of cooling towers in each year. The average denominator populations were as follows: 404 431 people lived more than 1 km from a cooling tower, 116 339 lived between 0.75 and 1 km away, 114 886 lived between 0.5 and 0.75 km away, 84 466 lived between 0.25 and 0.5 km away, and 27 884 lived less than 0.25 km away. Adapted from Bhopal *et al. British Medical Journal* (1991), **320**, pp. 378–83, with permission from the BMJ Publishing Group.

Legionnaires' disease, but this pattern was not present for travel-associated disease or lung cancer (data not shown; available in referenced paper). The data supported this hypothesis. This work, therefore, provided a general explanation for the phenomenon of clustering, but it did not provide a specific explanation for each of the many clusters, that is, which cooling tower was involved for each cluster. That is often the best that can be accomplished.

3.6 Applications of observations of disease variation

Variations in disease patterns are of practical value in helping to guide the clinician in both diagnosis and management of disease. For example, the diagnosis of myocardial infarction (heart attack) is much more likely to be correct in a man of 70 years complaining of chest pain than in a woman of 30. Clinicians can also make use of seasonal variations and of variations by ethnicity, geographical origins, occupation, and pattern of travel. So, for example, diabetic Muslim patients are most likely to have problems with control of their disease when fasting during daylight hours in the month of Ramadan than at other times of the year. Most infections have a distinct seasonal pattern; for example, influenza is more common in winter and gastroenteritis in summer. Outbreaks and clusters alert clinicians to otherwise rare diseases. Long-term trends are important to clinical practice; for example, the changing nature and decline of tuberculosis over the last hundred years has led to a change in the differential diagnosis (the preliminary list of possible diagnoses) of symptoms such as coughs and fever. It is likely that within 10–20 years, assuming that the recent rise and decline in coronary heart disease continues, the differential diagnosis of chest pain will also alter. Certainly, doctors in India and other industrialized countries, where CHD is on the rise, will be much more alert to this diagnosis than hitherto.

For health policy decisions, disease variations over decades (known as secular trends) are of special importance in setting priorities and for evaluating whether health objectives have been achieved. Variation in disease by place and by socioeconomic status is a guide to the level of inequity in health status. The healthcare planner uses disease variations to match resources to need. The simplest example is the prediction that in winter emergency admissions to hospital will rise, especially in an epidemic of influenza, and hence there will be fewer beds available for elective, non-emergency admissions.

The health promotor can tailor both the timing and the content of interventions. For example, an educational campaign on the perils of drinking and driving could be timed using information on alcohol consumption patterns by day of week, week of year, and information on the peak incidence of road traffic accidents. In the UK there is usually such a campaign before Christmas. Spatial variations in health behaviour and disease patterns can help in assigning staff and resources to particular places; for example, health visitors may be encouraged to spend more time in geographical areas with low breastfeeding rates.

Analysis of disease variation is vital in epidemiology and is the prime source of hypotheses on causation. As we have discussed and will continue to do throughout this book, variations are also at the heart of applied epidemiology.

3.7 Epidemiological theory underpinning or arising from this chapter

Disease variation arises because of either (a) changes in either the host, the agent of disease, or the environment; or (b) changes in interaction between the host, agent, and environment. As these changes occur at a different pace in different places and sub-populations, disease variations are inevitable. In studying these variations in epidemiology we are seeking to uncover the natural forces that caused them. The first step, however, is to ensure that variations are not merely artefacts.

3.8 Conclusion

The interpretation of change in disease frequency is difficult. Erroneous conclusions arise easily. Therefore, to avoid the twin and opposite pitfalls of false alerts or missed clusters, outbreaks and epidemics a systematic approach to the collection and analysis of data is necessary. The approach outlined here provides a structure for the investigator's thoughts. It places heavy emphasis on artefactual causes of changes in disease incidence. These artefacts are developed in the next chapter. Chapter 5 then develops the epidemiological approach to judging cause and effect when the association is not an artefact.

Summary

Diseases wax and wane in their population frequency. The underlying reasons are often difficult to detect and may remain a mystery. There are three principal reasons for investigating variations in disease frequency. First, to help bring under control an apparent abrupt rise in disease incidence (a suspected outbreak or cluster, the commonest public health emergency). Second, by understanding the factors which changed the disease frequency, to gain insight into the causes of disease. Third, to use the knowledge of the disease trend and its causes to make predictions about the future, both in terms of health policy and health care, and the frequency of disease. Disease variations are often, however, illusory, and arise from data errors and artefacts. A systematic approach to the analysis of variation in disease begins by differentiating artefactual change from real change. For real change which results from changes in host susceptibility, in the agent's capacity to cause disease, and in the influence of the environment, the epidemiological challenge is to pinpoint the causal factors. The principles behind the investigation of clusters, outbreaks, and epidemics and long-term variations both of communicable and non-communicable diseases, are similar.

Chapter 4

Variation
Role of error, bias, and confounding

Objectives

On completion of the chapter you should understand:

◆ that error in measurement, inevitable in all sciences, is crucially important in applied sciences such as epidemiology, based on free-living populations;

◆ that bias, considered as an error which affects comparison groups unequally, is particularly important in epidemiology;

◆ the major causes of error and bias in epidemiology, analysed based on the chronology of a research project;

◆ that bias in posing the research question, stating hypotheses, and choosing the study population are relatively neglected but important topics in epidemiology;

◆ that errors and bias in data interpretation and publication are particularly important in epidemiology because of its health policy and healthcare applications

◆ that confounding is the mis-measurement of the relationship between a risk factor and disease and arises in comparisons of groups which differ in ways that affect disease;

◆ that different epidemiological study designs share most of the problems of error and bias.

4.1 **Introduction** Accepting the null

> Man approaches the unattainable truth through a succession of errors.
>> Aldous Huxley

An error is by definition an act, an assertion, or a belief that deviates from what is right. In mathematics an error is the difference between a computed or measured value and a true or theoretically correct value. For example, a metre is a length fixed by agreement, but in different ways at different times: as a fraction of the length of the quadrant of the Earth's meridian through Paris, as the distance between two marks on a metal bar, and now as the path travelled by light in a vacuum in a particular time. In other words the true length of a metre is arbitrarily decided by agreeing a definition.

The difference between a 'correct' metre stick and an erroneous one can be accurately measured. In the arena of health and disease the truth is usually unknown and cannot be defined or computed. If not recognized, errors generate false knowledge, which only time and deeper study will show to be wrong. Error should be considered as an inevitable and important part of human endeavour, as captured in the quotation above. These ideas have particular importance in epidemiology for reasons discussed below. Before reading on reflect on the exercise in Box 4.1.

Box 4.1 **Error and bias**

Reflect on the word bias. What is the difference, if any, between error and bias? Why might error and bias be particularly common and important in epidemiology?

A bias is a more subtle matter than error and is a preference or an inclination, especially one that inhibits impartial judgment or that leads to an unfair act or policy stemming from prejudice. In statistics a bias is an error caused by systematically favouring some outcomes over others. In science, including epidemiology, error and bias are frequently used as synonyms. Bias is the usual term applied to a range of errors in science (usually excepting random statistical error). *Last's Dictionary* defines bias as a deviation from the truth. In this usage the word adds nothing to the concept of error, but it does free science from producing erroneous results, only biased ones! In this book bias in epidemiology is conceptualized to be error which applies unequally to comparison groups. Bias may be intentional or unintentional.

Error is common in science, contrary to popular view. Whether science is estimating the age of the Earth, calculating the speed of light, achieving cold fusion in the laboratory, or assessing when humans first started using weapons, errors and corrections are the norm. Epidemiology proves no exception to this tyranny of error. Indeed, the widely supported Popperian view is that science progresses by the rejection of hypotheses (by falsification) rather than the establishment of so-called truths (by verification) (Popper 1989).

Biological research is difficult because of the complexity and heterogeneity of living things, and because of the variations which occur in biological measures; for example those arising from circadian and other natural rhythms. In addition measurement techniques are usually limited by technology, cost, or ethical considerations. In human studies, especially those using large community-based populations, these difficulties are compounded by the necessarily strict rules on what measurement is permissible ethically and what humans are willing to give their consent to. To take an example, the best way to make a diagnosis of Alzheimer's dementia is brain biopsy, and this is usually done after death. Occasionally, in instances of extreme diagnostic difficulty a brain biopsy may be needed in the living patient. This 'gold standard' test would not be possible in an epidemiological study to measure the prevalence of the disease in the population. We accept the error inherent in other methods of diagnosing Alzheimer's disease, mainly based on clinical assessment and brain imaging, and forgo the brain biopsy test.

Experimental manipulation to test a hypothesis is usually done late in the process of human research, and observation, without deliberate intervention by the investigator, is the dominant mode of investigation in epidemiology. Moreover, epidemiology is interested in health and disease in human populations living normally in their natural environment.

Most discussions of error and bias in epidemiology focus on factors which can be categorized under the headings of (a) selection (of population), (b) information (collection, analysis, and interpretation of data), and (c) confounding. The broader and equally important question of whether error and bias are inherent in the process of developing research questions and hypotheses is seldom raised. For example, are the questions of sex or racial differences in intelligence, disease, physiology, or health erroneous, biased, or unethical questions? A long history of misleading and damaging research would have been avoided if questions about racial and sex differences had either not been posed at all, or not posed in the way they were. The Tuskegee Syphilis Study of the US Public Health Service (see Jones 1993), for example, followed up 600 African American men for some 40 years, to assess the natural history of disease. The underlying question was: does syphilis have different and, particularly, less serious outcomes in African Americans than European origin Americans? The investigators deliberately denied the study subjects treatment even when it was available and curative (penicillin). The study was based on a premise which has guided so much research on race and health: that races are biologically different in regard to a broad range of diseases. This premise has repeatedly been shown to be in error. In retrospect the study question and design was unethical. The question of whether the general process of defining research questions is biased, which lies in the domain of the ethics of science, deserves more attention in consideration of errors and bias.

Much of epidemiology is concerned with population subgroups and comparison between them. Even when an epidemiological study is of a single group, its interpretation usually rests on an understanding of, and inference about, how the group compares with the population from which it was selected. The scientific value of the work, in the sense of generating understanding about disease patterns, arises from its generalizability. Furthermore, to make sense of studies where the data have only been collected from a fraction of the population of interest, sometimes due to non-response by study subjects, the interpretation rests on the assumption that the results apply, by and large, to the whole group as originally chosen. The choice of population group is, therefore, a crucial matter in avoiding error and bias.

One concept of bias which is particularly useful in epidemiology, and which is close to the everyday perception and usage of the term (discrimination against the interests of individuals and groups because of prejudice), is error which either:

◆ affects population or study subgroups unequally; or

◆ results from the inappropriate generalization of study data to another population which differs from the population actually studied.

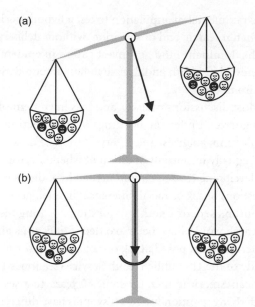

- Error is normal in science
- Researchers have their human foibles
- In epidemiology bias is unequal error in comparison populations
- Bias creates false patterns and misjudgements - either differences where none exist (a) or failure to detect differences (b)

Fig. 4.1 Bias: a symbolic representation of unequal errors in compared populations. (a) Error is unequal in one of these groups leading to a false interpretation of the pattern of disease—falsely detecting differences. (b) Error is unequal in one of these groups leading to a false interpretation of the pattern of disease—here failure to detect differences. (Each circle is a person—shaded circles represent cases of a disease.)

In this usage, bias is an error which affects one group more than another. Figure 4.1 uses the scales of justice to symbolize and illustrate the concept of bias as unequal error in compared populations, which may lead to both wrong and unfair conclusions.

Bias results in false understanding about differences between groups and generates misleading patterns of disease. Bias is, arguably, even more important than random errors which affect all comparison groups equally. However, even errors which affect groups equally (non-differential errors) can generate misleading conclusions. Misclassification errors are discussed later to illustrate this point. Error control requires awareness and good scientific technique. Bias control needs equal attention to error control in all the population subgroups. But as error and bias cannot be fully controlled the most important need is for systematic, cautious, and critical interpretation of data (Chapter 10, Sections 10.10–10.12).

4.2 **A classification of error and bias**

Epidemiologists have been particularly creative in identifying and naming biases. The result, however, has been long lists of unconnected biases. It is neither necessary nor appropriate for the student (or this book) to attempt to cover all possible biases, rather to develop an understanding of the nature and effects of bias. Errors and biases can be analysed logically by using the concepts above and a framework. As there is no

Box 4.2 **Towards a classification of errors and biases**

Think through the main steps of a research project and consider how error and bias might arise at each step. Develop a set of three or four broad categories for all the errors and biases you list. In doing this you can consider in what ways two groups of the population might be unequally affected in terms of:

◆ choice and phrasing of the study question;

◆ choice of the study population;

◆ participation of individuals in a study;

◆ baseline assessment of disease and factors which could cause disease;

◆ follow-up of participants;

◆ assessment of outcome;

◆ analysis, interpretation, presentation, and publication of data.

standardized classification it is a good idea for each reader to think through this matter. Before reading on try the exercise in Box 4.2, using the chronology of a research project for ordering your thoughts.

As stated above, one useful grouping of biases consists of selection bias, information bias, and confounding, but it is incomplete. In Table 4.1, this classification is shown in the context of a broader set of categories as discussed below: question/hypotheses bias, selection bias, confounding, information bias, intervention bias, interpretation bias, and publication bias.

4.2.1 **The research question, theme or hypothesis**

Science is done by human beings who often have strong ideas and views, generated both through and independently of their research. Science is as much about generating imaginative ideas and collecting data to test them as about looking to data to inspire ideas. Scientists develop and become attached to ideas which they hope to support (and if necessary reject) through their research. As human beings they share in the social values and beliefs of their era, including those which may in retrospect be considered unworthy such as class, racial, and sexual prejudice.

It is worth reflecting on whether a scientific question or research theme can be inherently biased. In epidemiology, a biased question would adversely affect one group more than another. The question 'Are men more intelligent (or healthy) than women?' could be considered a biased question, for there is a presupposition in the way the question is written which points out that there is a case to be answered. Otherwise the question could have been whether women are more intelligent than men. The

Table 4.1 A classification of error and bias based on the chronology of a research project

Potential cause of bias	Example	Specific terminology	Broad general category of bias
1. Research theme, question or hypothesis is biased	Choosing a research theme or posing a question or hypothesis in a way which shows one population in a poor light, and creating a sense of superiority and inferiority	None	The terms assumption or conceptual bias are close matches. My preferred term is research question bias
2. Choice of populations is biased	Sampling based on convenience, or cultural preferences of researcher	Population bias (volunteer bias, sex, race, or age bias)	Selection bias
3. Participation in a study	Hospital populations studied where two or more associated problems increase the chance of hospitalization	Berkson's bias	Selection bias
	Unequal time and effort spent in the invitation leading to unequal participation	Response bias	
	Unequal interest or motivation		
4. Comparing populations which differ	Study population is older or poorer than the comparison population, leading to a false interpretation of the reason for differences in disease rates	Confounding	Confounding
5. Mis-measurement: assessment of disease, and factors which could cause disease	Diagnostic effort, skill, facilities unequal	Measurement error	Information
	Measurement imprecise or unequal	Measurement error	Information
	In reporting, there is unequal memory of the problem in minds of doctors or patients	Recall bias	Information

	Effort, skill, facilities to collect data unequal in comparison groups	Workup bias	Information
	Interviewer extracts information differently in different groups	Interviewer bias	Information
	Factors unequally memorable for respondent	Recall bias	Information
	Deception by study subject, investigator, or diagnostician	No specific name but it is scientific misconduct if the investigator or professional is involved	Misconduct
Measurement at follow up and outcome	Unequal effort made to maintain contact by investigator or subject	No specific name	Selection
	Unequal proportion of subjects drop-out	No specific name	Selection
	Intervention in health care not equal	No specific name	Intervention bias
	Participation in study alters behaviour unequally in different groups	No specific name	Participation bias may be appropriate
Analysis and interpretation of data	Preferred outcome in mind of investigator	No specific name	Interpretation or presentation
Selected findings reported	Reporting interesting findings, usually findings of difference between groups (i.e. positive results) Reporting publishable findings	Various	Publication
Interpretation, judgement and action by readers and listeners	Reader and listener interpret data in a way that suits them	No specific name	Interpretation

apparently neutral hypothesis here would be that there are no gender differences in intelligence. If the underlying values of the researchers are that men are more intelligent than women (a view that has been widely held through much of history and is now deeply undermined) then the bias will remain. These values are likely to be revealed at the analysis and interpretation stage by biased interpretation. Researchers' beliefs and hopes do influence the conduct of research.

To quote Ruth Hubbard:

> The mythology of science asserts that with many different scientists all asking their own questions and evaluating the answers independently, whatever personal bias creeps into their individual answers is cancelled out when the large picture is put together. This might conceivably be so if scientists were women and men from all sorts of different cultural and social backgrounds who came to science with very different ideologies and interests. But since, in fact, they have been predominantly university-trained white males from privileged social backgrounds, the bias has been narrow and the product often reveals more about the investigator than about the subject being researched.
>
> Ruth Hubbard, Mary Sue Henifin and Barbara Fried (1979) (ed.)
> *Women look at biology looking at women.*

This issue demands more attention in the ethics of epidemiology particularly as this discipline is founded on population level differences. It is problematic to describe difference without conveying a sense of superiority and inferiority. This is discussed further in Chapter 10.

4.2.2 **Choice of population**

Bias can result from the choice of populations to be studied. This is known as selection bias. Investigators will sometimes pick populations of convenience rather than representative ones. In particular, volunteers are a popular choice. The problem is that volunteers tend to be different in their attitudes, behaviours, and health status compared with those who do not volunteer. Men have been selected more often than women, for example, in studies of coronary heart disease. Sometimes investigators want to avoid the ethical problems posed by the possibility of pregnancy, at other times the problem under study is seen as less relevant to women. Ethnic minority groups are much more likely to be excluded from major studies than the ethnic majority, leading to a policy from the main USA research funding agency (NIH) requiring investigators to include women and ethnic minority groups or provide a reasoned justification. Investigators are prone to exclude individuals and populations for reasons of convenience, cost, or preference rather than for neutral, scientific reasons.

In many studies selection bias is an inevitable result of the chosen source of a study population. For example, the telephone directory and the register of licensed drivers are both popular in the USA. Those without a telephone and without a driver's licence are selected out of the study. In the UK, the registers of electors and those registered with a general practitioner in the National Health Service are popular, but exclude those not eligible to vote (or unwilling to divulge their details) or those not registered

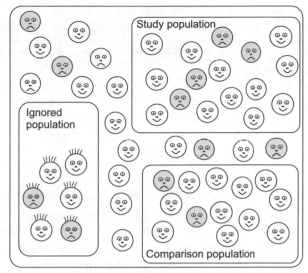

- Ignoring populations
- Questions harming one population
- Measuring unequally
- Generalizing from unrepresentative populations

Study population

Ignored population

Comparison population

Fig. 4.2 Bias in epidemiology: population concept.

with the NHS, respectively. Figure 4.2 illustrates these points. In addition to the ignored population (e.g. those who do not speak English or are not on the list from which the sample is drawn), there are others who are missed either inadvertently or because they actively do not participate. Population biases occur from bypassing populations, posing questions that harm sub-populations, measuring populations unequally and generalizing from unrepresentative data.

Work colleagues, and 'captive' populations such as those in institutions (schools, prisons, universities, hospitals) are popular choices for study. Some captive populations may be fairly representative of their age group (e.g. schoolchildren), others not at all (e.g. university students). The attention given to such captive populations means that research effort is deflected away from other populations which may be less accessible. While these choices would not cause a bias if the investigator made no claim that the results were generalizable beyond the population actually studied, extrapolation of results is the norm rather than the exception. Indeed investigators may even explicitly compare populations derived in different ways. One example is the ground-breaking survey of health and health behaviours by the Health Education Authority (1994), which studied ethnic minority groups in the UK. Typical results are given in Table 4.2.

The ethnic minority groups were shown to be different compared with the UK population in a wide range of indicators. The emphasis in interpretation fell on those issues where the ethnic minority groups were worse off, thus leading to widespread perceptions that the health of ethnic minorities was seriously impaired, a view propagated in professional journals and newspapers. The comparisons were, however, invalid because the ethnic minority groups were drawn from small areas (enumeration districts) where at least 10 per cent of the population was born in six overseas areas of

Table 4.2 Selected data, standardized for age and sex, on health and related factors from the HEA's report on black and minority groups (figures are percentages)

Topic	African Caribbean	Indian	Pakistani	Bangladeshi	UK population
Describe health status as poor	17	16	20	29	8
Suffered high blood pressure	16	8	8	10	14
Current smokers	22	10	16	22	28

From Health Education Authority 1994; *Health and Lifestyles*—see Permissions.

the world (e.g. India, the West Indies). Such areas would almost invariably be in inner city areas, where the poorest people live, while the comparison 'UK' population included all areas, not just inner city ones. The design, therefore, excluded those ethnic minority populations who lived in suburban areas. Irrespective of this error the study remains of value and interest, but the interpretation is biased in the sense that it is likely to show the ethnic minority groups as being worse off than they actually are. This example illustrates a population selection bias, interpretation bias, and publication bias.

Berkson's bias is an example of how subtle bias can be. It specifically refers to a bias in the interpretation of hospital-based case-control studies (see Chapter 9). It arises because hospitalized cases of a disease are not usually a true and representative sample of cases. In fact they tend to be the more complex ones, often with other health problems and risk factors. For example, a man with influenza is more likely to be admitted to hospital if he has diabetes or chronic bronchitis or is a heavy smoker.

Selection bias matters much more in epidemiology than in biologically based medical sciences. Biological factors are usually generalizable between individuals and populations, so there is a prior presumption of generalizability. For example, if an anatomist describes the presence of a particular muscle, or cell type, based on one human being it is likely to be present in all human beings (and possibly all mammals), for the number of models of life are few. The anatomist is likely to check that the finding applies to a few other individuals and if so will rapidly conclude that it applies universally. By contrast, epidemiological findings usually concern the interaction of social and biological factors. Since societies are made up of highly variable individuals and population groups, the outcome of the biology/environment interaction is variable and context dependent. The result is crucially dependent on the choice of study population and the interpretation depends on proper understanding of its circumstances. For example, in nearly every population the blood pressure rises with age. It would be easy to conclude that this is a generalizable finding, possibly based on the biology of the ageing process. But, this assumption and generalization needs serious qualification for in nomadic populations living in traditional ways in rural areas of countries such as Kenya there is little or no association between age and blood pressure.

4.2.3 **Non-participation**

Some of those subjects chosen for a study do not participate. This is non-response bias which is a sub-category of selection bias. In studies of randomly sampled populations the non-response is typically 30–40 per cent, and sometimes much higher. It is likely that these non-responders differ from those who respond; for example, in a written questionnaire study the literate may be more likely to respond than those who have difficulty in reading and writing. The effect of this bias can be understood if some information is available on those not participating, such as their age, sex, social circumstances, and why they refused. Investigators should seek this information as a high priority. Usually, this information is not available, enticing investigators to assume that the responders were not atypical of non-responders. A similar problem arises in studies of health records when the records of a subject are lost or otherwise inaccessible to the investigator. Without information on non-responders generalization is difficult. The problem is compounded when the non-response differs greatly in two populations that are to be compared; for example, men and women, groups in different social classes or ethnic groups.

Investigators should ensure that time and effort made in recruitment should be equivalent in relation to need, and that comparison populations are given equivalent opportunities to generate interest and motivation. The strategies for recruiting comparison populations may well differ but, ideally, the outcome in terms of the type of people participating and the level of non-response would be similar. A degree of non-response bias is an intrinsic limitation of the survey method and hence of epidemiology.

4.2.4 **Comparing disease patterns and risk factor-disease outcome relationships in populations which differ (confounding)**

Confounding is a difficult idea to explain and grasp (and the reader may wish to return to this section again, after reading the remainder of the book). In essence, it is the error in the estimate of the measure of association between a specific risk factor and disease outcome, which arises when there are differences in the comparison populations other than the risk factor under study. These other characteristics may not have been measured at all or they may have been measured imprecisely. The word confounding is derived from a Latin word meaning to mix up, a useful idea, for confounding mixes up causal and non-causal relationships. The word's meaning in everyday language, to confuse or puzzle, is also helpful.

Confounding is a major cause of bias in epidemiology, and arguably the most difficult one to understand and counteract. The potential for it to occur is there whenever the cardinal rule 'compare like-with-like' is broken. This rule is a counsel of perfection that is rarely, and perhaps never, attained except in experimental research. Comparing like-with-like may be achieved in experimental studies where subjects can be randomly allocated to one group or another, a technique which employs the laws of chance to create comparable groups. If the experimental study is large the randomized populations will tend to be similar. Even with randomization there is no certainty that the groups are comparable, especially in subgroup analysis (Chapter 9). The concept of confounding is best explained by examples (Table 4.3) and by illustrations as in Figs 4.3 and 4.4. Before examining these tables and figures reflect on the next three paragraphs and the questions following in Box 4.3.

Imagine that a study follows up people who drink alcohol and observes the occurrence of lung cancer. A group of people who do not drink and are of the same age and sex provide the comparison group. The study finds that lung cancer is more common in alcohol drinkers; that is, there is an association between alcohol consumption and lung cancer. Is it likely that alcohol causes lung cancer? In what other important ways might the study (alcohol drinking) and comparison (no alcohol drinking) populations be different? Could the association between alcohol and lung cancer be confounded? What might be the confounding variable?

In a study of mortality rates, investigators find that mortality rates in an English seaside resort are much higher than in the country as a whole. Why might this be so? Is it something to do with living in the resort or is there another explanation? In what ways might the population of the resort differ from the country as a whole and in a way that reflects mortality?

African Americans were demonstrated to be more likely to use crack cocaine than white Americans (see Lillie-Blanton *et al.* 1993). Is this a racial or ethnic difference in attitudes or behaviour in relation to this drug? Does the causal factor lie in racial or ethnic characteristics? In what ways relevant to this observation might the two populations differ from each other? Do the exercise in Box 4.3 before reading on and looking at Table 4.3, and Figs 4.3 and 4.4.

Box 4.3 **Some questions to assess confounding**

In each of the above examples ask these questions:

- Have the investigators compared like-with-like?
- In what important characteristics that impinge on disease occurrence might the two comparison populations differ?
- What are the potential explanations for the findings other than the self-evident ones (alcohol causes lung cancer, living in an English Seaside resort is a risk, and African Americans are prone to the crack cocaine habit)?
- What is the confounding factor? What is the confounded, non-causal factor? How can we check out that our understanding is correct?

[Handwritten annotation: Alcohol / Exposure → Lung / Outcome — Smoking / (Confounder)]

Table 4.3 Examples of confounding

The confounded association	One possible explanation	The confounded factor	The confounding (causal) factor	To check the assumption
(a) People who drink alcohol have a raised risk of lung cancer	Alcohol drinking and smoking are behaviours which go together	Alcohol, which is a marker for, on average, smoking more cigarettes	Tobacco, which is associated with both alcohol and with the disease	See if the alcohol-lung cancer relationship holds in people not exposed to tobacco: if yes, tobacco is not a confounder (stratified analysis Chapter 7)
(b) People living in an affluent seaside resort have a higher mortality rate than the country as a whole	A holiday town attracts the elderly, so has a comparatively old population	Living in a resort is a marker for being, on average, older	Age, which is associated with both living in a resort and with death	Look at each age-group specifically, or use age standardization to take into account age differences (see Chapters 7 and 8)
(c) African Americans are heavier users of crack cocaine than 'white' Americans	Poor people living in the American inner city are particularly likely to become dependent on illicit drugs	Belonging to the racial category 'African American'	Poverty and the pressures of inner-city living, including the easy availability of drugs	Use statistical techniques to adjust for the influence of a number of complex socio-economic factors (see Chapter 8)

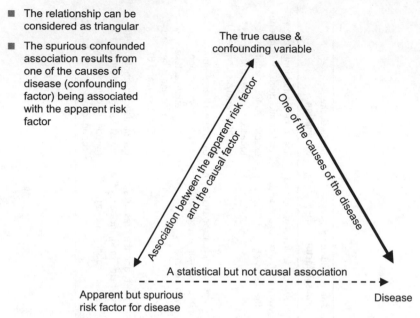

Fig. 4.3 Confounding variable: a pictorial representation.

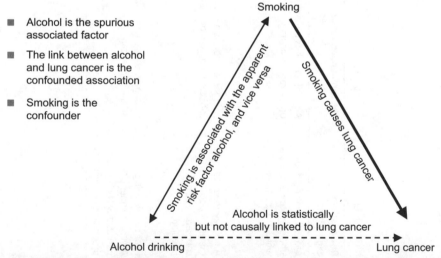

Fig. 4.4 Confounding variable, a pictorial representation: the example of alcohol and lung cancer.

The first key analysis in all epidemiological studies is to compare the characteristics of the populations under study, paying particular attention to factors which are known or suspected to influence disease causation. The details of the study hypotheses determine the characteristics which ought to be similar. Simply because the groups are similar on the characteristics actually measured does not imply they are similar on all relevant characteristics. For example, two groups may be comparable on age, sex, smoking, and exercise habits but differ in the type of housing they live in, a variable on which data are often not collected. If the study is of accidents, infections, or respiratory disease, for example, differences in housing may matter greatly. In a study of breast cancer or eczema, say, the type of housing may not matter. This same principle applies to all subgroup analysis. For example, a comparison of two populations may show that they are virtually identical in age structure. The investigator may wish to examine the disease experience of men and women separately. The age structure of each of the sexes must now be shown to be similar and this must not be assumed. Serious problems with confounding are likely if it is not considered at the stage of designing the study, analysing the data, and interpreting the findings. A combination of methods is usually applied to handle confounding depending on the needs of the study. In recent years the trend has been to control for confounding at the analysis stage but it is best to consider it at each stage and take one or more of the appropriate actions as shown in Table 4.4. Whatever is done the possibility of confounding can rarely be dismissed and, along with chance, it remains an alternative interpretation of epidemiological findings.

Figure 4.3 offers a pictorial representation of confounding. The relationship between disease, the associated apparent risk factor, and the confounding factor is shown as a triangular one. The confounding factor, shown at the apex of the triangle in Fig. 4.3, is a true causal factor, associated both with the apparent (confounded) risk factor and the disease. The right hand line is shown in bold to signify the clear causal nature of this link. Note that the arrow on the left-hand line points in both directions, showing a relationship in both directions. The arrow in the right hand line points in one direction because the causal (confounding) factor causes the disease, but not vice versa. The arrow at the bottom is a broken line to symbolize the non-causal nature of the relationship. Figure 4.4 illustrates this with the example of alcohol, smoking, and lung cancer. The link between the confounding (smoking) and confounded (alcohol) factor is also causal but in a complex and two-sided relationship. Do the exercise in Box 4.4 before reading on.

Box 4.4 **Pictorial presentation of associations in Table 4.3**

Analyse the associations (Table 4.3) between living in a seaside resort and high mortality, and between being African American and using crack cocaine, using the approach shown in Figs 4.3 and 4.4. What is the nature of the relationship between confounding and confounded factors here?

In the association between living in the resort and mortality, age (confounding factor) would be at the apex and living in the resort at the left-hand angle. In the association between African American race and crack cocaine use, socio-economic status would be at the apex and race at the left-hand angle. It is important to note these are

Table 4.4 Possible actions to control confounding

Possible Action	Example	Benefit	Cost/Disadvantage
Study design: Randomize individual subjects or units of populations e.g. schools	To determine the effectiveness of sex education in schools in reducing the incidence of teenage pregnancy, half of the schools in a city could be in the intervention group, the other half in a control group. The allocation of the group would be determined by chance (see Chapter 9, Section 7)	Selection biases bypassed	Limited to research questions where randomization is possible, and acceptable to subjects and professionals
			Avoids schools selecting themselves into the intervention group for they would be different from those which chose the control group
			Comparability may not be achieved, especially in small samples
			Effective in large studies
Study design: Select comparable groups/restrict entry into study	Study only subjects who are 35 years of age	Vagaries of chance and selection bias bypassed	Creates extra work in finding the chosen population
	Study non-smokers only e.g. in studying the health effects of air pollution		Findings may not apply to populations not studied
			Erroneous conclusions may be reached e.g. air pollution has no effect on health when it might affect smokers but not non-smokers
			Practical applications of findings in health policy etc. are reduced
Study design: Match individuals or whole populations	Select subjects and controls on pre-determined criteria e.g. age, sex, race, smoking	Investigators' judgements and knowledge of confounding factors is used	The result is not a population sample so there are problems of representativeness

Select populations on basis of population statistics e.g. unemployment levels, type of housing		Practical applications of data may be less Needs statistical analysis designed for matched populations Overmatching can lead to false conclusions
Analysis: Analyse subgroups separately	Compare disease experience of each age group, sex, race etc. separately (stratified analysis)	Makes assimilation of results difficult In most studies, there are insufficient subjects to make detailed stratification possible
Analysis: Adjust data statistically	Use techniques to amalgamate results of stratified analysis e.g direct or indirect standardization (Chapter 8), Mantel Haensel technique and multiple regression modelling (consult a statistics textbook)	Direct control and observation of possible confounding factors Summary measures possible Computers and statistical software make this relatively quick to do	Hard for non-statisticians to understand and do well Actual data are hidden behind summary figures Outputs are not easily used for health care policy and planning May lead to false sense of complacency that confounders are controlled

alternative and simplified explanations of a complex reality and, in turn, need to be subjected to test.

Risk or effect modification, in contrast to confounding, occurs when two causal factors, or one causal and one protective factor, interact to reduce or enhance risk. The risk of lung cancer in smokers who are exposed to asbestos is, for example, much higher than in those not so exposed. In this case both smoking and asbestos are causal factors, and neither are confounders. Failure to measure accurately and control confounding factors can lead to spurious findings of risk modification (see below in section on misclassification bias) and failure to seek or notice risk modification can lead to false measure of overall risk. Some actions to control confounding are summarized in Table 4.4.

4.2.5 **Measurement**

Measurement errors and biases fall into the huge general category of information bias. Before reading on you may wish to reflect on the questions in Box 4.5 on why measurement errors are likely to be common and important in epidemiological research.

Box 4.5 **Measurement errors in epidemiology**

Why are measurement errors in epidemiology likely to be more common and more important than in other scientific disciplines, say, physics, anatomy, biochemistry, or animal physiology?

Unlike measuring the length of a red cell, an atom, or even the orbit of the moon, assessing the presence of disease in living human beings requires a judgement. It is a subjective matter, aided by imprecise measures of biological indicators and information provided by the patient or study subject. After death the precision of the diagnosis can be improved by autopsy but the patient is no longer available for questioning and some tests, particularly dynamic ones (e.g. an exercise ECG or an intravenous pyelogram), are no longer available. A combination of clinical and autopsy data is sometimes essential to reach a diagnosis.

Similar problems apply to most measurements of exposures thought to be causing the disease in free-living humans, and to confounding factors. For example, measuring socio-economic circumstances, ethnic group, cigarette smoking habits, or alcohol consumption are complex matters. Even measures such as height, weight, and blood pressure are difficult to get right, particularly in the context of large studies where numerous people may be making measurements in different places. Accuracy in biochemical and other laboratory tests, though easier to achieve than disease or physical measures, is still problematic with issues such as the quality of the specimen and the changing laboratory reagents and techniques coming into play. In many instances, particularly for environmental exposures such as air pollution, past circumstances will need to be estimated, sometimes from contemporary measures.

Variation arising from measurement problems is compounded by biological variation, which is not error but may easily be confused with it. To take an example, blood pressure varies from moment to moment in response to physiological needs related to activity, in a 24 hour (circadian) cycle with lowered pressure in the night, and with the ambient temperature. To examine the relationship between blood pressure and disease we need a valid, that is meaningful and true, summary estimate of the blood pressure. There is, however, no such estimate. The compromise that is usually adopted is taking the blood pressure in standard conditions, measuring it on several occasions, and taking an average of the readings. The value obtained is valuable in clinical practice and epidemiology, for it is predictive of disease outcomes, but it is in no way an accurate summary of the constantly varying blood pressure.

Biological variations can cause bias. Imagine two populations with identical blood pressure under standard conditions. If blood pressure measurements on one population were made in the morning and in the other in the evening, or for one population in a hot room and for the other in a cold one, the average blood pressure in the two populations would be perceived to be different when it is not. For some variables the natural variation is so great that making estimates is extremely difficult, for example, in diet, alcohol consumption, and the level of stress.

Measurement errors include those arising from machine imprecision and inaccurate observation by the investigator or diagnostician. In measurement of the hypothesized causal factors and of confounding factors, information is often obtained from the subject alone, whereas information on the disease is obtained from a combination of the patient's account, the physician's examination, and laboratory tests. Measurement errors in the former, therefore, are more likely to be overlooked than in the latter.

Measurement errors which occur unequally in the comparison populations are, here, considered as epidemiological biases, and they can irreversibly destroy a study. For example, in a study where one population is interviewed face-to-face and the comparison population completes a self-completion questionnaire, the results are unlikely to be comparable. Inequality in follow-up arising from unequal interest by subjects or from the investigators, can lead to both selection and information bias, and will compound the problem of confounding. The investigation and follow-up of subjects is in itself an intervention which may have both educational and placebo effects. These effects are likely to be different in people with a disease than in people without. The study processes, then, may alter future measurement of risk factors and disease in a biased way.

Unequal measurement errors in comparison groups, called differential misclassification errors or bias, may be hard to discern but the damage they do is self-evident. Measurement errors which are equal in all comparison populations, or non-differential errors or biases, may be perceived as comparatively benign but this may not be so, as discussed in the section below.

4.2.6 **Misclassification bias**

Misclassification error (or bias) occurs when a person is put into the wrong category (or population subgroup), usually as a result of faulty measurement. For example, imagine a survey of hypertension in two towns. Inevitably, but particularly if an inadequately trained person is measuring blood pressure, some people who are hypertensive will be misclassified as normal, others who are normal will be misclassified as hypertensive. It may be that the misclassification is essentially random, with as many being misclassified in one direction as the other. If the same person is measuring blood pressure in both towns, the end result in terms of the prevalence of hypertension may be about right. This error is known as a non-differential misclassification bias, in that it affects all subgroups equally (non-differentially). Imagine that the sphygmomanometer in one of the two towns is faulty and is underestimating the blood pressure by 10 mmHg. In this town, many people who are hypertensive will be misclassified as not hypertensive, and very few the other way round. This is a systematic error, known as a differential misclassification bias. The degree to which a measure leads to a correct classification can be quantified using the concepts of sensitivity and specificity, and these are discussed in Chapter 6 in relation to screening tests.

Misclassification is inevitable because measurements are imperfect. The consequences of misclassification can be severe in both clinical practice and in the application of epidemiology. Clinically, misclassified persons will be treated wrongly. It is a common custom that information from epidemiological surveys is conveyed with the permission of the study subject to the personal physician. Epidemiological mismeasurements can, therefore, trigger off unnecessary clinical investigations and treatments, or falsely convey that there is no problem. If individually based clinical information from epidemiological research is conveyed to either the study subject or the subject's physician misclassification errors are always important. If not, small-scale non-differential errors are unlikely to alter the study's conclusion dramatically.

Differential errors, by contrast, deeply undermine epidemiological studies. If differential misclassification errors occur the study may need to be abandoned, unless the extent of the error can be quantified and data corrected. In the example in the first paragraph above, if we can reliably ascertain that the sphygmomanometer in one town always measured blood pressure 10 mmHg too low then we could add 10 mmHg to the recorded values. A correction can often be made for measures of physical attributes and for laboratory test measures. It is more difficult to correct for misclassification in social information collected by questionnaire or interview, and it is usually impossible for diagnostic information collected from medical records.

The effect of non-differential misclassification is more subtle than for differential error, and therefore more likely to be overlooked, particularly if there is little or no effect on the final prevalence figure. In measuring the strength of associations between exposures and disease outcomes, however, non-differential misclassification error has an

Table 4.5 Imaginary study of cardiovascular outcome and pill use: no misclassification

True classification of pill use status	Cardiovascular disease		Total
	Yes	No	
Yes	2000	8000	10 000
No	1000	9000	10 000
	3000	17 000	20 000

important and not always predictable effect. If the misclassification only applies to disease outcome then the strength of the association is always reduced, so the main problem is failing to find associations that, in reality, exist. Misclassification, however, affects exposure and confounding variables, and the combined effect of the mixture of misclassifications is not so predictable. This is best illustrated with an example.

Imagine a study of 20 000 women, 10 000 on the contraceptive pill and the rest not. Our interest is in the occurrence of new cases of cardiovascular disease over 10 years (incidence of disease). Say that over 10 years 20 per cent of those on the pill develop a cardiovascular disease (CVD) compared with 10 per cent of those not on the pill. The rate of disease in the oral contraceptive group is doubled (relative risk = 2). Table 4.5 shows the true results, given no misclassification at all in either the measurement of pill use or disease outcome.

Let us assume that misclassification in exposure occurs 10 per cent of the time, so that 10 per cent of women actually on the pill were classified as not on the pill, and that 10 per cent who were not were classified as on the pill. We also assume that there is no misclassification of disease outcome, and the disease incidence remains the same. Table 4.6 gives the results.

The risk of CVD in the 'pill users group' with 10 per cent misclassification is 1900/10 000, and in the 'not on the pill group' is 1100/10 000, so the relative risk is

$$\frac{1900/10\,000}{1100/10\,000} = 1.7$$

This illustrates the general principle that when the misclassification is of exposure then the strength of the association (measured here by the relative risk) is reduced. Misclassification will, inevitably, also arise in measurement of the disease outcome. Let us now assume that there is 10 per cent misclassification bias there. Table 4.7 gives the results. The total number of 'cases' is 1800 plus 800 = 2600 in the pill users group and 1800 in the not on the pill group.

Now the relative risk is

$$\frac{2600/10\,000}{1800/10\,000} = 1.44$$

In practice there will be misclassification in both measurement of exposure and in disease and this will distort the results even more. Generally, non-differential

Table 4.6 Pill and cardiovascular disease: 10% misclassification of pill use

Classification of pill use status	Cardiovascular disease		Total
	Yes	No	
Yes, classified right (on the pill so incidence rate is 20%)	1800	7200	9000
Yes, classified wrong (actually not on the pill so incidence rate is 10%)	100	900	1000
Subtotal	1900	8100	10 000
No, classified right (not on the pill so incidence rate is 10%)	900	8100	9000
No, classified wrong (actually on the pill so incidence rate is 20%)	200	800	1000
Subtotal	1100	8900	10 000
Total	3000	17 000	20 000

Table 4.7 Pill and cardiovascular disease: 10% misclassification in measurement of disease outcome

Oral contraceptive	Cardiovascular disease				Total
	Yes		No		
	Yes correctly classified as CVD	No CVD, misclassified as yes	CVD, but misclassified as no	No CVD, correctly classified	
Yes	1800	800*	200**	7200	10 000
No	900	900***	100****	8100	10 000
	2700	1700	300	15 300	20 000

* 10% of 8000 (row 1, column 3, Table 4.5).   ** 10% of 2000 (row 1, column 2, Table 4.5).
*** 10% of 9000 (row 2, column 3, Table 4.5).   **** 10% of 1000 (row 2, column 2, Table 4.5)

misclassification bias lowers the relative risk. This general principle may break down when misclassification occurs in confounding variables as well. The demonstration of this is beyond this book but there is a reference to a paper by Greenland giving access to the literature.

4.2.7 Analysis and interpretation

In virtually every project the potential for data analysis is far greater than that actually done. The choice of which data to analyse, the way to analyse them, and how to present the findings are usually left to the investigator. Clearly, the choices will be informed by the prior interests (and biases) and expertise of the researcher.

There is no easy solution to this problem. External scrutiny by objective advisers at an early stage of the research protocol, including the plan for data analysis and interpretation, is one important safeguard. Another step, one more difficult to achieve, would be the inclusion of objective, uninvolved people in the research team at the data analysis and interpretation stage. As a minimum, investigators should ensure that their analysis is driven by hypotheses, research questions, and an analysis strategy prepared in advance. One controversial proposal is that investigators should make public their data collection proforma, such as the questionnaire, their data, the analysis strategy, and other information required to replicate the analysis. Some scientific journals do require that authors of submitted manuscripts reporting original research make available the data on request. In practice, this requirement is rarely imposed, and is unlikely to be except in the case of suspected fraud.

4.2.8 **Publication**

The pressure to make choices is intensified at the stage of publication, particularly in scientific journals. The article will usually need to be written in 1500–5000 words (the most prestigious journals are usually at the shorter end of the spectrum). Research submitted as a short report may need to be in 500–700 words, and as a letter to the editor, even shorter. Choices on the data to be presented will be combined with choices on emphasis and interpretation. Convention dictates that the authors indicate their preferred interpretation, and that data are never published without discussion (the ultimate but impractical solution to the problem of bias in interpretation). Editorial guidelines usually indicate that originality, interest, and readability will be key criteria for publication. Researchers write accordingly, by highlighting the points of interest to themselves, editors, and readers. In epidemiology the usual point of interest, as determined by the dominant paradigm, is the difference in the pattern of disease between compared populations, and the potential to understand disease causation. Other interpretations are usually secondary. Similarities between populations are seldom commented on. Manuscripts showing interesting findings (positive results in trials, differences in disease patterns in most epidemiology) are most likely to be published in widely read journals, others are often left unpublished or published in specialist journals or as reports to the funding agency. The result is a biased understanding of the differences and similarities in the disease patterns of populations and an exaggerated view of the importance of associations between risk factors and disease outcomes.

4.2.9 **Judgement and action**

Finally, the data and interpretation are examined by those who need to make decisions, whether the population as a whole, politicians, industrialists, policy makers or researchers. It is likely that controversial interpretations, especially those which involve change that may threaten powerful interests, will be contested. Interpretation is a matter of judgement and judgement will depend on the prior values, beliefs, and interests of the observer. A pattern which is seen by one observer as clear evidence of the detrimental effect of smoking on respiratory health may be seen by another with different values and interests as due to error, bias, confounding, or another cause such as air pollution. According to Thomas Kuhn (1996), a key characteristic of science is that the scientist and the peer group are the sole arbiters of the meaning and validity of the theory and data. Epidemiology differs from other physical and biomedical sciences in that the data are usually of direct interest to a wide range of people and, moreover, are much more amenable to interpretation. As a result epidemiologists are not the sole arbiters of the theory and data. Epidemiologists have, therefore, the dual responsibilities of minimizing the impact of their own biases and preventing the misinterpretation of data and recommendations by those with vested interests.

4.3 A practical application of the research chronology schema of bias and error

The above 'research cycle' based discussion of bias in epidemiology is illustrated by reference to the study of the possible impact of industrial air pollution in Teesside on the health of populations living close by. Box 4.6 gives the title and abstract of the study. Using the list of potential causes of bias in column 1 of Table 4.1, analyse the information in Box 4.6. Do this exercise before reading on. The reference for this paper is given at the end of the chapter for readers who wish to read about it in more detail. Unusually, this study was followed by a formal examination of the impact of the research; again interested readers may wish to read how the study report was perceived. Table 4.8 provides some answers.

Box 4.6 **Analysis of an environment and health study based on the research cycle approach to bias**

Title

Does living close to a constellation of industries impair health? A Study of Health, Illness and the Environment in North East England.

Study objective

To assess the justification for public and professional concerns that industrial air pollution from a constellation of petrochemical and steel industries in Teesside, North-East England, was an important determinant of previously demonstrated poor health, particularly high mortality rates.

Design

Populations which were similar on a broad range of census indicators of social and economic circumstances, but which varied in the distance of the home from major

Box 4.6 (*continued*)

industries were compared on a broad range of health indicators including mortality, morbidity and self-reported health, health-related lifestyles, occupational histories, social circumstances, and attitudes to industry. The underlying hypothesis was that respiratory health in particular, would show gradients with the worst health in those populations living closest to industry.

Setting

Twenty-seven housing estates, 19 in Teesside and 8 in Sunderland, two conurbations in the North-east of England, were the focus of the study, but self-reported data (18 estates); and general practice data (11 estates) were on subsets of these estates. The estates were aggregated, on the basis of distance and direction from industry, into zones (designated as A, B and C in Teesside where A is closest to industry, and S in Sunderland).

Main measures

Census data (1981 and 1991), mortality (1981–1991), cancer registration (1983–1994), birthweight, and stillbirth (1981–1991) and fetal abnormality (1986–1993) statistics were compiled for all 27 areas. General practitioner consultation data (1989–1994) were studied in 2201 subjects in 12 Teesside estates. A population-based sample survey in 1993 based on self-completion questionnaires of 9115 subjects provided data on social, lifestyle, occupation, and health status. Current pollution levels were estimated by air quality measures and computer modelling of emissions from industrial, road traffic, and other sources; estimates of past exposure were made from a twentieth century land-use survey and historical pollution data.

Main results

The estates chosen for study were extremely economically deprived and comparable on a broad range of indicators including residential histories and unemployment, especially when grouped into zones. Mortality rates were high but there were no consistent and statistically and epidemiologically significant differences in all cause, or all age mortality, or for most causes. Lung cancer in women was, however, highest closest to industry (Zone A SMR = 393, Zone B = 251, Zone C = 242, Zone S = 185). A less striking gradient was observed for respiratory disorders. Lung cancer registration ratios were consistent with mortality data.

There were no associations between proximity to industry and birthweights, stillbirths, fetal abnormality, and general practice consultation rates. On a broad range of measures of both respiratory and non-respiratory health, including asthma, there were no important variations across the study zones. Smoking habits across the populations compared were similar.

Box 4.6 (continued)

Land-use data showed prominent heavy industry in the Teesside area, and that the contemporary proximity of the housing estates to industry was echoed in the past. Air quality data indicated major improvements in air quality in the preceding 20 years. Levels of major pollutants were generally below guide values.

Conclusions

Living close to a constellation of major petrochemical and steel industries was not associated with most health indicators, whether mortality or morbidity, including disorders such as asthma which had been a cause of concern to health professionals. Lung cancer in women was an important exception, and to a lesser degree respiratory mortality in women. In the absence of plausible explanations based on differences in social and lifestyle factors, exposure to past industrial pollution is the prime explanation. Further research and monitoring of lung cancer rates is warranted.

Note: This abstract is similar to that in Bhopal *et al.* 1998, *Occupational and Environmental Medicine*, 55, pp. 812–22, published with permission from the BMJ Publishing Group.

4.4 **Conclusion**

Error is inevitable in all sciences but is particularly important and likely in those studying human subjects. Bias, in an epidemiological sense, arises when errors affect comparison groups unequally. Since this is often the case, bias is a central issue in epidemiology, which is founded on comparison. As Chapter 9 on study design discusses, most epidemiological studies have similar problems in controlling error and bias and mostly these are inherent in the survey method, which underlies epidemiology. When epidemiological data are applied to provide health advice to individuals and to shape public health policy, error and bias are especially important. Epidemiology has successfully identified errors and biases, and hundreds have been listed. The epidemiological approach has been pragmatic rather than theoretical, such that problems have been identified and solutions developed. I am not aware of an epidemiological theory on why error and bias occur. To develop such a theoretically based understanding, one might start with social science perspectives on these topics. One of the most fundamental observations of social sciences on the nature of science is that the scientific endeavour is not wholly objective but open to the influence of society and context. This view helps to explain many scientific actions that lead to error and bias, e.g. the Tuskegee Study mentioned above and discussed in Chapter 10.

In studying and classifying bias this chapter has promoted the framework provided by the chronology and structure of a research project. The main principles which apply to all studies and help to minimize these errors include: develop research questions and hypotheses which benefit all the population and will not lead to harm; study a representative population; measure accurately and with equal care across comparison

Table 4.8 The research cycle framework for bias in epidemiology and the Teesside Study of health and the environment

Bias	Examples of source of bias
Research question	The question focused on industrial air pollution, the interest of the investigating team and the people of Teesside, but not of the local industry and local authority who would have preferred a focus on road traffic pollution, or a focus on all forms of pollution
Choice of populations	The study questions focused on one population living closest to industry (the population of interest living in Zone A). Another population was included because of the interests of the local authority, but investigators chose certain parts of the area Zone B in which this second population lived to maximize comparability with the population living closest to industry. Other populations were chosen on their comparability to the population of interest (living in Zones C and S).
Participation in a study	Unequal interest in the issue of industrial air pollution was reflected in unequal response rates with higher response in the three Teesside areas than in the comparison area in Sunderland (Zone S).
Comparing populations which differ	While the populations were very similar on a wide range of relevant indicators it would be impossible to show they were comparable on all potentially important exposures, say living near an asbestos plant 30 years before the study.
Assessment of disease	The comparison rests on the assumption that the diagnostic effort, skill, facilities were equal in the areas studied: a reasonable assumption in this case.
	The assumption is that subjects close to industry do not report health problems with more diligence; an assumption which cannot be accepted without testing
	In view of funding and time constraints, general practice records were not studied in the Sunderland area
Assessment of factors which could cause disease	As for assessment of disease
	Misinformation is a potential problem for, arguably, the populations living close to the industry have a vested interest in showing an association between pollution and ill-health while the local industries had the opposite interest.

Table 4.8 (*continued*)

Bias	Examples of source of bias
Follow-up	Not applicable
Outcome	Not an issue affecting the interpretation of the study
Analysis and interpretation of data	Many potential alternative analyses of the huge data set were avoided despite extreme pressures to veer away from the central hypotheses. A focus on the study questions was maintained by referring to the study proposal. While the investigators were trying to keep an open mind, for some the expectation and preferred outcome was an association between industrial air pollution and health, for others the opposite
	The analysis was searching, with detailed subgroup analysis going beyond the stated hypotheses, to seek such associations
Selected findings reported	The study report was comprehensive but analysis was confined to the study questions
	The first paper submitted for publication concerned the positive findings on lung cancer, deemed to be the most interesting and important finding
Interpretation by readers and listeners	The complex findings were interpreted by industry as showing no causal association
	Health and local authorities preferred to focus on the issue of poverty rather than on air pollution
	Most of the researchers interpreted the data as showing that air pollution from industry was important to health and that more research was warranted

groups; compare like-with-like; and check for the main findings in subgroups before assuming that inferences and generalizations apply across all groups. The findings of a single study should rarely be accepted at face value. In interpreting associations first consider artefact. (In Chapter 3, on variation in disease, a framework was provided to aid the analysis of associations.) A critical attitude is essential.

Summary

Epidemiological studies are prone to error, because they usually study human populations in natural settings and not in laboratory conditions. The large size of many epidemiological studies imposes time and cost constraints which may encourage errors. Bias in epidemiology may be thought of as error which affects comparison groups unequally or leads to inappropriate inferences about one group compared with another. Error and bias may be inherent in the research question and the hypothesis, a relatively neglected matter. Three broad problems confront epidemiologists: selection of population, quality of information, and confounding. Confounding causes an error in the assessment of the association between a disease and a postulated causal factor. It results from comparing groups which differ in characteristics other than the postulated causal factor under study.

The different epidemiological research designs have similar problems with error and bias, which are mostly inherent in the survey method. Principles which apply to all studies and help to minimize these errors include: construct research questions and hypotheses carefully, so as to benefit all the studied populations equally; study representative populations; measure accurately and with equal care across groups; compare like-with-like; and check before assuming that inferences and generalizations apply across groups. The chronology and structure of a research project offers a natural framework for systematic analysis of error and bias.

Chapter 5

Cause and effect
The epidemiological approach

Objectives

On completion of the chapter you should understand

• that the purpose of studying cause and effect in epidemiology is to generate knowledge to prevent and control disease;

• that cause and effect understanding is difficult to achieve in epidemiology because of the long natural history of diseases and because of ethical restraints on human experimentation;

• how causal thinking in epidemiology fits in with other domains of knowledge, both scientific and non-scientific;

• the potential contributions of various study designs for making contributions to causal knowledge;

• how to use a systematic approach which checks for error, chance and bias before reaching judgements on cause and effect;

• that epidemiological approaches to, and criteria for, causality are not a checklist and therefore conclusions must be carefully judged and tentative;

• the need to synthesize data from epidemiological studies and other disciplines before reaching conclusions.

5.1 Introduction: causality in science and philosophy

Cause and effect understanding is the highest form of achievement (the jewel in the crown) of scientific knowledge, and epidemiology is no exception. Causal knowledge permits rational plans and actions to break the links between the factors causing disease, and disease itself. Such actions may alter the natural history of disease in individuals and the course of disease in communities (Chapter 6). Cause and effect knowledge can help to predict the outcome of an intervention and help to treat disease. To quote Hippocrates 'To know the causes of a disease and to understand the use of the various methods by which the disease may be prevented amounts to the same thing as being able to cure the disease' (see Chadwick and Mann 1950).

The object of study of epidemiology, the natural phenomenon of disease, and the aim of understanding causes and effects, gives it the status of a science. As in sciences such as physics and chemistry, epidemiological understanding of cause and effect does not have to be 100 per cent complete or accurate to permit useful application. Arguably, more so than in other sciences, in epidemiology partial understanding must be applied as quickly and effectively as possible for it may be a life and death matter. There is, therefore, an ethical responsibility to apply knowledge even when, from a scientific point of view, further research is advised. Yet, this ethical imperative may turn out to be perilous.

Early application of theory and knowledge sometimes has devastating effects and sometimes beneficial effects. Sylvia Tesh (1988) gives two examples. The public health endeavours of the nineteenth century, including the building of sewers, the delivery of clean water, and the improvement of the sanitary conditions of the home and work-place, were driven by the 'miasma' theory of health and disease, which presumed noxious air to be the cause of most of the prevalent diseases including cholera. Though wrong, the miasma theory worked in this case. By contrast, according to Tesh, the contagion theory was both correct and dominant in explaining the occurrence of plague. Jews were incriminated in a poorly understood causal pathway of contagion and thousands were executed to control plague. Tesh gives a figure of 16 000 Jews killed in Strasbourg alone. (Roy Porter gives a figure of 2000 Jews slaughtered in Strasbourg and 12 000 in Mainz.) Though the contagion theory was widely accepted, it was only partially understood, and its application was ineffective and outrageous.

The effective application of incomplete knowledge requires the art, as well as the science, of medicine and of public health. Epidemiology is one of the principle sciences that public health policy draws upon. Recent examples of major policy decisions requiring the application of incomplete data include these: whether to ban consumption of beef products in the light of the epidemic of bovine spongiform encephalopathy in cattle; what action to take in the light of evidence that living near a nuclear power plant increases the risk of childhood leukaemia; what proportion of daily energy intake should be consumed as fat; what is the recommended daily salt intake; and whether women taking the pill have an increased risk of breast cancer and other adverse outcomes.

To the study of causality, epidemiology has contributed a philosophy of health and disease, models which illustrate that philosophy, frameworks for interpreting and applying the evidence, study designs to produce quantitative evidence for cause and effect, and information on the relationships of numerous factors and diseases. The first of these contributions is discussed in Chapters 1 and 2, the second and third are the subject of this chapter (continuing a theme introduced in Chapters 3 and 4), the fourth is the subject of Chapter 9, and the last is a recurrent theme.

Scientific modes of reasoning and methods are usually orientated towards turning empirical observations into theories and hypotheses that permit generalizable cause and effect judgements. This applies equally to many disciplines; for example, physics, microbiology, philosophy, and economics. Epidemiological reasoning on cause and effect is embedded in the observations of disease variation, the statement of association between putative causes of the variation and the disease pattern, and the ways of testing hypotheses. Epidemiology draws upon the reasoning of other disciplines including philosophy and microbiology, in reaching judgements. It is important to understand the historical context within which epidemiological reasoning has developed and appreciate that epidemiology shares similar problems of disentangling cause and effect relationships with other disciplines (particularly those mainly reliant on observation of naturally occurring events). Solutions to problems are likely to arise from sharing of ideas among such disciplines. This understanding helps to counter the criticism that epidemiological reasoning of cause and effect is empirical and atheoretical. On a pragmatic note, epidemiological debates on cause and effect are often in the public eye and, more so than most other sciences, non-epidemiologists become involved in the interpretation of data and making judgement on their meaning. This requires that epidemiological approaches to analysis of cause and effect are easy to understand.

The first and difficult question is, what is a cause? Before reading on you may wish to reflect on this apparently obvious question. In simple terms, a cause is something which has an effect, that is, it brings about or produces something. In epidemiology a cause can be considered to be something that alters the frequency of disease, health status, or associated factors in a population. These are pragmatic definitions, but it is worth knowing more about the broader debates and controversies on cause, and where such simple ideas fit.

Philosophers have grappled with the nature of causality for thousands of years (Cottingham 1996). Aristotle, for example, held a broad view that there were four elements to cause, which have been re-considered in the context of a house by John Dreker: the material (the stone, brick, or wood), the formal (the plan), the efficient (the thing which puts it into effect, here the builder), and the final (the purpose being to create a comfortable home). In Aristotle's view we have knowledge of something only when we find its primary cause(s) and he foresaw the same thing could have several causes. The material cause is the substance from which the object comes into being; for example, the bronze is the cause of the statue. In health terms, the tobacco plant can be considered as the cause of the cigarette. The formal cause is the form of a thing—its essence. What kind of thing is this? A cigarette could be said to be a device to efficiently transport constituents of tobacco to humans. The efficient cause is the primary source of something changing; for example, the father is the cause of the child. In our health analogy the nicotine in the cigarette is the cause of the addiction to tobacco, and other products, like tar, the cause of the cancer. Aristotle's final cause is the purpose of something. Aristotle asks, why do we walk? And answers, for the purpose of being healthy. Why are there cigarettes? We may guess the answer is complex but it will include, the giving of pleasure and the making of money. The cause of Legionnaires' disease is, at its simplest, exposure to the causal bacteria. From an Aristotelian point of view the four causes would be the existence of living bacteria (material), the essence of the nature of the relationship between bacteria and humans (the formal), the delivery of an infective dose by some mechanism, such as a cooling tower (the efficient), the need for bacteria to survive (they cannot do so for long in aerosol) and the human quest for efficient industrial processes and human comfort (final) that leads to complex water systems such as cooling towers.

David Hume's philosophy has also been influential. Hume's view that a cause cannot be deduced logically from the fact that two events are linked, but needs to be experienced or perceived, is crucially important to epidemiology. Just because thunder follows lightning does not mean thunder is caused by lightning (indeed, it is not as we discuss later). When we flick a light switch the light may go on but this does not prove that the one act causes the other. This perspective is echoed in the axiom 'association does not mean causation'. Cause and effect deductions need more than observation alone; they need understanding. This is close to Hume's view that causes need to be perceived and experienced. This idea's modern epidemiological counterpart is the debate on black box epidemiology. The black box metaphor comes from the increasing availability of technology as a closed unit, not amenable to easy opening and exploration. The unit works, or if it does not it is discarded and replaced, without regard to which components are or are not working. This has become an apt metaphor for epidemiological research based on the study of associations (risk factor epidemiology) and the evaluation of complex packages. The late Petr Skrabanek described it as epidemiology where the causal mechanism behind an association remained unknown but hidden (black) but the inference was that the causal mechanism was within the association (box). Skrabanek considered such epidemiology to be an embarrassment. He argued that the purpose of science is to open and understand the black box, which epidemiology too often failed to do.

The contribution of another philosopher, John Stuart Mill, captured in his canons, is so similar to the modern empirically based ideas of epidemiology that it is discussed in detail in the section on criteria for causality. Philosophical discussion on the nature of causality, questioning whether causes can be stated definitively or only as a matter of probability, is of central importance to epidemiology but further discussion of this is beyond the scope of this book.

5.2 Epidemiological causal strategy and reasoning: the example of Semmelweiss

The epidemiological idea is simple: that diseases form patterns, which are ever changing. Over short time periods the changes are largely, but not exclusively, caused by environmental changes. Over long time periods genetic variation also changes the pattern of disease. Clues to the causes of disease are inherent within these pattern. These patterns, therefore, can be studied both to generate ideas on causation and to test out ideas developed in other fields of enquiry. The combination of epidemiological and other types of observation is particularly potent.

The epidemiological mode of reasoning is illustrated by the discovery by Ignaz Semmelweiss of the cause of puerperal fever. Semmelweiss (1818–1865) was training in obstetrics in the teaching hospital in Vienna when he observed that the mortality from childbed fever (now known as puerperal fever) was lower in women attending clinic 2 run by midwives than it was in those attending clinic 1 run by doctors. He also noted the surprising finding that women who gave birth in the street, or prematurely, had a lower mortality than those in clinic 1. The statistics he collected are given in Table 5.1. Do these figures spark off any ideas of causation in your mind? Reflect on this question before reading on. He also noted that while the cases in clinic 2 were sporadic, in clinic 1 a whole row of patients would be sick. Semmelweiss was deeply perplexed but resolved that the pattern he observed meant an endemic cause, that is, the cause lay within the clinic itself. He tried, unsuccessfully, to solve the problem by delivering the mothers from the lateral rather than the supine position.

A year or so later, in 1847, his colleague and friend Professor Kolletschka died following a fingerprick with a knife used to conduct an autopsy. Kolletschka's autopsy showed inflammation to be widespread, with peritonitis and meningitis. Semmelweiss's mind was alert and he connected the disease in women with that of his friend. He wrote

> Day and night I was haunted by the image of Kolletschka's disease and was forced to recognise, ever more decisively that the disease from which Kolletschka died was identical to that from which so many maternity patients died.

Semmelweiss was 'compelled to ask' whether cadaverous particles had been introduced into the vascular systems of maternity patients as in the case of his friend.

Semmelweiss's inspired idea was that particles had been transferred from the scalpel to the vascular system of his friend and that the same kind of particles were killing maternity patients. He foresaw that the particles could be transferred from the hands of medical students and doctors to the women during pelvic examinations. If so, something stronger than ordinary soap was needed for handwashing. He introduced chlorina liquida, and then for reasons of economy, chlorinated lime. The maternal mortality rate plummeted, reaching the level of the midwives' clinic. Semmelweiss's discovery was resented in Vienna. He returned to his home in Budapest after failing to convince Viennese hospital authorities of the need for sterile conditions. He did, however, enforce antiseptic practices in the obstetric ward of Budapest's St Rochus Hospital. He died an unhappy man in a mental asylum.

Although Semmelweiss was not the first to link puerperal fever to lack of hygiene, his contribution was huge, particularly because of the systematic evidence he accumulated and the way he tested his ideas (hypotheses). The epidemiological observations

Table 5.1 Births, deaths, and mortality rates (%) for all patients at the two clinics of the Vienna maternity hospital from 1841 to 1846

First clinic (doctors)			Second clinic (midwives)		
Births	Deaths	Rate	Births	Deaths	Rate
20 042	1989	9.92	17 791	691	3.38

Extracted and adapted from Semmelweiss as reprinted in Buck et al. (p. 47).

outlined the problem and prepared the mind to seek a solution, itself inspired by clinical and autopsy observation, and tested by experimentation and epidemiological monitoring.

Two great principles are illustrated by this work. First, deep knowledge lies in the explanation of disease patterns, rather than in their description. The questioning mind may solve the riddle inherent in the pattern. Second, inspiration is needed, and may come from unexpected sources, as here from Kolletschka's autopsy. Such inspiration is considered to be a scientific hypothesis if it can be tested by scientific observation or experiment, as by Semmelweiss's intervention of handwashing with chlorinated lime.

Most disease patterns remain unexplained, despite lengthy study, and others are never explored. Those that are explained usually lead to profound insights. Epidemiology does not, however, have the tools to empirically demonstrate disease mechanisms. Whether the cause is biochemical, as in scurvy, or social, as in the rise of suicide in populations hit by unemployment, epidemiologists are reliant on other sciences, laboratory or social, to be equal partners in pursuit of the mechanisms. Epidemiology is best conducted as a multidisciplinary endeavour.

Action cannot always await understanding of the mechanism. A contemporary example of this is the use of epidemiological data to show that lying an infant on its front (prone position) to sleep raises the risk of 'cot death' or sudden infant death syndrome. Yet, the prone position was long advocated as a means of avoiding the potential danger of infants inhaling their own vomit. A campaign to persuade parents to lay their infants on their backs has halved the incidence of cot death. The mechanism is yet to be fully explained.

5.3 Models of cause in epidemiology

5.3.1 Interplay of host, agent, and environment

The idea that disease is virtually *always* a result of the interplay of the environment, the genetic and physical make-up of the individual, and the agent of disease, is one of the most important of the cause and effect ideas underpinned by epidemiology. This theory applies both to diseases said to be multi-factorial (e.g. cancers or heart disease) and to diseases which are by their definition a result of a single cause, such as tuberculosis, a drug side-effect or an overdose.

Diseases attributed to single causes are invariably so by definition. For example, tuberculosis is a disease which has many manifestations. It is characterized by a multiplicity of diffuse signs and symptoms which affect nearly every part of the body, and diagnostic test results which overlap with other diseases. Some diseases, for example sarcoidosis, are often indistinguishable from tuberculosis clinically, while the histological finding in Crohn's disease looks very similar to tuberculosis. In some ways tuberculosis is a number of distinct diseases (e.g. pulmonary tuberculosis, cutaneous tuberculosis, tuberculous meningitis), some of which are indistinguishable from other diseases. The fact that 'tuberculosis' is 'caused' by the tubercle bacillus is a matter of definition. In fact the causes of tuberculosis are many, including malnutrition and overcrowding. This view will be developed below.

This idea is captured by several well-known disease causation models, such as the line, the triangle, the wheel, and the web. These models help to organize ideas about causes and about strategies to prevent and control disease. Figure 5.1 illustrates the idea of the line of causation. First, an arbitrary division is made between genetic and all other causes, called by convention, environment. The line conceptualizes causes as lying on a spectrum from being wholly caused by genetic factors or by environmental ones. Although the interaction of the genome and the environment is the key to understanding causation, the gene—environment dichotomy, though artificial, is widely used as a simple first step in analysing the causes of disease. At one extreme lie diseases which are almost entirely genetic, such as Down's syndrome (trisomy 21). At the other extreme lies injury, say, arising from a road traffic accident or a fire. Most diseases lie in between. One of the early judgements required on diseases of unknown cause is the likely relative importance of genetic and environmental factors, for the preventive or control strategy will be fundamentally different. Try the exercise in Box 5.1 before reading on.

Box 5.1 **Exercise on gene/environment interaction**

Think about three or four health problems or diseases that you or your friends or relatives have had. Place them on the line of causation. (Use these diseases for the following exercises too.)

Think through the cause of disease X using this model (Box 1.6, Chapter 1). What is your judgement? Is disease X likely to be genetic or environmental? Why?

Figure 5.2 shows how epidemiology can help to make judgements on the question in Box 5.1. Diseases where the incidence varies rapidly over time or is much different in genetically similar groups are strongly influenced by environmental factors, while diseases which have a stable incidence or are clustered in blood relatives are more likely to have strong genetic influences. Figure 5.3 places some diseases on this spectrum.

The triangle, wheel and the web are more complex versions of the same concept as the epidemiological line, and they lead to more complex analysis. Each model has its strengths and limitations for helping to clarify causal thinking. Each model is, however, a simplification. In analysing causes it is advisable to move from simple to complex models.

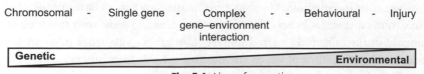

Chromosomal - Single gene - Complex - - Behavioural - Injury
gene—environment
interaction

| Genetic | Environmental |

Fig. 5.1 Line of causation.

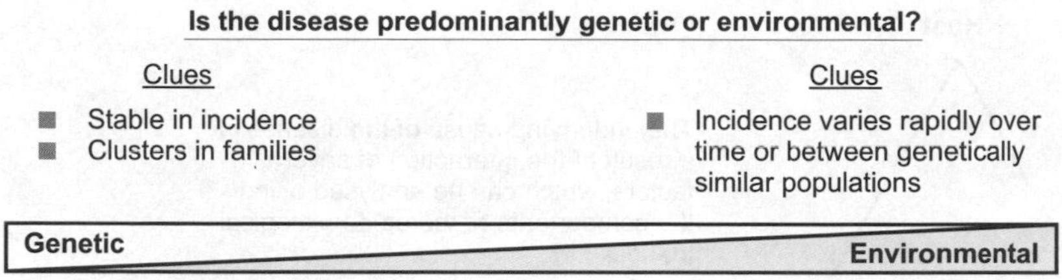

Is the disease predominantly genetic or environmental?

Clues	Clues
■ Stable in incidence	■ Incidence varies rapidly over
■ Clusters in families	time or between genetically
	similar populations

| Genetic | Environmental |

Fig. 5.2 Line of causation: clues to environment or genetic causation.

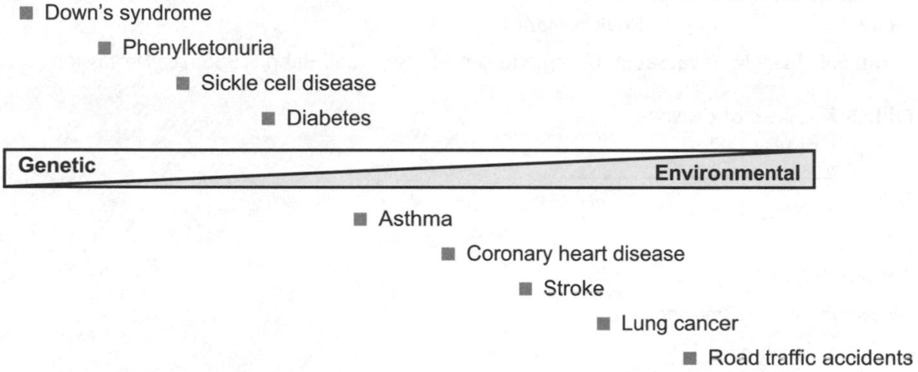

■ Down's syndrome
  ■ Phenylketonuria
    ■ Sickle cell disease
      ■ Diabetes

| Genetic | Environmental |

    ■ Asthma
      ■ Coronary heart disease
        ■ Stroke
          ■ Lung cancer
            ■ Road traffic accidents

Fig. 5.3 Line of causation: examples of diseases.

The categories of host, agent, and environment (Fig. 5.4) are arbitrary. While the meaning of the words host and agent of disease are self-evident, or can be illustrated with simple examples (Tables 5.2 and 5.3), the same is not the case for the environment which has an immensely broad meaning (Table 5.4). The host and agent are, of course, both part of the environment. The environment, in this context, is arbitrarily defined to mean factors external to the host and the agent of disease. The environment, in particular, can be split to some benefit into several categories, such as the chemical or physical environment.

Tables 5.2, 5.3 and 5.4 list some of the many host, agent, and environmental factors which are generally important causes of human disease. Of the factors listed in Table 5.2, age is the most powerful, and for many diseases, particularly of the reproduction tract, sex equally so. In using epidemiological comparisons to spark *new* understanding of disease causation, therefore, it is essential that the populations compared are alike in *known* causal factors, of which age and sex are the most important. Hence the almost automatic use of age and sex matching or adjustment techniques in causal epidemiology (Chapter 7). This said, even for variables such as age and sex, the causal effects and mechanisms are complex and cannot usually be specified in detail. For example, at any age, women have a lower incidence of cardiovascular diseases such as myocardial infarction. This sex difference is well characterized but the exact mechanisms cannot

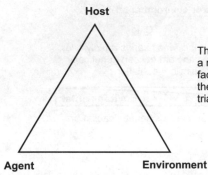

The underlying cause of the disease is a result of the interaction of several factors, which can be analysed using the components of the epidemiological triangle

Fig. 5.4 Triangle of causation (Adapted from Mausner and Bahn, 1985; see Permissions).

Table 5.2 Causes of diseases: examples of host factors

Age
Sex
Previous disability
Behaviours (such as smoking)
Genetic inheritance
Height and weight

Table 5.3 Causes of diseases: examples of agent factors

Virulence of organism
Serotype of organism
Antibiotic resistance
Cigarette—tar content
Type of glass in motor car windscreen

Table 5.4 Causes of diseases: examples of environmental factors

Home overcrowding
Air composition
Workplace hygiene
Weather
Water composition
Food contamination
Animal/human contact
Cooling tower use

be specified and are likely to involve a mix of genetic, behavioural, and social factors. Mostly, host factors in disease causation are well characterized in epidemiology and usually fairly well understood. It is worth noting that the exception to this is genetic inheritance, but that the human genome project is likely to lead to rapid growth in understanding. Before reading on do the exercise in Box 5.2.

Box 5.2 **Analysing disease using the triangle of causations**

Reconsider your chosen health problems (Box 5.1) using the triangle of causation (Fig. 5.4). Also, think through the cause of disease X (Box 1.6, Chapter 1) using this model.

The triangle is a useful model for analysing interactive causal relationships and to derive public health strategies as shown in Figs 5.5 and 5.6, for example, for the control of Legionnaires' disease. In this and other infectious diseases the concept of the disease agent is central to causation, and usually a specific agent can be identified or assumed.

In explaining population differences in the pattern of disease, agent factors, examples of which are in Table 5.3, arguably receive less attention than they deserve. This is possibly because in infectious disease epidemiology characterizing the virulence of organisms is difficult and sometimes impossible, and in other diseases conceptualizing the cause as an agent is not easy. The issue of agent virulence should be considered more carefully.

The change in the pattern of diseases associated with streptococci is partly attributable to antibiotics and partly to a decline in their virulence. The reason for this decline in

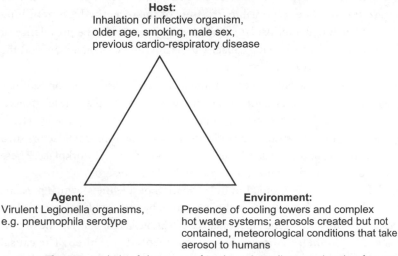

Fig. 5.5 Analysis of the cause of Legionnaires' disease: triangle of causation.

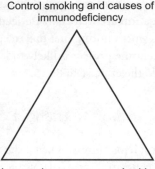

Control smoking and causes of immunodeficiency

Minimize growth of organisms and factors which enhance pathogenicity, e.g. algae

Avoid wet type cooling towers, look for a better design and location, separate towers from population and enhance tower hygiene

Fig. 5.6 Analysis of the control of Legionnaires' disease: triangle of causation.

virulence is not known. The sequencing of the microbial and human genome promises to revolutionize understanding of both human susceptibility to disease and the virulence of micro-organisms. The bacterium *Helicobacter pylori* is associated with severe inflammation and duodenal ulceration in 89 per cent of infections with the VacAsla strains and 20 per cent of infections with the vac s2 strain. Virulence genes can be identified and can be removed to create organisms that are not pathogenic to humans. An outbreak of Legionnaires' disease may be associated with virulent serotypes colonizing a water system and replacing avirulent ones.

Traditionally the concept of the disease agent has been applied to infections but it works well with many non-infectious agents; for example, cigarettes, motor cars, and alcohol can be considered as the agents of disease and injury. A reduction of the tar content of cigarettes could be responsible for some of the recent reduction of lung cancer incidence, which may not just be caused by the decrease in the prevalence of smoking. The idea of virulence, varying capacity to harm, can be extended beyond the microbe to inanimate agents of disease.

The interaction of the host, agent, and environment is rarely understood. For example, the effect of cigarette smoking is substantially greater in poor people than in rich people. The reason is unclear. It may be that there is an interaction between the agent (cigarettes), susceptibility due to host factors such as nutritional status, or environmental factors such as air quality in the home, in the residential neighbourhood or in the workplace. These ideas are illustrated below in the context of Legionnaires' disease.

Legionnaires' disease is a pneumonia (an inflammation of the lungs) which presents with some atypical features. It results from the inhalation by susceptible people of virulent organisms belonging to the genus Legionellacae (legionellas for short). The organisms which cause Legionnaires' disease are environmentally acquired. The causal micro-organism is found in most natural waters and is usually harmless. It is, therefore, a simplification to say that this normally harmless bacterium is the cause of Legionnaires' disease; and this could lead to erroneous action to control this disease through attempts to eliminate this widely distributed organism from water.

The underlying cause of Legionnaires' disease lies in the creation by humans of water systems which permit the organism to thrive and be aerosolized at sufficient concentration to cause human disease. The ageing of the population, the presence of immunocompromised people and of people who impair their lung's defence mechanisms by smoking are also important causal factors. The bacterium, which is not normally a human pathogen, finds itself interacting with humans in this environment. The triangle of causality provides a framework for this type of reasoning as illustrated in Fig. 5.5. An understanding of the range of causes permits the development of rational preventive strategy as shown in Fig. 5.6. Before reading on do the exercise in Box 5.3.

Box 5.3 **Reflection on the value of models**

Consider how your thinking on the cause of Legionnaires' disease has changed as a result of the analysis in Figs 5.5 and 5.6.

In a systematic analysis based on a model as shown in Figs 5.5 and 5.6, attention is deflected from the micro-organism as a specific cause, to the environment, host, and agent as interacting causes. This thinking broadens the control strategy. On current thinking the most effective approaches are to design better complex water systems, and to use hygiene and chemical measures to inhibit bacterial growth.

Table 5.5 shows how the epidemiological triangle can be combined with the schema of the levels of prevention to devise a comprehensive framework for thinking about possible preventive actions. Primary prevention is action to prevent the disease or problem from actually arising, secondary prevention is the early detection of the problem to prevent its damaging effects, and tertiary prevention is to contain, and if possible reverse, the damage already done. It is worth re-emphasizing that these frameworks are there to aid analysis and not to make choices, or set priorities. Before reading on do the exercise in Box 5.4.

Table 5.5 Control of Legionnaires' disease: triangle and levels of prevention

	Agent	**Host**	**Environment**
Primary	Design and hygiene	Smoking and general health	Use and location of cooling towers
Secondary	Hygiene	Nil	Separate people from source once outbreak has occurred e.g. in a hospital ward
Tertiary	Nil	Medical therapy	Close cooling towers; repair

Box 5.4 **Combining causal models and the levels of prevention**

Think about the control of the three or four health problems you picked and disease X (Chapter 1, Box 1.6) using the triangle and the levels of prevention.

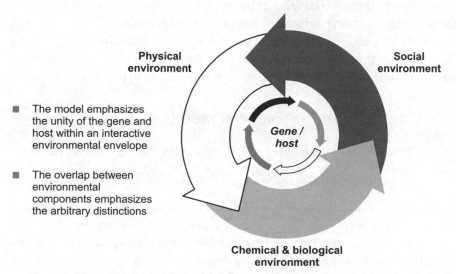

Physical environment

Social environment

Gene / host

- The model emphasizes the unity of the gene and host within an interactive environmental envelope

- The overlap between environmental components emphasizes the arbitrary distinctions

Chemical & biological environment

Fig. 5.7 Wheel of causation (Adapted from Mausner and Bahn, 1985; see Permissions).

Figure 5.7 shows the wheel of causation. The principles behind this model are as for the triangle, but it emphasizes the unity of the interacting factors. The genetic make-up of the individual and its expression in the body (phenotype) is shown as the hub of the wheel, but enveloped within an interacting environment. This version of the model emphasizes the fact that the division of the environment into components is somewhat arbitrary.

In Fig. 5.8 the model is applied to phenylketonuria, the archetypal genetic disorder. Phenylketonuria is an autosomal single gene disease. Phenylalanine hydroxylase, an enzyme required to metabolize the dietary amino acid phenylalanine and turn it into tyrosine, is deficient, and so phenylalanine accumulates in the blood. Brain damage is the outcome. Early diagnosis, usually through screening, and dietary manipulation can prevent the disease. The cause of this disease could be said to be a faulty gene. More accurately, and to clinical and public health benefit, the cause of the disease could be considered as a combination of a faulty gene, exposure to a chemical and biological environment which provides a diet containing a high amount of phenylalanine (about 15 per cent of the protein of most natural foods), and in the case of failure of diagnosis and dietary advice, a social environment unable to protect the child from the consequences of a gene disorder.

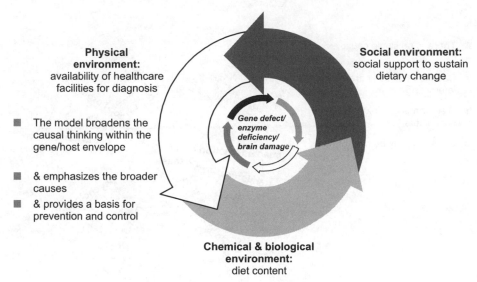

Fig. 5.8 Wheel of causation applied to phenylketonuria.

For many disorders such as coronary heart disease, and many cancers, our under-standing of the causes is highly complex. Either the causes are truly complex, or equally likely, our understanding is too rudimentary to permit clarity. These disorders are referred to as multifactorial or polyfactorial disorders. As argued earlier all disorders have several causes and where that is not the case, it is simply a matter of our causal definition. In disorders with multifactorial causation often no specific causes are known, many factors appear to be important, and mechanisms of causation are not apparent. The complexity of these diseases is not adequately captured by the line, wheel, and triangle concepts (which remain useful nonetheless) and is better portrayed by the metaphor of the spider's web. In some portrayals the web is shown as a highly schematized diagram, more like an electronic circuit or an underground transport map. Such portrayals tend to underestimate the complexity and overestimate the state of understanding. The web, as shown in Fig. 5.9, emphasizes the interconnections among the postulated causes. This model, more than the others, indicates the potential for the disease to influence the causes and not just the other way around. For example, lack of exercise may be one of the causes of heart disease and osteoporosis but these diseases can also cause people to stop exercising (reverse causality). The metaphor of the web permits the still broader causal question: where is the spider that spun the web? (After Krieger, 1994.) The question can be answered at a number of levels, for example, evolutionary biology, social structures, and role of industries. The relatively simple analysis of heart disease causation using the web concept begins to illustrate the great complexity of this disease (see Fig. 5.10).

- There is no single cause

- Causes of disease are interacting

- Disentangling is nigh impossible

- Causality may be two way

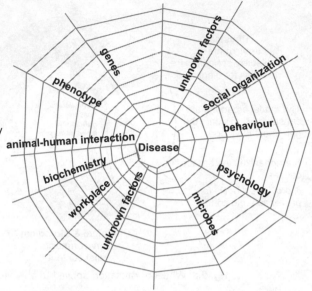

Fig. 5.9 Web of causation.

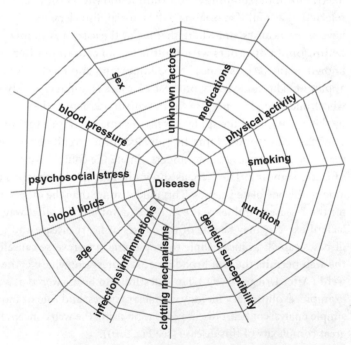

Fig. 5.10 Web of causation and coronary heart disease.

Box 5.5 **Analysing disease using the wheel and web models**

Review the health problems or diseases that you picked and disease X (Chapter 1, Box 1.6) using the wheel and web models.

The purpose of models is to simplify reality and make it easier for the mind to grasp the essence of the issue. The web permits us to grasp the complexity of multifactorial diseases but the line, triangle and the wheel help us to focus on their essentials. Before reading on do the exercise in Box 5.5.

These models provide a means of analysing causal pathways and a foundation for the application of epidemiological knowledge to public health action. Narrow causal thinking based on single causes, in contrast, can mislead epidemiologists into prematurely believing that a problem has been resolved and can seriously distort public health action. These causal models also help us to understand the ideas of necessary or sufficient causes.

5.3.2 **Necessary and sufficient cause**

Epidemiological thinking on causality has been deeply influenced by the concepts of necessary and sufficient cause, which are easily confused. The fourth edition of *Last's Dictionary* tells us that a necessary cause is 'A causal factor whose presence is required for the occurrence of the effect.' *Last's Dictionary* defines sufficient cause as a 'minimum set of conditions, factors or events needed to produce a given outcome'. A sufficient cause does not require any other determinant for a disease to occur. A factor, or a group of factors, whose presence leads to an effect is a sufficient cause, so some causes of diseases are said to be sufficient in themselves to induce disease while others are said to be necessary components in a larger jigsaw of causes. To take a simple example, the tubercle bacillus is required to cause tuberculosis but, alone, does not always cause it, so it is a necessary, not a sufficient, cause. In other words, a single factor does not cause this disease. This is, of course, the key message of the causal models discussed in the previous section.

The problem is that rarely, if ever, does a cause on its own induce a disease except in the case of extremely serious genetic defects. The model has theoretical value for analysing causes, but in epidemiology, as Susser (1977) points out, most causal factors are neither necessary nor sufficient, but contributory.

Consider the causes of Down's syndrome (trisomy 21), sickle cell disease, tuberculosis, scurvy, phenylketonuria, and lung cancer. If the cause is sufficient its presence, alone, would induce the disease and if it is necessary, in its absence the disease would not occur. (The reader may wish to reflect on this matter before continuing.)

Down's syndrome is the name given to a disorder where a person has a highly characteristic appearance (leading to the previous name, mongolism), and who will inevitably be mentally retarded because he or she has three copies of chromosome 21 instead of two (trisomy 21). This genetic feature is a sufficient cause of Down's syndrome. In other words, this chromosome abnormality alone will lead to the characteristics that define Down's syndrome.

Sickle cell trait (one sickle cell gene allele per cell) and sickle cell disease (two sickle cell gene alleles per cell) are genetically inherited conditions. The position is not quite the same as for Down's syndrome because the word disease leads to an expectation that the person has, or will develop, a health problem. The presence of two sickle cell genes per cell alone is a necessary cause. In milder cases especially, external stimuli such as infections are required to cause clinical disease. Here we have another example (phenylketonuria was discussed earlier) of genes being necessary but not always sufficient causes.

Scurvy occurs when there is insufficient vitamin C in the diet to maintain health, usually due to lack of fruit and vegetables. This does not occur in natural circumstances, but does when a restricted diet is taken, as in the past by sailors, and nowadays by food faddists or the mentally disturbed. Vitamin C insufficiency is a necessary and sufficient cause of scurvy. By definition, other diseases, several of which look like scurvy, are not so unless there is a lack of vitamin C. And yet, dietary insufficiency of vitamin C is unnatural, so other factors, in practice, come into play.

For tuberculosis, exposure to the bacillus is necessary but alone is insufficient in most people to cause disease, and in many people the organism lives harmlessly in the host. For both tuberculosis and scurvy contributory causes include poor nutritional and socio-economic conditions which increase both the risk of exposure to the necessary cause and, for tuberculosis, increase the likelihood of the organism actually establishing a clinically important infection. A diagnosis of tuberculosis may, in clinical practice, sometimes be made without demonstrating the presence of tubercle bacilli.

For phenylketonuria, the necessary cause is a genetic defect and that together with a diet containing phenylalanine is sufficient (Fig. 5.8). For lung cancer tobacco smoke is neither necessary nor sufficient, for there are many other causes. Some smokers do not develop the disease and some non-smokers do.

The above analysis begins to show the strengths and weaknesses of the necessary/sufficient cause concept. When a specific cause of disease is well known it can be incorporated into its definition (as in Down's syndrome, sickle cell disease, and vitamin C deficiency). At that point the specific cause becomes necessary by definition. For complex multifactorial diseases, at least at present, there are no necessary causes. The example of lung cancer illustrates this well. In practice, except for unusual or unhelpful scenarios (e.g. a bolt of lightning, or falling off a cliff), there are no single sufficient factors that inevitably lead to chronic diseases or death. Old age (or perhaps birth!) is probably the only sufficient cause of death. The concept of sufficient causes has, therefore, veered from single causes to group causes.

Rothman's interacting component causes model (Fig. 5.11) has emphasized that the causes of disease comprise a constellation of factors and has broadened the sufficient

Each of the three components of the interacting constellations of causes (ABC, BED, AEC) are in themselves sufficient and each is necessary

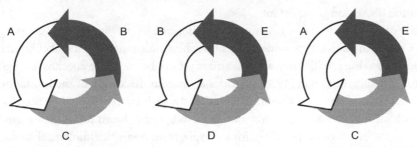

Fig. 5.11 Interacting component causes (Adapted from Rothman and Greenland 1998; see Permissions).

cause concept to be a minimal set of conditions which together inevitably produce the disease. Different combinations of these factors may together cause the disease. Figure 5.11 is a simplified version of Rothman's ideas. Three combinations of factors (ABC, BED, AEC) are shown here as sufficient causes of the disease. Each of the constituents of the causal 'pie' is necessary, and hence contribute to 100 per cent of the risk of disease attributed to that particular combination of causes. The factors are conceived to act in a biological sequence which determines the period between the beginning of causal action and the initiation of disease. It follows that control of the disease could be achieved by removing one of the components in each 'pie' and if there were a factor common to all 'pies' the disease would be eliminated by removing that alone. In this case removing factor A would remove all the disease caused by the first and third constellation of causes. This mode of reasoning, and model, is hard to apply to specific diseases but has considerable theoretical value.

5.4 Guidelines for epidemiological reasoning on cause and effect

5.4.1 Comparison of epidemiological and other concepts of causal reasoning

Turning epidemiological data into an understanding of cause and effect is challenging. To convince colleagues and the public alike, epidemiologists need an explicit mode of reasoning. There is a view that there is no room for subjectivity in science, but in practice scientists, like all other human beings, rely on intuition in evaluating evidence and making judgements. For instance, Einstein intuitively understood the theory of relativity years before he published and before there was empirical evidence to support the predictions. The theorems of the mathematical genius Srinivasan Ramanujan were intuitive to him and many of them have yet to be resolved, though they are generally accepted as correct on the basis of experience of his work. Subjective judgements on cause and effect in epidemiology should not be dismissed. Epidemiologists place much more emphasis on the evaluation of empirical data, and have devised (and adopted from other disciplines) so-called criteria for causality. Before discussing these, some background discussion is important.

The use of a set of criteria for reaching causal judgements in epidemiology is controversial. Criteria for causality provide a way of reaching judgements on the likelihood of an association being causal. They are not, and must not be used as, a checklist or algorithm for causality. Rothman (1998) provides a vigorous discussion of the limitations of causal criteria as stated by Bradford Hill. Clearly, such criteria should be seen as a framework for thought, applied before making a judgement, based on all the evidence available to the investigator including, for example, from non-epidemiological studies. One simple rule is that it is unwise to infer cause and effect from a single study though in exceptional cases where the need is urgent, and other evidence is not forthcoming easily, this may be necessary.

The epidemiological mode of causal reasoning comes under frequent attack, particularly from people and organizations who do not agree with particular research findings. Of the criticisms, the more serious ones are that epidemiologists' reasoning lacks a theoretical basis and it falls short of the rigorous modes of causal thinking in the physical sciences. These criticisms are unhelpful and perhaps unjustified. Epidemiology is predominantly an observational and not experimental science. The limitation is shared with many other sciences including demography, geology, evolutionary biology, palaeontology, and archaeology. The subject matter of epidemiology is far more complex than that of most sciences. The scope for experiment in epidemiology is strictly limited by ethical constraints on human research. Causal thinking in epidemiology draws upon the principles of other disciplines including philosophy, the laboratory sciences, and the social sciences and is theoretically grounded, though it may not be obvious. Epidemiology has, moreover, contributed new ways of thinking about causality when experiment is not possible. Epidemiological criteria are, however, designed for thinking about the causes of disease in populations and not in individuals. When applied to the individual, as in the courtroom, they may naturally be found wanting. Epidemiology has made its mode of reasoning on cause and effect open, because of the need to explain the findings to other professionals and the public.

Table 5.6 summarizes some of the principles of cause and effect thinking in the disciplines of microbiology, health economics, philosophy, and epidemiology. It is evident that there are commonalities in the mode of reasoning. The approach to establishing causality in the experimental medical sciences is illustrated by the Henle–Koch postulates (Table 5.6, column 1). Jacob Henle (1809–1885) was a German pathologist and one of the first people to publish the view that many diseases were caused by microorganisms. His ideas on how to confirm this fact were developed by Robert Koch (1843–1910), a German bacteriologist who established the bacterial cause of many infectious diseases, including anthrax (1876), tuberculosis (1882), conjunctivitis (1883), and cholera (1884).

First, the organism must be present in every case. This is, however, impossible to show for many bacterial diseases including tuberculosis. (In clinical practice a trial of anti-tuberculosis therapy is common when the patient has a clinical picture of tuberculosis but the organism cannot be grown in the laboratory.) Second, the organism must be grown in pure culture. Viral organisms are particularly hard to grow, and so are some bacteria such as the mycobacteria causing leprosy. Third, when inoculated into a susceptible animal the specific disease should occur. Animal models are sometimes not available, and even when they are the induced disease may be very different from the human version. Fourth, the organism must be recovered from the animal. If the animal can be infected this is usually possible. Clearly, there are ethical constraints in demonstrating the third and fourth criteria in humans.

The Henle–Koch postulates are a counsel of perfection and too stringent even within the field of microbiology. Evans (1978) points out that even when they were developed it was recognized that they were not to be applied rigidly, and that Koch himself believed that the cholera bacillus was the cause of cholera even though the postulates were not achieved. According to Evans, leprosy, typhoid fever, syphilis, malaria, mycoplasma pneumonia, and *Chlamydia trachomatis* infection are among the microbial diseases which have causes that still do not meet the criteria. Further, with new technologies such as antibody tests and DNA sequencing available the postulates are being superseded. Epidemiologists need to be aware of such criteria, even if only as a standard to incorporate into their own work.

Linking cause to effect has preoccupied philosophers and some of their ideas were considered in Section 5.1. John Stuart Mill (1806–73) was a British philosopher and economist who succinctly offered a practical interpretation of causal thinking in philosophy, the nub of which is now known as Mill's canons (Table 5.6, column 2). The principles so enunciated are of paramount importance to epidemiology and are essentially incorporated into its own widely used criteria.

The method of concomitant variation corresponds to current ideas on correlation and association; the method of agreement to the search for a factor in common (e.g. in an outbreak of Legionnaires' disease all those sick may have been to a particular air-conditioned hotel); the method of difference is at the core of epidemiological thinking (e.g. why do some people get heart disease and others of the same age and sex do not); and the method of residues echoes modern ideas of experiments of preventive action, to establish what proportion of disease can be prevented, or where this is not possible, calculations of attributable risk (see Chapter 8). (Readers should note that the order in which the canons are presented in Table 5.6 does not correspond to Mills's numbering of his canons, e.g. the method of concomitant variation is the fifth in his list.)

Economics also evaluates associations in similar ways (Table 5.6, column 3). Even more so than epidemiology, health economics relies on observation and modelling, with the scope for experiment being extremely limited. According to Charemza and Deadman (1997), the operational meaning of causality in economics is more on the

Table 5.6 A comparison of four modes of thinking about causality

Microbiology: Henle–Koch's postulates	Philosophy: Mill's Canons[1]	Economics[2]	Epidemiology: criteria for causality[3]
The micro-organism causing the disease can be demonstrated in every case of the disease	Method of concomitant variation: the phenomenon which varies when another phenomenon varies in a specific way is either a cause, an effect, or connected through some fact of causation	The future cannot predict the present	The cause precedes the effect (temporality)
The organism can be isolated and grown in pure culture	Method of agreement: if there is only one circumstance in common in instances of the phenomenon, then the common circumstance is the cause of effect	The effect (y) can be predicted more accurately by using values of the cause (x) than by not using them	The disease is commoner in those exposed to the cause (strength)
Animals (or humans) exposed to the cultured organism develop the disease	Method of difference: if there is only one difference in the circumstances when a phenomenon occurs compared with when it does not occur, that difference is part of the cause or effect	Instantaneous causation does not exist, since there is a time difference between independent actions. If A, itself, causes B, and A did not exist, B would not have occurred	The amount of exposure relates to the amount of disease (dose-response)
The organism can be grown from the experimentally exposed animal (or human)	The method of residues: remove from the phenomenon any part known to be the effect of known antecedents (causes), and the remainder is the effect of the remaining antecedents	One cause can have many effects and one effect many causes	The causes are linked to diseases in specific and relevant ways (specificity)

Altering the amount of exposure to the cause leads to change in the disease pattern (experiment or natural experiment)

Different types of studies reach similar conclusions (consistency)

The putative cause A may have an effect by itself or be a part of the cause

[1] Note: Mill's canons have been paraphrased from original quotations given in Susser (pp. 70–71).

[2] The discussion of causal thinking in economics comes from Charemza and Deadman (1997) and from Hicks (2001).

[3] The criteria for causality have been reduced to six by the author, for simplicity. The seventh criterion biological plausibility is discussed in the text and is, strictly, not an epidemiological criterion.

lines of 'to predict' than 'to produce' (an effect). A scan of the third and fourth columns show the similarity in concept, if not details, between economics and epidemiology.

The nub of epidemiological reasoning (Table 5.6, column 4) is that the cause must precede the effect, should raise the incidence of the disease in a population, should have a greater effect in greater quantity, be associated with specific and relevant effects, and the cause/effect relationship should show consistent effects across a number of studies. These epidemiological ideas are similar to Mill's canons and to thinking in health economics. Evidence from experiment, natural or by design, on humans or animals, may show that manipulating exposures changes the disease or may elucidate the mechanisms by which this happens. The cause–effect relationship should make biological sense. These latter ideas are those of the other biological sciences, including the Henle–Koch postulates. The epidemiological criteria for causality are not simply an idiosyncratic epidemiological invention. Their validity has not, however, been assessed empirically.

In the modern era an amalgam of epidemiological and basic science criteria are adopted as the standard for causal thinking as shown in the example in Box 5.6 and in the ensuing examples. Can you, the reader, discern the links between the evidence in Box 5.6 and causal criteria in Table 5.6?

In the case of Kaposi's sarcoma (Box 5.6) the first and second items of evidence derive from the ideas underpinning the Henle–Koch postulates. The third and fourth are based on epidemiological concepts (strength of association) and the data could be converted to a measure of strength such as relative risk (see Chapter 8). The fifth item is a mixture of microbiology (distribution in tissues) and epidemiology (transmission). The sixth item is, again, epidemiology, as is the seventh (temporality).

Box 5.6 **Aetiology of Kaposi's sarcoma (Beiser, BMJ, 314, p. 581): Evidence cited for a herpesvirus as the cause**

- Viral sequences (DNA) can be detected in sarcoma tissues in most cases.
- Such sequences are rarely detected in other tissues.
- Virus is detected in blood cells in 50 per cent of cases but not in controls.
- HIV positive patients who had the virus in blood cells had a greater risk of developing sarcoma than comparable patients without the virus.
- The virus is probably sexually transmitted and is found in semen and other genital tissues of healthy adults.
- Antibody levels in blood correlate with presence of sarcoma.
- Antibody levels rise before Kaposi's sarcoma appears.

  Conclusion: Kaposi's sarcoma is caused by a herpesvirus.

The emergent principle for epidemiology is this: causation is established by judgement on the basis of evidence from all disciplines. Failure to meet some criteria (with the exception that the cause must precede the effect, which is not easy to establish conclusively) does not dismiss causality and achievement of some criteria does not ensure it.

Epidemiology establishes causes in populations but this information applies to individuals in a probabilistic way, which does not prove cause and effect at the individual level even though causality at the population level is unequivocal. If 90 per cent of all lung cancer in a population is due to smoking, what is the likelihood that in an individual with lung cancer the cause was smoking? The answer is that we do not know. If the person is a non-smoker the cancer may have arisen from passive exposure to tobacco but is more likely to be due to other factors, and if the patient is a smoker the cause is most likely smoking, but may result from other factors such as exposure to radiation or asbestos. There is no way to distinguish a lung cancer resulting from smoking from a lung cancer arising from another cause. A drug or public health intervention may be effective in a population but harmful to an individual. For example, exercise may be good generally but lead to collapse and death in some individuals. Some people are harmed by alcohol and others benefit and the net effect on the health of the population as a whole is unclear. In contrast, the net health effect of tobacco consumption is overwhelmingly negative.

Epidemiological data are difficult to apply in legal cases about individuals. To quote Evans discussing the issue of causality in the USA (1978 p. 194)

> Legal requirements are concerned with the risk in the *individual*, the plaintiff, and whether the preponderance of evidence supports the conclusion that *that* exposure 'more likely than not' resulted in *that* illness or injury in *that* person.

Evans contests that a higher order of proof and specificity is required in legal proof than in epidemiological proof, concluding that epidemiological evidence is often inapplicable in this context. One perspective is that epidemiology is a science based on studies of groups and cannot be directly applicable to individuals, and this is an inherent limitation. Equally, a factor demonstrated to cause a disease in an individual, by a science of individuals, say toxicology or pathology, may not be demonstrable as harmful in the population, either because the effect is too small or because harmful effects are balanced by beneficial ones. This is an inherent limitation of a science of individuals. The problem lies not with epidemiology itself, but with those who apply epidemiology in these circumstances. (The law too will extrapolate from population data to the individual.) The standard of proof in epidemiology is not of a lower order than in law, it is of a different order. We now consider how epidemiological criteria for causality help to analyse the causal basis of associations.

5.4.2 Application of criteria to associations

The association (or link or relationship) between disease and postulated causal factors lies at the core of epidemiological thinking. Mostly, such associations are found by observing that disease varies with time, place, or person in observational data. An association rarely reflects a causal relationship, but it may. The preceding chapters on variation and error showed how to separate the probably not causal association from the possibly causal one. Table 5.6 begins and Table 5.7 further develops the questioning and reasoning process used in epidemiology to make the difficult judgement on whether an association may be causal. These six criteria are a distillation of, or at least echo, the ten Alfred Evans postulates in *Last's Dictionary of Epidemiology* (4th edn) and the nine Bradford Hill criteria.

Temporality

Did the cause precede the effect? If the effect is simultaneous with or precedes the proposed cause the association is definitely not causal in the direction postulated. If there is no clear answer the judgement will be tentative, irrespective of other data. If the effect follows the action of a proposed cause the association may be a causal one and the analysis can proceed. This matter of timing is referred to as temporality. Demonstrating that this criterion is satisfied does not establish causality. Before reading on, do the exercise in Box 5.7.

Box 5.7 **The deduction of cause and effect from the linkage of events**

Reflect on whether the linkage of two events provides convincing evidence on cause and effect. For example thunder follows lightning. Does lightning cause thunder?

If you flick a switch and a light goes on, can you deduce that you and your action cause the light to go on? If you observe this once or a thousand times does it make a difference? What other explanations might there be?

Thunder follows lightning but is not caused by it, for both are generated by an electrical discharge, the later appearance of the thunder is simply a result of the slower speed of sound than of light. Without an understanding of the nature of thunder and lightning erroneous conclusions about cause and effect are likely. To take another electrical analogy, we repeatedly observe that the action of flicking a light switch is the cause of the bulb lighting up. Empirical observation convinces us of this truth. However, this empirical observation alone does not show cause and effect. Other theoretical explanations can be generated, albeit with some difficulty. Far-fetched though it may seem, there may be other mechanisms of cause. For example, there may be an infrared or other detector that detects your hand moving to the switch and puts on the light. You may be being observed, and someone else is actually putting on the light as you flick the switch. Generating alternative explanations is a good discipline in epidemiology. Our alternative explanations can be put to the test. If the act of flicking similar switches in other settings turns on the light we are likely to accept a cause and effect relation on empirical grounds. The observation has no explanatory power for exceptions, when

Handwritten margin notes:

Hill's Cr
1) Strength →
2) Consistency →
3) Specificity → ☐
4) Temporality ✓
5) Biological ○

Table 5.7 Questions underlying the criteria for causality and implications of evidence for interpretation of associations

Question underlying criterion	Label for criterion	Evidence:		
		Unsure	No	Yes
Does the supposed cause precede the disease (or other effect)?	Temporality	Judgement premature	Not causal	Causal relation possible
Does exposure to the cause raise the incidence of disease?	Strength of association	Judgement premature	Not causal in the population context but does not rule out causal effects in individuals	Causal relation possible
Does varying exposure lead to varying amounts of disease?	Dose response	Not critical	Causal relation still possible if there is a threshold effect	Strengthens case for a causal judgement
Is the association between risk factor(s) and disease(s) limited in range	Specificity	Not critical	Not critical but added caution	Strengthens causal claim
Is the association consistent across different studies and between subgroups?	Consistency	Defer decision, and await further research unless an immediate judgement is essential	Judgement will require explanation for inconsistent results	Strengthens causal claim
Does manipulating the level of exposure to the cause change disease experience?	Experimental confirmation	Not always possible, so not critical	Caution needed for a causal claim	Strong confirmation of a causal relation
Is the way that the cause exerts its effect on disease understood?	Biological plausibility	Not critical	Not critical but great caution needed for causal claim	Causal judgement strengthened

the light does not go on e.g. a break in the wiring, or when it goes on even without the switch being flicked to the on position e.g. water penetration. When there is a deeper understanding of the nature and action of electrical circuits the same association may be agreed as causal and it explains exceptions. This is reasoning analogous to Hume's views on causality and has relevance to risk factor (black box) epidemiology. Just because B follows A does not, of itself, confirm a causal relation. Deeper understanding, or opening the black box, is essential.

Strength

Does exposure to the cause change disease incidence? If not or we are unsure, there is no epidemiological basis for a conclusion on cause and effect. The failure to demonstrate this does not, however, disprove a causal role. Reflect on Box 5.8 before reading on.

Box 5.8 **Epidemiology fails to uncover a cause**

Can you think of circumstances when exposure to a causal factor does not change disease incidence?

The cause may be so rare that there are insufficient cases available to reach a conclusion. Epidemiology is not good at demonstrating causal links when the rise in disease incidence is low, for example 10–20 per cent excess. Alternatively, there may be some people in the population in whom the cause is operative while in others it has no effect or even an opposite effect, leading to the view that there is no association. In this circumstance it would be reasonable to say that the cause was operative in raising or reducing disease in individuals or even subgroups but not in whole populations. Alternatively, the cause may be operative on everyone. If oxygen is the cause of, say, pancreatic cancer we cannot show this epidemiologically (or even possibly in any other way). The most usual way of measuring the increase in incidence is the relative risk. The technical name for this criterion is the 'strength of the association'. The greater the relative risk, the greater the strength of the association as will be discussed in Chapter 8.

Dose–response

Does the disease incidence vary with the level of exposure? If yes, the case for a causal relation is advanced (for in most known causes of disease this in indeed the case) but, if not, we need to be aware that the effects may be independent of the amount of exposure. It is difficult to find examples to illustrate this. Allergy is one example where trivial doses of substances such as peanuts can cause life-threatening hypersensitivity reactions. For most exposures the relationship with disease is not linear but the principle that more exposure leads to more disease tends to hold. For high blood pressure there is a threshold above and below which adverse effects arise. Above the threshold the dose–response concept applies. For weight and alcohol consumption, there is an adverse effect at both low values and high values (called a J shaped distribution). The dose–response relation is also measured using the relative risk (Chapter 8) so this can be considered as a development of the concept of the strength of the association; that is, does the strength of the association vary with the level of exposure?

Specificity

Is the effect of the supposed cause specific to relevant diseases and are diseases caused by a limited number of supposed causes? This idea is called specificity. Imagine a factor which was linked to all health effects. Why would that be so? Unless the links to a broad range of diseases can be explained, the case for causality is weakened for non-specificity is characteristic of spurious associations (e.g. underestimating the size of the population denominator; Chapter 7). Some factors do have broad effects, for example poverty and less so smoking. However, even these are not associated with more of every health problem. In the UK, poverty is associated with less malignant melanoma, an observation which makes sense. While specificity is not a critically important criterion epidemiologists should take advantage of the reasoning power it offers.

Consistency

Is the evidence within and between studies consistent? It is wise to be tentative if it is not. Unless the inconsistency can be explained the case is weakened. Consistency is linked to generalizability of findings. Experience tells us that causal effects tend to be widely applicable, while spurious associations are often local.

Experiment

Does changing exposure to the supposed cause change disease incidence? This is experimental confirmation. Sometimes there have been natural experiments, with changes over time in exposure to risk factors. For example a spill of a pollutant into a water supply, the closure of a factory, the availability of a new product, or a change of policy (e.g. putting fluoride into a water supply). These can be vitally important. Often there is no such evidence, and some form of deliberate experimentation will be necessary. The problem is that human experiments or trials are sometimes impossible on ethical grounds and always difficult to organize. Ethically, the individual involved must have the potential to benefit. For risk factors, as opposed to protective factors, there may be no such benefit. Then the experimental approach requires a valid 'in-vitro' or animal model. Causal understanding can be greatly advanced by laboratory and experimental observations. But such data must be integrated with epidemiological observations, to ensure that the theoretically predicted effects do occur in free-living populations.

Biological plausibility

Is there a biological mechanism by which the supposed cause can induce the effect? This is the criterion of plausibility. If there is plausibility the case for a causal effect will be easier to advance. For truly novel advances, however, the biological plausibility may not be apparent. For example, it is biologically plausible that lying an infant on its back to sleep may lead to it inhaling vomit. Therefore, it is better to lie the infant on its side or front. This biologically plausible theory has been overturned by the biologically implausible observation that lying a child on its back halves the risk of cot death. The mechanisms are still being worked out. That said, biological plausibility remains important particularly in confirming causality. The analogy is with the light switch; when there is understanding of the electrical circuit the causal basis of flicking the light switch is confirmed.

Judging the causal basis of the association

The investigator can now proceed to a conclusion but the interpretation ought to be tentative for judgements on cause and effect are not universal and lasting truths. An association which meets many or even all of the criteria may, at least theoretically, be non-causal. George Davey Smith (1992) has shown that the association between ciga-rette smoking and suicide meets many (but not all) of the criteria for causality includ-ing temporality, strength, and dose–response. Yet, he argues, the association is not causal. The criteria are particularly valuable in exposing the lack of evidence for causal-ity, for indicating the need for further research and for avoiding premature conclusions. This said, sometimes firm judgements are possible, and at other times forced upon us, even in the face of limited evidence. A judgement may be essential when policy is to be made. Using either this (or an alternative causal framework) makes the judgement explicit. Table 5.7 indicates how the questions implicit in causal criteria can be applied to weigh up evidence.

Three examples of the case for causality (illustrating the need for a systematic mode of analysis) are shown in Table 5.8: diethylstilboestrol as a cause of adenocarcinoma of the vagina (Herbst *et al.* 1971), smoking as a cause of lung cancer (Doll *et al.* 1956), and residential proximity to a coking works as a cause of ill-health (Bhopal *et al.* 1994). Before reading on reflect on the exercise in Box 5.9. Readers are invited to read the original studies (listed in References).

Box 5.9 **Reaching a judgement on cause and effect**

Reflect on the evidence in Table 5.8 and deliver a verdict on whether the associations between smoking and lung cancer, diethylstilboestrol and adenocarcinoma of the vagina, and living close to a coking works and ill-health are causal.

At the time that the key studies referred to in Table 5.8 were published the authors claimed that the smoking–lung cancer association was causal (many remained uncon-vinced), that diethylstilboestrol had caused adenocarcinoma of the vagina (this was accepted), and that residential proximity to a coking works had caused respiratory morbidity but not mortality (the case was not, however, accepted as rock-solid, though it was the best that was achievable).

Table 5.8 Three examples of applying the criteria for causality

Question	Smoking and lung cancer	Diethylstilboestrol and adenocarcinoma of the vagina	Living near a coking works and ill-health
Does the supposed cause precede the disease (effect) (temporality)	Yes, clearly so	Yes, maternal exposure to diethylstilboestrol preceded the disease in the offspring	Yes, the coking works was functioning before most people in the study were born
By how much does exposure to the, cause raise the incidence of disease? (strength)	Greatly and as much as 20 to 30 fold in smokers of 20 or more cigarettes per day	Greatly, as estimated from the first case-control-study	The excess of disease is modest, varying for each problem but is rarely more than 30–50% greater than expected
Does varying exposure lead to varying disease? (does-response)	Yes, there is clear relationship and more smoking causes more disease	No clear evidence	The evidence is suggestive that the closer the residence to the coking works the greater the effect on health
Does the cause lead to a rise in a few relevant diseases? (specificity)	No, numerous diseases show an association with smoking	Yes	Yes, the association is restricted, mainly, to some respiratory diseases
Is the association consistent across different studies and between groups?	Yes, the association is demonstrable in men and women, and across social groups	Yes	There are no directly comparable studies, but it fits with understanding of the role of industrial air pollution
Is the way that the cause exerts its effect on disease understood? (biological plausibility)	Only partly. The tar in cigarettes contains important carcinogens	At the time of the discovery, no	Generally, yes, specifically no. Coking works produce complex mixtures of emissions. Most knowledge is on single components of air pollution, not mixtures

Table 5.8 (continued)

Question	Smoking and lung cancer	Diethylstilboestrol and adenocarcinoma of the vagina	Living near a coking works and ill-health
Does manipulating the level of exposure to the cause change disease experience? (experimental confirmation)	Yes. Reducing consumption of cigarettes reduces risk. Persuading people to smoke more would be unethical. Tobacco is carcinogenic to animals	Yes	Don't know. An experiment is not possible, but the plant closed during the research, producing a natural experiment. Closure of the coking plant was not linked to changes in consultation with a general practitioner, but on days when pollution levels were high the consultation rates were high

5.4.3 **Interpretation of data, study design, and causal criteria**

Causal knowledge is born in the imagination and understanding of the disease process of the investigator; data can fuel the imagination and understanding. Scientific data do not, in themselves, offer knowledge. Indeed, the same data can be interpreted in quite different ways depending on the way of thought of the investigator. For example, a data set which to one scientist, Morton, indicated clear differences by 'race' in cranial capacity and hence brain size (and ultimately intelligence), to another, Gould (1984), indicated that there were no noteworthy differences. The opposite conclusions drawn from the same data set arose because of differences in the way of seeing the world (including the research world) of the two investigators. This way of seeing the world is often referred to as the paradigm. The paradigm within which epidemiologists work will determine the nature of the causal links they see and emphasize. There is a strong case for researchers to make explicit in their writings their guiding research philosophy (see also Chapter 10).

Causal thinking and study design (discussed in Chapter 9) are distinct, though interlinked, issues. No epidemiological design confirms causality and no design is incapable of adding important evidence. In all studies there are limitations and pitfalls. There are differences among the various study designs in both the type of pitfalls and their likelihood (see Chapter 9). While a single observation may spark off causal understanding it would be wise to exercise great caution until further observations confirm or refute the idea.

Table 5.9 indicates the potential contributions of various study designs to the epidemiological criteria for causality. Note that with the exception of consistency, to

Table 5.9 Potential contributions of study design (see Chapter 9) to causal criteria

Criteria	Case-series	Cross-sectional	Case-control	Cohort	Trial
Temporality	Sometimes	Sometimes	Sometimes	Often	Usually
Strength or dose-response	Sometimes	Sometimes	Often	Always	Always
Experimental confirmation	Sometimes, in the case of natural experiment	Sometimes, in case of repeated studies, following an intervention	Seldom	Sometimes, following natural changes	Always
Specificity	Sometimes	Sometimes	Yes, for disease	Yes for the risk factor(s)	Yes for the risk or preventive factor
Biological plausibility	Not directly	Not directly	Not directly	Not directly	Not directly
Consistency	Yes	Yes	Yes	Yes	Yes

which all designs contribute, and biological plausibility, to which no designs contribute directly, all epidemiological studies contribute to some but not all criteria.

5.5 **Epidemiological theory illustrated by this chapter**

Several theories underpin epidemiological causal thinking. First and foremost, is the theory that diseases arise from a complex interaction of genetic and environmental factors. Second, there is a theory that causes of disease in individuals may not necessarily be demonstrable as causes of disease in populations and vice versa. The third (and pragmatic) epidemiological theory of causation is that reliable cause and effect judgements are achievable through hypothesis generation and testing, with data interpreted using a logical framework of analysis, which draws on multidisciplinary perspectives.

5.6 **Conclusion**

The most important aim of epidemiology is to generate and use cause and effect theories to break the links between disease and its causes and to improve public health. The application of erroneous theory may have serious repercussions including deaths on a mass scale, while the proper application of sound theory can transform the control of disease. It is difficult to achieve trustworthy causal knowledge because of the complexity of diseases, the long timescales over which many human diseases develop, and ethical restraints on human experimentation. Nonetheless, there is an imperative to act, even when our knowledge is incomplete, for lives depend on our science. In the words of Bradford Hill (1965):

> All scientific work is incomplete—whether it be observational or experimental. That does not confer upon us a freedom to ignore the knowledge we already have, or to postpone the action that it appears to demand at a given time.

A rigorous analysis of all the scientific data available is essential, though to quote Bradford Hill again, 'this does not imply crossing every "t", and swords with every critic, before we act'.

Epidemiology engages with policy makers and planners who are ultimately the users of much of the work. Rothman (1986) has helped to open up the prickly question, posed by Lanes, of whether epidemiologists (as scientists) ought to be engaged in choosing between theories of causation or whether they should simply present the evidence and the theory options to policy makers and leave the choices to them. Clearly, the latter approach would go counter to current practice. Readers need to ponder on this question and form their own views. Whatever viewpoint prevails, epidemiology has a responsibility both to understand the theories of causation used by other disciplines, particularly those with which research collaborations or health interventions take place, and to educate others about the mode of thought in epidemiology. Simplistic notions of causality, for example a cause is something which raises the incidence of disease, are not particularly helpful in persuading sceptical others of the strength of the epidemiological evidence. Demonstrating to the skeptics' satisfaction that a cause raises the disease incidence is complex and requires detailed understanding by both parties of causal reasoning in epidemiology. Developing effective actions, a difficult challenge usually achieved in cross-disciplinary partnerships, is also demanding in epidemiological knowledge.

Epidemiology provides a broad perspective on the causes of disease which contrasts with the narrower one of the physical and most biological sciences. The causal models reinforce this perspective and provide a framework to organize ideas. The concept that virtually all diseases are caused by the interplay of genetic and environmental factors is crucial in epidemiology. The prevailing attitude in epidemiology, that all judgements of cause and effect are tentative, is both pragmatic and in line with modern thinking about the nature of scientific advances. The increasing understanding that the data do

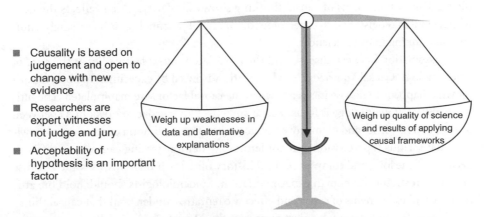

- Causality is based on judgement and open to change with new evidence
- Researchers are expert witnesses not judge and jury
- Acceptability of hypothesis is an important factor

Weigh up weaknesses in data and alternative explanations

Weigh up quality of science and results of applying causal frameworks

Fig. 5.12 Cause and effect: judgement.

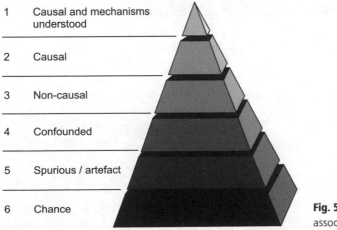

1 Causal and mechanisms understood

2 Causal

3 Non-causal

4 Confounded

5 Spurious / artefact

6 Chance

Fig. 5.13 Pyramid of associations.

not hold an unequivocal answer, and that the answers derived are dependent on human judgement (symbolized in Fig. 5.12), though apparently common sense, are harder to accept for they give space for subjectivity where science prefers objectivity. Epidemiologists should be alert for error, the play of chance, and the constant presence of bias, and should apply criteria for causality as an aid to thinking and not as checklist. Only rarely will causal mechanisms be understood as symbolized by the pyramid of associations in Figure 5.13. Finally, epidemiology should seek corroboration from other scientific disciplines in terms of both data and scientific frameworks for cause and effect.

Summary

Cause and effect understanding is the highest form of scientific knowledge, for it permits prediction and generalization, one of the main purposes of science. Understanding of cause and effect has also been a preoccupation of philosophy. A comparison of epidemiological and other forms of causal thinking shows similarity, which reflects the debt which epidemiologists owe to other, older disciplines. Epidemiology is increasingly influencing thinking in other sciences.

An association between disease and the postulated causal factors lies at the core of epidemiology. Causal knowledge can be greatly advanced by experimental observations on what happens to disease incidence when the causal factors are manipulated. The ultimate aim of epidemiology is to use cause and effect knowledge to break links between disease and its causes and to improve public health. The application of erroneous knowledge has serious repercussions. In epidemiology demonstrating causality is difficult because of the long and complex natural history of many human diseases and because of ethical restraints on human experimentation. Epidemiologists should: hold the attitude that all judgements of cause and effect are tentative; understand that causal thinking demands a judgement; be alert for error, the play of chance, and bias; utilize the power of causal models that broaden causal perspectives; apply criteria for causality as an aid to thinking and not as checklist; and look for corroboration of causality from other scientific frameworks for assessment of cause and effect.

Chapter 6

Natural history, spectrum, iceberg, population patterns, and screening
Interrelated concepts in the epidemiology of disease

Objectives

On completion of this chapter you should understand:

- that the natural history of disease is the unchecked progression of disease in an individual;
- that natural history ranks alongside causal understanding in importance for the prevention and control of disease;
- that the technical and ethical challenges posed to medical sciences, including epidemiology, in elucidating the natural history of disease are great, particularly where the time between exposure to the causal agents and the onset of disease is long;
- that the changing pattern of disease in populations over time and the spectrum of the presentation of disease are related to natural history, yet are separate concepts;
- that the 'iceberg of disease' is a metaphor emphasizing that for virtually every health problem the number of cases ascertained (those visible) is outweighed by those not discovered (those invisible);
- how the iceberg of disease phenomenon thwarts assessment of the true burden of disease, the need for services and the selection of representative cases for epidemiological study;
- that screening is the application of tests to diagnose disease (or its precursors) in an earlier phase of the natural history of disease (often in well people) than is achieved in routine medical practice;
- that the key to successful screening is a simple test which can be applied to large populations with minimum harm and has a high degree of accuracy (high sensitivity, specificity, and predictive powers) in separating those who need more detailed investigation from those who don't;
- that the potential of screening is vast but there are important limitations such as the inability to influence the natural history of many diseases, and the need to balance the costs and benefits of earlier diagnosis.

6.1 **Natural history of disease**

The natural history of disease is the uninterrupted progression in an individual of the biological development of disease from the moment that it is initiated by exposure to the causal agents. Do the exercise in Box 6.1 before reading on.

Box 6.1 **Potential effects of an exposure to a causal agent**

Reflect on the possible outcomes in an individual of exposure to a causal agent. The causal agents to consider include microbes (say those causing Legionnaires' disease or tuberculosis) and inanimate ones (say particulate air pollution or tobacco smoke).

There are four main types of response to such an agent. First, the exposure may have no discernible effect at all. The exposure may have had no effect because the dose was too low or the recipient was not susceptible. There may, however, have been an effect but one too small to notice. Strictly speaking, then, for such individuals there is no 'history of disease' or even precursors of disease. Nonetheless, from an epidemiological and public health perspective this type of response is important, because we may learn how to protect those individuals who do develop disease with this level of exposure. Second, there may be demonstrable damaging effect of the exposure which may be repaired. Microbiological, immunological, biochemical, or pathological studies may be able to demonstrate inflammation, tissue change, and repair. This type of response is likely to lead to some illness, possibly non-specific symptoms and signs such as tiredness and fever. Third, the effect may be an illness that is rapidly contained by the body's defence mechanism. In this case there will usually be a short illness. In the case of tuberculosis there may be a fever which subsides. The tuberculosis bacilli are contained though they remain alive. Particulate air pollution may lead to a bronchial illness that is soon resolved. Fourth, the illness may progress until it leads to continuing long-term problems, irreversible damage, or death. This progression may be curtailed by treatment (but then it no longer represents the natural history of disease). The outcome will depend on the interactions of host, agent, and environmental factors. For example, an elderly person with cardiorespiratory diseases may die on exposure to smog on a cold wintry day, when similar exposure in summer of a younger person (in the same amount of smog) would have no important adverse effect. The natural history, as outlined in these four responses to exposure, is a biological and clinical concept of great importance to all medical sciences, including epidemiology.

Figure 6.1 provides an idealized view of the concept. The idea here is that individuals start life healthy or at least disease free. As they age they are exposed to disease-causing agents which, cumulatively, increase their susceptibility to disease and burden of ill-health, some of it chronic. In the early years, exposure to disease agents causes little lasting harm. This cumulative burden eventually leads to death. With the exception of

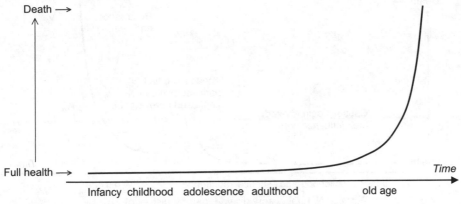

Fig. 6.1 Natural history of disease, idealized.

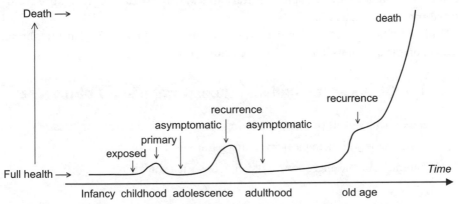

Fig. 6.2 Natural history disease: outcome of untreated tuberculosis.

the period *in utero* and early infancy, which are perilous times in terms of health risks, this idealized picture is becoming true in the affluent parts of the world, where the pattern of health, ill-health, and death generally follows that shown. The burden of serious ill-health is being 'compressed' into the later part of life. The same concept can be applied to individual diseases.

Tuberculosis provides an excellent example, illustrated in Fig. 6.2, which shows the natural history in one hypothetical individual in a simple way. This man was exposed to the tubercle bacillus in early childhood but the primary tuberculosis which followed hardly impaired his health. He harboured this illness through childhood but it recurred in adolescence (possibly because of other health problems at that time) with recovery, but then a second recurrence in early old age led to death. Figure 6.3 shows a typical path for the natural history of coronary heart disease (CHD). The causes exert their effect in early life and the development of atheroma usually begins in adolescence (or earlier). Disease may not be manifest until adulthood (often middle age). The first

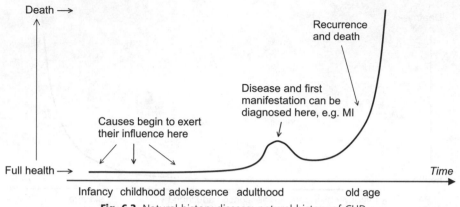

Fig. 6.3 Natural history disease: natural history of CHD.

clinical occurrence may be angina or heart attack, with partial recovery, until recurrence and death in later life.

While of vital importance, information on natural history is very hard to obtain. Reflect on the questions in Box 6.2 before reading on.

Box 6.2 **Obstacles to studying the natural history of disease**

+ What difficulties can you see in studying the true natural history of disease?
+ Would you be willing to participate in a natural history study?
+ What might be the effect on you of being in such a study?

In practice, the natural history of diseases such as tuberculosis is interrupted as soon as possible either by treatment or immunization with BCG. It would be ethically unacceptable *anywhere in the world* to set up a study to observe the natural history of tuberculosis. As a medical diagnosis is essential to studies designed to define the natural history of disease, the truth about the natural history of most diseases is seldom known for two major reasons. First, the mere act of diagnosis and follow-up by a physician may initiate changes in the disease process, for example, through the placebo effect, or by changing the behaviour of the person observed. This principle is clear in the case of psychological disorders, say depression or anxiety, but probably applies to all diseases in a more subtle form. For example, the observation of the natural history of CHD by repeat electrocardiogram or Rose Angina Questionnaire is likely to raise awareness of the disease and induce some modifications of lifestyle. Second, the scientific objective of observing the natural history of disease clashes with the ethical medical imperative to act to alleviate, contain, or treat the disease. It would be unethical for any investigator to observe patients with tuberculosis, for treatment is curative and cheap. For medically qualified epidemiologists the ethical imperative is clear, but it is less so for non-medical ones, for there is no widely agreed and enforced ethical code for science. In cases of doubt, such epidemiologists should ensure that their work is cleared by an ethical committee. Defining the natural history of most diseases in the modern world is, therefore, problematic.

Studies of the natural history of disease are potentially ethically explosive. One infamous example was the US Public Health Service's Tuskegee Syphilis Study (see Jones 1993), where 600 'negro' men with syphilis in the state of Alabama in the USA were followed up for a period of about 40 years. They were actively shielded from treatment by the investigators. The investigators believed that the scientific value of their observations exceeded the right of their subjects to therapy. There was no informed consent by the subjects. Even if there had been the study would still be unethical, because it clashes with the medical ethical imperative to do good and not harm (this example is also discussed in Chapter 4 in relation to bias and in Chapter 10 in relation to epidemiological ethics).

The ethical principles for epidemiological studies of natural history are that these studies can only be done on informed individuals; studies are only permissible when there is no known effective therapy; if an effective therapy becomes available (after the study starts) then the study will need to be modified or abandoned. The placebo group in some clinical trials is, potentially, an important source of information on the natural history (see Chapter 9). The emerging principle for trials is that the control group should receive the best available therapy, and not placebo, so this source of data on the natural history of disease may dry up.

Follow-up, or cohort, studies are needed to define the natural history of disease (see Chapter 9 for a discussion of cohort studies). Repeated observation of the same individuals is usually necessary in chronic diseases. Ideally, a disease-free population would be observed closely and repeatedly, until either the population is no longer at any risk of the disease or until death. For example, in an ideal study of the natural history of gestational diabetes a representative sample of pregnant women would be followed, with observations to include tests of blood sugar levels. For those who did not develop diabetes in pregnancy, the observations could stop until the next pregnancy. For those who did develop diabetes, follow-up would continue after pregnancy, to assess whether it resolves and whether there are long-term adverse outcomes. In the latter case the follow-up may be measured in decades, and in those with continuing diabetes and complications, until death. With this information we can decide whether gestational diabetes is a harmful phenomenon, and develop appropriate health services, on appropriate timescales. To take one simple question: does gestational diabetes herald type 2 diabetes in later life? If not, after pregnancy the woman need not be followed up, at least in relation to diabetes. If yes, such women may need to be followed up. In practice such cohort studies are rare, and long-term observations may prove costly or impossible. The natural history is usually pieced together from a mixture of observations, including those from single individuals (case reports) or from case series observed by clinicians, rather than in formal epidemiological studies.

The period of time between exposure to the agent and the development of disease is called the incubation period. It varies greatly in individuals but in populations the pattern can be defined both for broad categories of disease and for specific diagnoses. Diseases that have long incubation periods, usually measured in years and sometimes decades, generally have a long clinical course and, if so, by convention they are called chronic diseases. An example of a chronic disease is chronic bronchitis. This disease is likely to have been caused by prolonged exposure to a mixture of agents including respiratory infections in childhood and adulthood, air pollution, and tobacco smoke. Chronic bronchitis is likely to run a clinical course measured in decades and the damage is usually irreversible. Other examples of chronic diseases include rheumatoid arthritis, CHD, diabetes, and most cancers.

Some chronic diseases, paradoxically, lead to sudden and unexpected death (e.g. a stroke or heart attack); the diagnosis is then made postmortem. The label chronic disease is based on the natural history as defined in many individuals, not the clinical course in an individual. The opportunity to control and treat a chronic disease may be short, but the opportunity to prevent it will be prolonged.

Diseases with a short incubation period (days, weeks, and sometimes months) usually have a short course, and by convention are known as acute diseases. These include most infections and many toxic disorders e.g. influenza, food poisoning, and carbon monoxide poisoning. Paradoxically, the effects of acute disease may also be severe and prolonged, such as post-viral syndromes. Clearly, an acute disease can leave permanent (chronic) sequelae; for example, meningitis can lead to chronic deafness. The incubation period, together with minimal clinical information on the nature of the illness (e.g. a rash and fever), may be sufficient to identify the disease. This is particularly the case with infectious diseases. For example, vomiting within a few hours of eating a meal in a group of people is much more likely to be due to *Staphlyococcus aureas* food poisoning than salmonella.

Knowledge of the natural history is usually vital for disease prevention policies, particularly for secondary prevention based on screening, and provides the underlying rationale for all medical practice. Indeed, it would not be an exaggeration to say that the whole purpose of medicine is to influence the natural history of disease by reducing and delaying ill-health. Figure 6.4 illustrates this. When this is achieved through deliberate actions by societies the collective endeavour is public health.

The natural history concept applies to individuals but it has implications for thinking about disease in populations. First, changes in the natural history of disease in individuals do, of course, affect the population pattern. Improved general nutrition, for example, reduces the likelihood of an individual developing secondary tuberculosis. In turn this reduces the risk of person-to-person transmission, and hence the incidence of clinical tuberculosis and death. Second, the various paths to progression in individuals can be aggregated to produce a portrait of what alternatives may happen in a population. This is shown in Fig. 6.5 and will be discussed in Section 6.3.

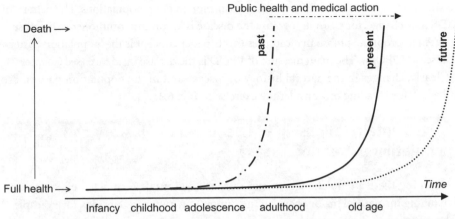

Fig. 6.4 Natural history of disease: giving purpose to public health and medicine.

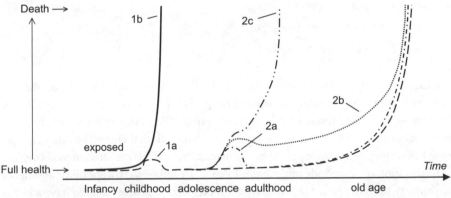

Fig. 6.5 Natural history of disease: pathways in tuberculosis. 1a: primary infection with complete remission (death from other causes); 1b: Fatal tuberculous meningitis; 2a: recurrence with successful treatment (death from other causes); 2b: TB with residual disability (and TB contributory or actual cause of death); 2c: recurrence with fatal outcome.

6.2 **The population pattern of disease**

The concept of the natural history of disease should not be (but is) confused with the changing pattern of disease in populations over time, for example, the decline in recent decades of gastric cancer, stroke, heart disease, and tuberculosis, or the rise of AIDS, asthma and childhood leukaemia. There is no widely agreed word or phrase to capture this concept, though the 'secular trend' in disease (secular in the sense of long term) is sometimes used. The secular trend is, however, a limited concept; it does not capture the point that the incidence of the disease may not change much but the population pattern of disease occurrence may be radically altered. For example, the distribution of a disease across socio-economic groups may change as it has for coronary heart disease which has become less common in wealthy, and more common in poor, populations. The pattern of AIDS may change, for example, because the disease is becoming commoner in heterosexuals. An appropriate phrase that captures this broader concept is the 'population pattern of disease' (PPOD). The main measure of PPOD is the disease incidence (see Chapter 7).

Clearly, changes in the natural history of disease and in the population pattern are linked. Before reading on consider the exercise in Box 6.3.

Box 6.3 **Interrelationship between natural history and population pattern of disease**

Assuming there are no changes to exposure to the causal agent, what effect would changing the natural history have on the population pattern? Consider, for example, the effect of:

- reduced and enhanced susceptibility;
- a shorter or longer course of disease;
- a longer and shorter incubation period;
- a more severe or less severe disease.

Reducing the population's susceptibility would diminish the number of cases of overt, diagnosed disease, so reducing the disease frequency as measured by incidence, while enhanced susceptibility would have the opposite effect. The secular trend would change. If the changes in susceptibility were uneven across a population, there will be other changes in the PPOD too, for example the change in inequalities in CHD as referred to above.

The duration of an episode of disease is likely to be linked to susceptibility, and hence the capacity to fight against the disease. A shorter course is also likely to have a better outcome, with less long-term morbidity or mortality. While the disease incidence will not be affected, the prevalence and case fatality is likely to be (chapters 7 and 8).

The length of the incubation period can affect disease patterns. If the incubation period lengthens in a chronic disease from 20 to 30 years, then the disease burden will decline, at least for some time. The severity of the disease can also change either as a result of changed virulence of the disease agent or changed susceptibility of the host. This will alter the balance between diagnosed and undiagnosed cases and change the measured incidence and prevalence.

The idea that an exposure can lead to variants (and varying severity) of the same disease is the spectrum of disease (also an idea that is understandably confused with the natural history of disease). This concept can be combined with the natural history to enrich our understanding.

6.3 **Spectrum of disease**

The spectrum of disease captures the idea that disease may present with varying signs, symptoms, and severity. The role of epidemiology is to define the nature and causes of this variation, to quantify disease progression in aggregate populations, and to make reliable predictions on outcome at both the individual and the population level. For example if a hundred people are exposed simultaneously to an aerosol contaminated with the Legionnaires' disease bacillus, most (about 98 per cent) will have no perceptible problems. The remainder will have disease which varies from a mild influenza-like illness to a fulminating pneumonia. Of those who become ill about 10–15 per cent will die unless effective treatment is given. The mortality rate will be higher in some settings and population groups, such as in nursing homes or hospital outbreaks where the frail or elderly are effected. The period of time between exposure and first symptoms will vary from as little as 2 days in some people to as much as 10 days in others. The symptoms and signs of illness will vary greatly; some people have an illness dominated by neurological problems, others by chest problems. Among survivors, some will recover fully and others will be left with disability. This principle of variability of outcome applies to nearly all diseases whether infections, toxic problems, or cancers. This epidemiological picture is vital to responding appropriately to control disease.

Tuberculosis is another particularly good example and is illustrated in Table 6.1 and Fig. 6.5, which combines the natural history and spectrum of disease concepts. Figure 6.5 develops this idea from a population perspective where the collective observations on a number of individuals are summarized as possible pathways in the natural history. With some exceptions children develop a mild illness (or a sub-clinical problem) from which they recover. This illness is not usually recognized as primary tuberculosis, but as a febrile illness of childhood. This progression is shown by line 1a in Fig. 6.5. Rarely, this first exposure will lead to a serious infection which may be systemic (i.e. affects the whole body). Tuberculous meningitis is one of the rare, potentially fatal outcomes of such infection (line 1b). More usually, the primary tuberculosis is followed by a lifetime of cohabitation by the agent and host with living organisms sealed off in caseous lesions in the lymph glands of the patient (line 1a). In some cases, particularly when the natural defence mechanisms of the patient are weakened by other illnesses (e.g. AIDS, age, or other factors), the bacillus overcomes the defence mechanisms to cause secondary tuberculosis (line 2). The commonest form of this disease is respiratory, but it may be a more general illness with fevers and weight loss. In most instances the disease will respond to therapy (after which we are not observing the natural

Table 6.1 Spectrum of disease: tuberculosis

Primary tuberculosis	Secondary tuberculosis
No symptoms	Fever and weight loss
Minor self-limiting illness	Enlarged lymph glands
Grumbling illness with fevers	Persistent cough
Overwhelming illness such as tuberculous meningitis	Skin rashes Septicaemia (miliary tuberculosis)

history but the prognosis) or heal spontaneously (line 2a). Some people will be left with permanent disability (line 2b) while others will die (line 2c).

The spectrum of disease is, primarily, a population concept (while natural history is primarily a concept relating to individuals) with obvious and important implications for clinical medicine in that doctors who are not aware of the full spectrum of disease, particularly the less severe or rare forms, are likely to be misled. The spectrum of disease may differ in different population groups. For example, while pulmonary tuberculosis is the dominant mode of clinical presentation in European-origin residents in the UK, lymph node tuberculosis is the commonest form in UK residents of Indian subcontinent origin; and coronary heart disease is more likely to present as angina in women, and as a heart attack in men. In the elderly and in people with diabetes, in particular, coronary heart disease may present as a silent myocardial infarction, that is, a heart attack without chest pain. The diagnosis may be made, by chance, many years later on ECG. The spectrum of coronary heart disease is broad and ranges from no symptoms, signs, or disability to devastating chest pain and disability. The main recognized variants in the spectrum of coronary heart disease are: asymptomatic, angina, arrhythmia, heart failure, and myocardial infarction (heart attack).

Some diseases occur more than once. Presentation of the same disease may differ at different times. The first occurrence of malaria is likely to be far more severe than subsequent episodes. In chronic diseases, however, recurrences may be manifest in a characteristic way; for example, if a person develops pain in the tongue in one occurrence of angina, then that person is likely to have a similar pattern at recurrence, rather than, say, pain in the left arm.

The spectrum of disease is about the variability in the nature of disease while the natural history is about the progression of disease. The fact that diseases may be mild or even 'silent' are among the many explanations for undiagnosed disease in the community, even when people are served by an excellent health service, a phenomenon described by the metaphor of the iceberg of disease (see Last 1963).

6.4 The unmeasured burden of disease: the metaphors of the iceberg and the pyramid

Surprisingly, for most health problems and within all healthcare systems there are large numbers of undiscovered or misdiagnosed cases of disease. The exceptions to this generalization are the serious diseases which have obvious symptoms which lead to a rapid and accurate diagnosis. Lung cancer is an excellent example of an exception, while prostate cancer is illustrative of the generalization. While lung cancer has characteristic symptoms and, if untreated, spreads and is invariably fatal, prostate cancer may remain localized, with no signs or symptoms and in these circumstances poses little threat to health. Yet, prostate cancer may kill, and be diagnosed too late to cure. Serious and killing disorders such as diabetes, atrial fibrillation and hypertension are other good

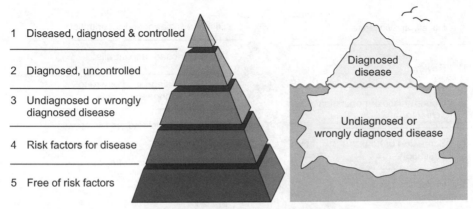

Fig. 6.6 Pyramid and iceberg of disease.

examples of this iceberg phenomenon. This principle applies alike to populations served by comprehensive, publicly funded healthcare systems and to those with private services only available to those who can pay. Obviously, the number of undiagnosed cases in relation to those diagnosed will be bigger where the healthcare system is poor.

An illustrative and commonly used metaphor for this phenomenon is the iceberg of disease and symptoms. Cases that have been correctly diagnosed can be likened to the tip of the iceberg, visible and easily measured. In most diseases, as with the iceberg, the larger presence lurks unseen, unmeasured and easily forgotten with potentially catastrophic consequences. Figure 6.6 illustrates this idea and develops the iceberg concept in the form of a pyramid of disease by using its clear structure and shape. At the tip of the pyramid are the cases which are diseased, diagnosed, treated, and controlled. The next block is the diagnosed but uncontrolled cases. The failure to control the disease arises from either technical or organizational factors or from the patient's preferences not to participate in therapy (so-called non-compliance). The third block comprises the patients with undiagnosed disease, which may be a reflection of the difficulties of making the diagnosis or the failure to access an appropriate level of health care. The fourth block is the population that harbours the causal factors for disease, but remains disease free. The final block is the population free of both disease and causal factors. Blocks 1 and 2 correspond to the iceberg above sea level and 3 to 5 below sea level. The pyramid comprises both the diseased population and those potentially diseased (i.e. it is a whole population concept), while the iceberg relates only to the diseased population.

There is a specific and minimal level of healthcare need at each level (Fig. 6.7). For block 1 the need is for vigilance and continuity of high quality care through follow-up. For block 2 there is a need for review and attempts to deliver effective and acceptable care. For block 3 there is a need for opportunistic or population screening for people with early disease. For block 4 there is a need for screening and health education. For block 5 there is a need for health promotion to maintain this desirable state for people.

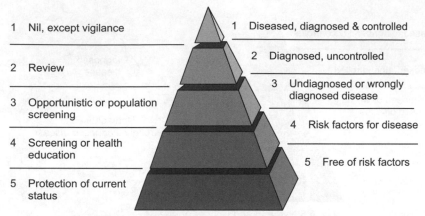

1   Nil, except vigilance

2   Review

3   Opportunistic or population
    screening

4   Screening or health
    education

5   Protection of current
    status

1   Diseased, diagnosed & controlled

2   Diagnosed, uncontrolled

3   Undiagnosed or wrongly
    diagnosed disease

4   Risk factors for disease

5   Free of risk factors

Fig. 6.7 Pyramid (iceberg) of disease: potential unmet need.

Epidemiology that forgets the iceberg phenomenon of disease, and merely counts the number of cases actually seen by clinicians and diagnosed, is weak and potentially misleading. Epidemiology reliant on statistics obtained from routine systems like hospital admissions is likely to be seriously compromised. The missing cases thwart efforts to assess the true burden of disease which in turn creates great difficulties in judging the priorities and assessing the need and demand for health services. There are no easy rules or formulae which can be applied to judge the true burden of disease based on those diagnosed. However, experience with diabetes indicates that about 50 per cent of the cases in the community are diagnosed at any point in time. The findings for hypertension are about the same. For less serious diseases (migraine, eczema, back pain) or those which tend to get less attention (thyroid disorders, chronic bronchitis, peptic ulcer, and osteoarthritis) the proportion diagnosed would be lower. It is reasonable for researchers and health planners to use these findings to predict that the true burden of disease is much higher than their data show, and unreasonable to reach conclusions on the burden of disease without reference to the iceberg phenomenon (as is too often the case).

Unidentified cases may be different from identified ones, in terms of both the natural history and the spectrum of disease. For example, people with undiagnosed prostate cancer are less likely to have urinary symptoms or pain compared with those diagnosed. Where symptoms and disease progression and outcome are related, the undiagnosed cases are likely to be less severe. For this reason a screening programme (see next section) may uncover not just cases of disease at an earlier stage of the natural history but also less aggressive and severe cases. This may mislead the evaluation of screening programmes. In contrast, when symptoms and signs are not evident in the early stages of disease, as in high blood pressure or chronic glaucoma, undiagnosed cases may be just as severe as diagnosed ones.

Epidemiological studies of the causes and consequences of disease should, ideally, be of representative cases. Studies based on selected cases from the tip of the iceberg may give an erroneous view. The study of the outcome of prostate cancer based on cases diagnosed in hospital would lead to the view that the disease is usually, if not always, progressive, whereas studies of unselected cases show that prostatic cancer can be a static, or slowly progressive phenomenon.

Patients who are at the tip of the iceberg are more likely to have multiple health problems than others because these diseases bring them to medical attention, which in turn increases the diagnostic activity. Their susceptibilities to various diseases, the causal pathway, and their outcomes may differ too. For example, people with cardiorespiratory problems and diabetes, and those living alone or in poverty, are more likely to be admitted to hospital. This is the basis of the bias known as Berkson's bias (Chapter 4).

6.5 **Screening**

The dictionary provides many meanings of the word screen, but the two that correspond to the epidemiological one are: to sift coarsely and to sort out by tests. The US Commission on Chronic Illness, according to Last (2001, p. 165) defined screening as:

> The presumptive identification of unrecognized disease or defect by the applications of tests, examinations or other procedures which can be applied rapidly. Screening tests sort out apparently well persons who probably have a disease from those who probably do not.

Screening is the use of tests to help diagnose diseases (or their precursor conditions) in an earlier phase of their natural history or at the less severe end of the spectrum than is achieved in routine clinical practice. In so doing, screening attempts to uncover the iceberg of disease. On the pyramid model in Fig. 6.7, screening is applied to block 3 and, less commonly, to block 4. The main aim is to reverse, halt, or slow the progression of disease more effectively than would normally happen. This is the only form of screening that is unequivocally ethical. Providing knowledge about the diagnosis, whether to the patient or professional, is insufficient reason for screening.

There are, however, some more controversial purposes of screening than a better outcome for individuals. Screening is also done to protect society, even though the individual may not benefit, or might even be harmed. Screening potential immigrants at the point at which a visa is issued or at the port of entry (for both contagious and chronic diseases) is an example. To gain information on the changing prevalence of HIV infection there has been anonymous screening of pregnant women attending antenatal clinics in the UK. Screening may be done to select out unhealthy people, for example, for a job. Screening is done routinely by most employers but it may be cursory, by self-completion questionnaire. The police, fire brigade, armed forces, and airlines are employers that screen potential employees in detail. Screening is sometimes done to help to allocate healthcare resources that are limited. The purpose of screening then is to sort out those with the greatest need, from those with lesser need. The most extreme example is the wartime practice of triage, when those unlikely to survive war

Box 6.4 **Aims of screening**

- Better prognosis/outcome for individuals
- Protect society from contagious disease
- Rational allocation of resources
- Selection of healthy individuals
- Research (natural history of disease)

wounds are left untreated. Screening may be done simply for research; for example, to identify disease at an early stage to help understand the natural history. In these circumstances, when the screening is not primarily for the benefit of individuals being screened, there are difficult ethical issues, and these are being sharpened by the advent of genetic screening.

The ethical viewpoint, that the natural history of disease must be influenced favourably, sets limits on the scope of screening, and poses important challenges to epidemiology and public health. To overcome this ethical constraint means that the natural history of the disease needs to be understood, there need to be effective interventions for treating or controlling the disease, and the screening test needs to detect the problem at a stage when the disease is not advanced beyond therapy. These aims of screening are summarized in Box 6.4.

Screening applies tests to people who have not actively sought clinical care or advice for the disease to be tested for. This is the feature that distinguishes screening from normal clinical practice where the patient has initiated the contact. The ethical basis of screening is hence fundamentally different from testing in clinical settings because who initiates the test and why is all-important. Other distinguishing features, for example, that screening is applied to large populations and that the tests are not usually diagnostic, are of minor significance.

Potentially, screening could be done for every disease for which there is a diagnostic test or diagnostic signs and symptoms. To guide the rational development of screening programmes there are criteria, usually variants of those of Wilson and Jungner (1968), as listed in Table 6.2.

These can be crystallized as six questions:

- Is there an effective intervention?
- Does intervention earlier than usual improve outcome?
- Is there an effective screening test that recognizes disease earlier than usual?
- Is the test available and acceptable to the target population?
- Is the disease one that commands priority?
- Do the benefits exceed the costs?

Table 6.2 The criteria of Wilson and Junger

1. The condition sought should be an important health problem
2. There should be an accepted treatment for patients with recognized disease
3. Facilities for diagnosis and treatment should be available
4. There should be a recognizable latent or early symptomatic stage
5. There should be a suitable test or examination
6. The test should be acceptable to the population
7. The natural history of the disease, including latent disease, should be adequately understood
8. There should be an agreed policy on whom to treat
9. The cost of case-finding (including diagnosis and treatment of patients diagnosed) should be economically balanced in relation to possible expenditure on medical care as a whole
10. Case-finding should be a continuing process and not a 'once for all' project

Adapted from Holland and Stewart 1990 (pp. 12–13) with permission (see Permissions).

If the answer to these six questions is yes then the case for screening is sound. From a public health stance it would be unethical not to advocate a screening programme in this context but the final decision will, as ever, depend on availability of resources and the priority of this programme in relation to others.

Screening programmes need more careful evaluation than clinical care. The reasons for this include the fact that screening is a professionally initiated activity; the beneficial outcomes of screening are not easily measured for they accumulate over long time periods; the acceptability of a programme may change with time; the performance of the test may change over time, particularly if the frequency of disease changes; and, pragmatically, screening is an expensive and difficult process which is hard both to put in place and to withdraw.

Screening for hypertension illustrates the above issues. Hypertension is a major causal factor in stroke, coronary heart disease, cardiac hypertrophy, heart failure, and in disorders of other organs, particularly the kidney. In most cases, perhaps 90 per cent or more, the cause of high blood pressure cannot be found, and this type of disease is called essential hypertension ('essential' is an alternative to the blunter, longer, but more accurate phrase 'of unknown cause'). In perhaps 5–10 per cent of cases there is an identifiable cause (e.g. severe kidney diseases lead to hypertension), and this form is known as secondary hypertension. Hypertension is not, strictly, a disease but a precursor of disease. Nonetheless, its importance and close association with diseases has led to it being considered, in practice, as a disease.

Hypertension usually occurs without symptoms and may present as a stroke or heart attack. The clinical and public health challenge is to reduce this morbidity and mortality and as some of the changes induced by hypertension occur at an early stage of the natural history and may be irreversible, this is best done through screening. Wilson and Jungner's criteria are met and the answer to the six questions above is, more or less, yes. The problem is a priority. Effective, acceptable treatments that improve long-term health outcomes are available. A screening test is widely available and acceptable though it has some problems. The benefits of screening for hypertension far exceed the costs. The screening test is measurement of the blood pressure, usually using a sphygmomanometer, on one or a small number of occasions. Sometimes two readings may be made, 5 to 30 minutes apart. The diagnostic test is, effectively, repetition of the same test on several occasions combined with a clinical history, examination, and other tests to check for other diseases, particularly those that cause specific forms of hypertension. A check is also made on whether the adverse consequences of high blood pressure have occurred. Additional tests of high blood pressure are possible but used infrequently, including 24-hour readings using equipment that permits measurement while the person is ambulatory. Blood pressure screening based on the sphygmomanometer is done in many settings: in routine clinical practice in primary care and hospital settings; in pre-employment physical examinations; in workplace health programmes, as part of a periodic check up; in well-woman/well-man clinics; and in antenatal clinics. As the equipment and expertise to do the test is so widespread there is little need for a specially designed population-based screening programme.

The ideal test would pick up all or most cases of hypertension in the population tested. This attribute of the test is known as high sensitivity (or true positive rate). Such a test would be sensitive to the presence of disease. Clearly, the ideal test would also correctly identify all people who do not have the disease, that is, the test is specific to those who have the disease. This attribute of the test is the specificity (or true negative rate). The ideal test would, therefore, correctly identify both cases and non-cases. In the ideal test, therefore, when cases go for more detailed clinical examination, the screening test result is confirmed. A positive test in ideal circumstances predicts with 100 per cent accuracy the presence of hypertension and, similarly, a negative test predicts its absence. These attributes are known as the predictive powers. There is, of course, no such perfect test, whether for screening or for diagnosis. The closer we can get to 100 per cent accuracy the better. As 100 per cent accuracy is not attainable with any test or set of diagnostic procedures we apply the best available means of diagnosis as the 'gold' standard against which the screening test is compared. The accuracy of a test is assessed by applying it to population groups and this places evaluation of screening tests in the domain of epidemiology rather than clinical medicine.

These four measures, sensitivity, specificity and predictive power of a positive and negative test, are the main way to assess the performance of a screening test. These and other measures of performance can be calculated from the 2 × 2 table as shown in Table 6.3. The rows of Table 6.3 show the results of the screening test, the columns the disease status. The disease status is said to be the true status of the person based either on a definitive ('gold' standard) series of tests or on observation, often made over long

Table 6.3 The 2 × 2 table: validating the screening test

Screening test	Disease (true/definitive test)		
	Present	**Absent**	**Total**
+ve	a	b	a + b
−ve	c	d	c + d
Total	a + c	b + d	a + b + c + d

Sensitivity or true positive rate = a/(a + c).   Predictive power of a +ve test = a/(a + b).

Specificity or true negative rate = d/(b + d).   Predictive power of a −ve test = d/(c + d).

time periods (possibly checked postmortem). As even the definitive test is never 100 per cent accurate the reader will appreciate that a screening test is being evaluated against another imperfect, albeit better, test.

Table 6.3 uses a standard notation and layout: the letter 'a' represents true positive results on the screening test, 'b' false positives, 'c' false negatives, and 'd' true negatives. The formulae for the four measures are in the table. The best way to understand these formulae and to interpret the data is through practice. Try the exercise in Box 6.5, before reading on.

Box 6.5 **Calculating sensitivity and specificity**

Five hundred patients known to have a particular disease were screened with a new test. Five hundred controls without this disease were also screened. Of the 500 patients 473 had a positive test. Of the healthy group without the disease seven had a positive test. Create a 2 × 2 table based on Table 6.3 and reflect on the interpretation of the data.

Calculate sensitivity and specificity of the test. Is this a good performance? What are the implications for those wrongly classified by the test?

The sensitivity (94.6 per cent) and specificity (98.6 per cent) of the test are very high, as shown in Table 6.4, and this level of accuracy is unusual in clinical practice. In other words, in these circumstances the test will correctly identify most people who have the disease (a), and also correctly identify most people who are disease free (d). Nonetheless, about one person in twenty who does have the disease will be misclassified as disease free (c), and hence wrongly reassured. Far fewer people without disease will be misclassified as having the disease (b). This is reassuring from a population perspective, but it is not exactly the information of direct interest to individuals and their doctors who

Table 6.4 Calculation of sensitivity and specificity based on data in Box 6.5

Screening test	Diseased (true/definitive test)		
	+ve	−ve	
+ve	473 (a)	7 (b)	480 (a + b)
−ve	27 (c)	493 (d)	520 (c + d)
	500 (a + c)	500 (b + d)	1000 (a + b + c + d)

Sensitivity $= a/(a + c) = 473/500 = 94.6\%$.   Specificity $= d/(b + d) = 493/500 = 98.6\%$.

want to know the implications of their individual results; this is given by predictive powers. Reflect on Box 6.6 before reading on.

Box 6.6 **Predictive powers**

If a man is positive on the screening test and asks what is his chance of having the disease once all the tests are done, what can we advise? Similarly, what do we advise if the test is negative on the screening test? From Table 6.4 calculate predictive powers.

The answer is that the predictive power of a positive test is $a/(a + b) = 473/480 = 98.5$ per cent; and of a negative test is $d/(c + d) = 493/520 = 94.8$ per cent. In other words, only 1 or 2 per cent of those testing positive will have this result overturned by the definitive test. More of those with a negative test, however, will have this result overturned. This excellent performance is, however, a result of the artificial nature of the population, in which 50 per cent have the disease.

The prevalence of the disease has a profound effect on the predictive powers. Imagine that the prevalence of a disease is actually zero. Then all screening test positive cases must, of necessity, be false positives (i.e. b in the notation in Table 6.4) and all screen negatives will be correct (i.e. d in the notation in Table 6.4). The predictive power of a positive test is zero since a is zero (and the predictive power of a negative test is 100 per cent).

If the prevalence of a condition is 100 per cent then, logically, all screen positive cases will have the condition (and screen negatives will all be false), so the predictive power of a positive test is 100 per cent (and of a negative test zero). Predictive powers vary with prevalence, as shown in Fig. 6.8. You can examine the effect of varying prevalence on predictive powers by doing the exercise in Box 6.7. In practice most diseases are uncommon, so the predictive power of a positive screening test tends to be low.

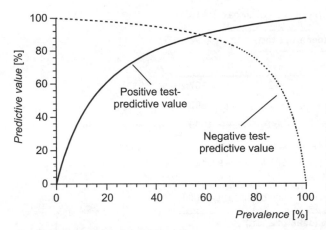

Fig. 6.8 Changes of predictive values with the prevalence of a disease (this example is calculated with a test sensitivity of 0.93 and a specificity of 0.85) (source: Mausner and Bahn, 1985; see Permissions).

Box 6.7 **Varying prevalence: impact on predictive power**

Assume that the test in Table 6.4 is applied to a population of (a) patients attending general practice, and that there the prevalence of the disease is 10 per cent; and (b) in a community setting where the prevalence is 1 per cent. Your populations are 1000 in each of these circumstances. The sensitivity and specificity is as in Table 6.4. Prepare two 2 × 2 tables, complete the cells starting with $(a + b)$, $(b + d)$, and $(a + b + c + d)$, and calculate the predictive powers. Now compare your answers with Tables 6.5(a) and 6.5(b).

As the prevalence declines, as Table 6.5(a) and (b) shows, the predictive power of a positive test declines, and the opposite is true for a negative test. When the prevalence is 1 per cent—a figure which actually represents a disease that is common in the community—the predictive power of this same test is 40.6 per cent, in other words, in 6 of 10 cases the screening test will be wrong, and the person will be subjected to unnecessary anxiety and tests.

It is generally the case, in theory, that the sensitivity and specificity of a test are independent of prevalence but in practice they are not. As the prevalence of the disease declines the vigilance of observers in making accurate measurements in screening and diagnostic tests is diminished, reducing the sensitivity (Fowkes, 1986).

The sensitivity and specificity are, however, profoundly affected by the 'cut-off' value of the measure at which a test is defined as positive. This is a very difficult decision. How do we make it? We could observe the disease outcomes over some years and see whether organ damage occurs. For blood pressure, for example, we could take any cut-off value that is associated with a higher risk of disease. Because, by and large, low blood pressures are better, this could mean a cut-off value less than 120/80 mmHg, this being the mean in most industrialized populations. The problem is that about half of the population would thereby be defined as hypertensive on sphygmomanometry, and for most people so defined the true additional risk of hypertensive disease would be very low.

Table 6.5(a) Predictive power (prevalence of disease = 10%)

Screening test	Disease (definitive test)		
	+ve	−ve	
+ve	94.6	12.6	107.2
−ve	5.4	887.4	892.8
	100	900	1000

Predictive power of positive test = $a/(a+b)$ = 94.6/107.2 = 88.2%.
Predictive power of negative test = $d/(d+c)$ = 887.4/892.8 = 99.4%.

Table 6.5(b) Predictive power (prevalence of disease = 1%)

Screening test	Disease (definitive test)		
	+ve	−ve	
+ve	9.46	13.86	23.32
−ve	0.54	976.14	976.68
	10	990	1000

Predictive power of a positive test = $a/(a+b)$ = 9.46/23.32 = 40.6%.
Predictive power of a negative test = $d/(c+d)$ = 976.14/976.68 = 99.9%.

Based on a low cut-off point, say 120/80 mmHg, and knowing that the prevalence of end-organ damage, and of disease incidence is low, the sensitivity of the test for true hypertensive disease would be very high, specificity low, the predictive power of a positive test low, and predictive power of a negative test high. If we took the hypertensive cut-off value as 180/120 mmHg few people would be defined as hypertensive and for those that were the target organ damage and incidence of disease would be high. Sensitivity for the hypertensive disease would be low, specificity high, predictive power of a positive test high and of a negative test low. There is a price to be paid for each choice of cut-off point. The lower cut-off picks up nearly all cases, but creates unnecessary anxiety and the risk of unnecessary treatment among those who were not destined to develop hypertensive end organ damage (false positives). The higher cut-off, however, misses cases (false negatives). Setting the cut-off point is a matter of difficult judgement, balancing the costs and benefits of false positives and false negatives. For blood pressure the agreed cut-off point has been reducing over the years from about 160/100 mmHg to 140/90 mmHg. This is partly to do with the availability of better therapies and better services and partly to reducing tolerance of the adverse effects of high blood pressure.

Screening will make blocks 1 and 2 in the pyramid of disease (Fig. 6.6) grow and block 3 shrink. The danger is that through false positive tests people in blocks 4 and 5 are wrongly placed in blocks 1 and 2, and through false negative tests people in blocks 1 and 2 are placed in blocks 4 and 5.

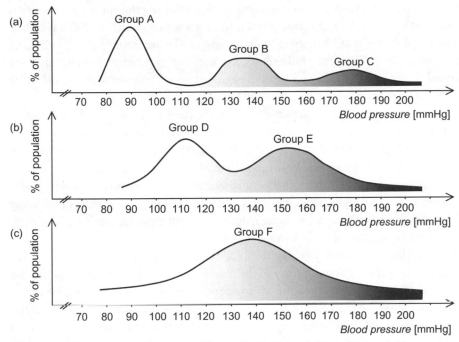

Fig. 6.9 Blood pressure: theoretical and actual distribution of values. Darker shading indicates higher level of risk of adverse outcome.

The underlying reason for the reciprocal nature of the sensitivity and specificity is that, for most diseases, cases and non-cases belong to one, not separate, distributions of values. This is illustrated in Fig. 6.9. In Fig. 6.9(a) there are three distributions which could be described as low, medium, and high blood pressure with varying levels of risk of hypertensive end-organ disease. The risk is indicated by the shading, darker shading meaning higher risk. If the objective were to separate Group A from C cut-off points are comparatively easy to set. A value of 155 mmHg systolic blood pressure would clearly separate the high (Group C) and low risk (Group A) groups with some overlap in the medium and other groups. The overlap is the cause of difficulties. Nonetheless, misclassification would be uncommon and, importantly, the classification of people in Group A as Group C and vice versa would be rare. At a cut-off of 140 mmHg one can see that a few people at highest risk of disease (shaded as grey) are missed; mostly they belong to Group B. Extremely few people who belong to Group A will be wrongly judged as at high risk of hypertensive disease (by being placed in Group B or rarely in Group C). Even with this artificial distribution—the screener's ideal—there is some error. Setting the cut-off higher will increase specificity (and positive predictive power) but reduce sensitivity.

Figure 6.9(b) shows a more realistic, so-called bi-modal (two peak), distribution. The distribution implies there are two groups of people—one with high blood pressure and high risk of disease (Group E) and one with low blood pressure and low risk of disease (Group D)—with overlap between them. Setting the cut-off point here is problematic. Setting it at 155 mmHg will lead to many people at risk of disease being missed, and setting it at 120 mmHg to many people who are actually at low risk being screened positive. This type of distribution is not common but it illustrates the idea behind screening. There is a natural, though not necessarily correct, cut-off value which divides Groups D and E at about 130 mmHg.

Figure 6.9(c), however, is the picture portraying the distribution of the risk factors for many common disorders including stroke and CHD (risk factor–hypertension), diabetes (risk factor–blood sugar), and glaucoma (risk factor–intraocular pressure). There is no natural separation between people at risk of disease and not at risk. The cut-off point is set solely on a judgement balancing the importance of avoiding false positives (achieving high specificity) versus avoiding missing true positives (achieving high sensitivity). For hypertension the judgement is not clear, for neither a false positive nor a false negative result is a trivial matter.

Three actions are essential to help to define the cut-off point. First, we need a clear understanding of the natural history of the disease (untreated) at each level of the risk factor. Second, we need to know the adverse consequences of treatment (by, for example, clinic follow-up studies). Third, we need to know the sensitivity, specificity, and predictive powers of the screening test in the population to be screened. A fourth action is desirable, and this is the definition of subgroups of the population according to their level of risk by screening for interacting risk factors. For example, it is unlikely that a blood pressure of 150/100 has the same consequence for everyone. It is likely to pose a greater risk of heart disease for a smoker, a diabetic, someone with high cholesterol, and someone who is genetically susceptible to coronary heart disease. In future, when the screening programme includes a scan of the genome for disease susceptibility genes, prediction of risk will be improved. A person's risk of adverse outcomes, shown as grey on the distribution curve (Fig. 6.9) is likely to be determined by a combination of environmental and genetic factors.

Unfortunately, our state of knowledge for most diagnostic and screening tests is limited, and interpretation of results is problematic. There are errors in measurement and true variations in the environment and the biology of the person. Errors also occur in the recording and interpretation of the result. Even when these problems are resolved the relation between a screening test result and the disease outcome may differ between populations. Some of these problems are illustrated in relation to hypertension, but these principles can be generalized to most screening tests.

Some of the problems with screening for hypertension based on sphygmomanometry are these:

♦ Hypertensive disease is a consequence of long-term raised pressure of blood inside a complex vascular system. In screening we measure the pressure at one or a few time points, using an indirect measure of the intra-arterial pressure at one place in the vasculature.

- Individuals and groups are differentially susceptible to the consequences of a particular level of blood pressure.

- Blood pressure is variable, changing from minute to minute in response to stimuli including smoking, external temperature, exercise, emotional stress, and posture. Blood pressure also shows a 24-hour (circadian) rhythm, and is much lower at night than during working hours. Finally, in most populations blood pressure rises with age. A measure at one time is no more than a snapshot of highly variable factors.

- The measurement of blood pressure by manual sphymomanometry requires some skill, including the ability to choose and apply the right cuff in the right way, release the pressure in the cuff and coordinate what is heard (Korotkoff sounds) while watching a falling column of mercury and taking the readings at the appropriate moment. Observer errors are common, ranging from crude ones such as those caused by deafness to the more subtle ones such as preference for particular numbers, usually those ending in 5 or 0, so causing rounding errors. (Automated methods also have problems.)

- Poorly maintained equipment is a common cause of measurement errors. Sphygmomanometers are robust instruments but they do go wrong, and need regular calibration and occasional repair.

These sorts of problems, which arise in many screening programmes and research projects, can be partially solved by following these principles:

- Study and quantify the relationship between the screening test (here blood pressure by sphygmomanometer) and the underlying measure of interest (here intra-arterial blood pressure). In this way you confirm whether, in principle, the screening measure is a good indicator of the underlying phenomenon to be measured.

- Study and quantify the relationship between the screening test and disease outcome in the population as a whole and in population subgroups.

- Standardize the measurement. For blood pressure, as a minimum in clinical practice, the person must be sitting, at rest for 5 minutes, and the cuff needs to be of specified and appropriate size. Ideally, the blood pressures would be taken at the same time of day, in a controlled physical environment, and the subject should not have smoked for at least 20 minutes. In a research context still more stringent criteria are necessary.

- Training needs to be provided in a standard way, and skills regularly updated and checked.

- Equipment needs rigorous quality checks.

Imagine that all this is in place for blood pressure screening. How good in practice is a population-based blood pressure screening programme? This question requires careful evaluation: a complex subject beyond the scope of this book. Table 6.6, however, gives a sketch of the main ways that screening programmes are evaluated, the designs usually

Table 6.6 Evaluation of screening programmes: in practice

Option	Design	Problem
Examination of trends in morbidity/mortality	Before/after screening programme comparisons	Natural fluctuations in disease over time occur making interpretation difficult
Geographical comparisons in trends in mortality and morbidity	Regional/international comparisons of places with and without screening	Variation in diagnostic and treatment practices between places makes interpretation difficult
Audit/surveillance of cases to assess the stage of disease when diagnosis is made	Case-series analysis over time (see Chapter 9)	Screened cases are probably self-selected volunteers, higher social class, at an earlier stage of disease (lead time bias) and may have less severe disease
Comparison of incidence, case fatality, and mortality in screened vs. unscreened populations within the same population at a particular time or time period	Population case series, case-control and cohort studies (see Chapter 9)	Differences between screened and unscreened groups are many; apparent benefits may be due to these. Unscreened cases are those missed by screening, refused uptake, lost to follow-up and cases picked up between screenings
Experimental implementation of screening	Trials (see Chapter 9)	The ethical, practical, and financial constraints of organizing effective, large trials

used, and some of the potential problems. This table provides a foundation for further reading.

There are three important biases (Table 6.7) that are vitally important in interpreting data from non-trial-based evaluations. The solutions given are only partial ones.

Screening programmes are often implemented before there is irrefutable evidence of benefit. The reason why this happens is not wholly clear but the fact that screening often seems good on common-sense grounds is possibly part of the story. Clinical practice, with screening on an ad hoc basis, may long precede the implementation of screening targeted at the whole population: a public health programme. This may make rigorous evaluation based on a randomized controlled trial (Chapter 9) impossible. Figure 6.10 illustrates why rigorous evaluation is essential; a vast amount of work is entailed in screening.

6.6 **Applications of the concepts of natural history, spectrum, and screening**

These concepts are directly applicable to health care. Health policies can be formulated and evaluated in terms of their expected influence on the natural history and spectrum

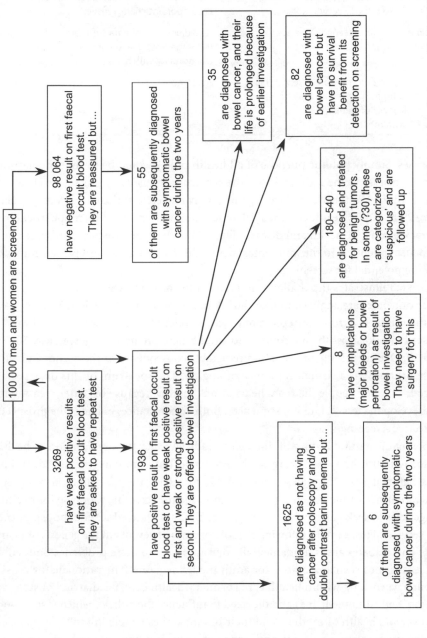

Fig. 6.10 Screening: example of colorectal screening based on faecal occult blood (reproduced from the *British Medical Journal* (2000) **320**, p. 872, with permission from the BMJ Publishing Group).

Table 6.7 Three biases and their solutions

Bias	Solution
Self-selection i.e. those accepting screening are different from those declining it	Match comparison populations for all the important characteristics
'Lead time' bias, i.e. screened cases are picked up at an earlier stage	(a) Adjust survival data for estimated lead time (b) Stage disease and compare morbidity/ mortality within stages
Speed of disease progression i.e. 'length bias': cases picked up by a screening may be less severe, and slowly progressive compared with others	Awareness

of diseases. Simply put, the purpose of all health policy would be to shift the natural history of disease to the right and alter the spectrum so disease is less severe (Figs 6.4 and 6.5). In the UK the idea of health gain, closely related to this concept, was popular in the 1990s. Public health and medical action can be seen as the force spearheading the attack against ill-health and disease (Fig. 6.4). The natural history of disease concept focuses attention to the long timescales in disease causation and prevention and hence the potential for screening.

Figure 6.3 illustrates the challenge in relation to coronary heart disease. The main adverse outcomes are angina and heart attack in middle and old age. But, as the causes exert their influence from conception onwards, a policy for heart disease control would necessarily work across the life course and would therefore need to be seen as a 50–75 year plan. One surprising and yet also predictable consequence of the decline in heart disease mortality is a rising prevalence of angina. The spectrum of this disease has changed; as fewer people die from heart attack mainly because of better treatment, more develop the less serious consequences. Both circumstances enhance the prospects for effective screening.

Knowing the natural history of disease can radically alter the organization of health care, for with this knowledge care can be proactive, both in managing the control of disease before it arises through screening and in managing the rehabilitation and long-term surveillance of the patient. It may also provide the scientific rationale for health-care agencies to seek partnership with other agencies such as education, housing, and social services. For example, knowing the role of early life events in the genesis of heart disease and diabetes alters fundamentally our approach to these problems. Suddenly, the disease is not seen as a matter for adult medicine alone. The rationale for cross-disciplinary working within health care (primary health care, paediatrics, obstetrics, nutrition, and adult medicine) and the need to influence the policies which foster good education and health of mothers and their infants unites people in multiple agencies involved in improving social and economic circumstances such as housing, employment, agriculture, and nutrition.

While the study of natural history of disease is itself a great challenge to science, the discovery that the period between exposure, pathogenic effect, and disease may be decades (indeed, sometimes the disease never occurs) makes the process of discovery of disease processes fraught with problems. Scientists studying people with disease now, may need to obtain information about the life circumstances of the patient in childhood and even *in utero* (the fetal origins hypothesis), as for coronary heart disease (Fig. 6.3). Information may be needed for the period even before conception! This strains most scientific methods. Epidemiological methods which require people to recall information on causal factors are severely limited by lack of quality data. How can we ask, reliably, a 60 year old patient with a heart attack about her life circumstances in infancy (e.g. birthweight) and in the teenage years, say on diet? This is leading to the development and testing of new methods such as the life-grid approach where questioning is linked to memorable life events e.g. smoking habits at the time of marriage or at the birth of the first child.

Prospective epidemiological methods entail delay, measured in the same order of time as the natural history of the disease. A cohort study (Chapter 9) to study the full range of known and postulated risk factors for coronary heart disease would need to last for about 70 years, and even then would not provide information about the causes and course of the disease in old age. Furthermore, the ethical basis of research that observes without intervening is increasingly questioned. For these reasons the natural history of most human diseases is patchily understood, and that of coronary heart disease will probably never be fully grasped.

Prevention of disease is dependent on understanding the natural history of disease. The timing of prevention interventions is critically important, for in some diseases the pathogenic effects are irreversible. Natural history of disease is also essential to diagnosis, therapeutics, and prognosis. For example, in managing the care of a child presenting for the first time with an epileptic fit, the physician needs to understand what the likely course of events is and whether this child is likely to have epilepsy long term or whether this episode is likely to be a single one. This knowledge will affect both therapy (are preventive drugs necessary?) and general care (can the patient be discharged from specialist care or does the patient need long-term review?). The parents and child will put great emphasis on the long-term outcome, which cannot be easily or accurately predicted for the individual but is usually based on the aggregated natural history in past patients.

The level of need for health services is often underestimated. New services designed to meet a quantified demand commonly find that new demands emerge to again outstrip supply. This may perplex and frustrate health planners who conclude that the demand for health care is infinite when the simple explanation is that some of the previously unidentified cases are coming to light as a result of the extra service, or cases are being identified at an earlier point in their natural history.

The iceberg of disease phenomenon underpins the idea that health policy should be based on a realistic estimate of the size of the unidentified population of cases and those at risk. Basing policy decisions on data showing the utilization of services is flawed, though pragmatic. This principle is easy to state but hard to implement. First, estimating the true size of the disease iceberg is not easy, and requires representative population-based surveys, which have their own limitations and costs. Some diseases, especially rare ones such as multiple sclerosis, or those with a very short natural history such as transient ischaemic attacks, are not suitable for study using survey methods, and rely on disease registers which can only list diagnosed cases. Second, not all those with identifiable disease in the context of an epidemiological survey will, in practice, ever be identifiable by a routine service. An example of this would be the number of people who have diabetes.

The WHO definition of diabetes requires a glucose tolerance test in standardized conditions. Such a test can be done in research conditions but is not suitable in routine practice. The results may change over relatively short periods of time, so a single test is insufficient in clinical practice. Some people with diabetes would not wish to avail themselves of the services even once the diagnosis is made. Basing services for diabetes on epidemiological surveys of the true size of the iceberg could, therefore, lead to over-provision. Population-based surveys are, therefore, complementary to information on service utilization.

By combining health utilization statistics, epidemiological survey data, and their own experience, clinical staff can assess the level of service needed. The district nurse or health visitor is likely to have a broader knowledge about the extent and impact of, say, venous ulcers of the leg in the population than is the general practitioner, who in turn will have a broader perspective than the hospital physician. The current structures of most health services place artificial boundaries between nursing and medical disciplines and between primary care and hospital care, which inhibits sharing of knowledge about disease patterns. The result is that the specialist's knowledge about a disease may be inapplicable to the primary care physician or nurse. Yet, the hospital specialist is a key source of education about the diagnosis and outcome of diseases.

Clinicians need to take an active approach to identifying cases in the submerged part of the iceberg and work both with epidemiologists in assessing the true population burden of the disease, and with primary care staff to understand the specific clinical requirements of these cases. Health promotion's primary role is to attack the submerged parts of the iceberg of disease. This is done by organizing society and the environment to protect the whole population, and by a combination of education and early detection of disease through screening targeted at blocks 3, 4 and 5 as conceptualized in the pyramid of disease (Fig. 6.7).

6.7 Epidemiological theory: symbiosis with clinical medicine and social sciences

In pointing to epidemiological theories underpinning this chapter, it would be futile to seek to disentangle them from other clinical sciences. Epidemiology has been pre-eminent in promoting the theory that many diseases are initiated by events acting years, or decades, before any clinical manifestation. Epidemiology has emphasized, and contributed greatly to, building the picture of both the natural history of disease, and the spectrum of disease. The spectrum concept has illustrated that diseases may manifest themselves in many ways, including asymptomatic yet damaging forms. Shifts in diseases' natural history and the spectrum partly underlie changes in population patterns of disease and help to explain the iceberg concept of disease. In trying to understand why some people with symptoms and signs of disease seek care, and hence are diagnosed, while others do not, epidemiology crosses to the social sciences, linking into theories of illness-seeking behaviour. These theoretical constructs have immense practical significance, both in terms of prevention, early detection, and management of disease, and in terms of managing health services, for example explaining why demand rises as health service capacity increases. Screening is an application of epidemiology, but it rests on other theoretical concepts, particularly the natural history of disease.

6.8 **Conclusion**

Understanding the interrelated concepts of the natural history, spectrum, and iceberg of disease and their relation to screening is crucial to the epidemiological public health and medical endeavour. Natural history is usually pieced together from an understanding of causes and their effects, and outcomes of disease, and hence lies at the heart of epidemiology. Rational health policy, health care, and health promotion require a knowledge of the natural history. The ethical and technical difficulties of studying natural history is a deterrent, however, and the necessary work is too rarely done. The model of the natural history of disease provides a unifying common purpose for all the medical sciences, and all branches of the healing and caring health profession: to influence the natural history of disease by reducing or delaying exposure to the causal agents, to promote resistance to these agents, to detect the pathogenic effects early while disease onset can be prevented or delayed (often through screening), and to manage disease onset to minimize complications and long-term effects including delaying death. This is a mission which engages everyone in the health professions.

Summary

The natural history of disease is the uninterrupted progression of disease from its initiation by exposure to the causal agents to either spontaneous resolution, containment by the body's repair mechanisms, or to a clinically detectable problem whether resolved or not. The natural history is seldom known, for the act of diagnosis and treatment influences it. Studies of natural history impose profound ethical difficulties. The pattern of disease progression may be distinctive. As the causes of some diseases act decades before the disease is diagnosed, often the only way of studying the natural history of disease is to do cohort studies. The impact of knowledge about the natural history of disease is often profound. For example, understanding that coronary heart disease, a killer in middle and old age, is influenced by factors acting in the uterine and early childhood environment significantly alters the strategy of prevention. The primary purpose of public health and medicine is to influence favourably the natural history of disease.

The natural history of disease is related to (and influences), but is not synonymous with, the changing pattern of disease in populations or the different levels of severity with which a disease may present (spectrum of disease).

For most health problems the number of cases identified is exceeded by those not discovered. An illustrative metaphor is the iceberg. Correctly diagnosed cases are represented by the tip of the iceberg visible above sea level, and undiagnosed ones by the larger presence below sea level. An alternative metaphor of the pyramid of disease develops this into a population concept. The iceberg phenomenon thwarts epidemiological efforts to assess the true burden of disease and creates difficulties in accurately judging the need and demand for services. Since unidentified cases are different from identified ones it is often impossible to identify truly unselected and representative cases for epidemiological studies.

Screening is the application of tests to diagnose disease (or its precursors) in an earlier phase of the natural history of disease (often in well people) or in a less severe part of the disease spectrum than is achieved in routine medical practice. Screening uncovers the iceberg of disease. Screening tests are not usually diagnostic but they may be, for example in screening for high blood pressure. The key to successful screening is a simple test that can be applied to large populations with minimum harm and a high degree of accuracy in separating those who need more detailed investigation from those who do not. The ideal test would have high sensitivity (i.e. it picks up cases) and specificity (i.e. it correctly identifies non-cases). A person positive on the screening test would have a high probability of being confirmed as a case. A person negative on the screening test would have high probability of being confirmed as problem free. The potential of screening is vast but there are important limitations such as the inability to influence the natural history of many diseases, either because of lack of effective intervention or lack of services to deliver them, and the need to balance the benefits of earlier diagnosis against penalties such as engendering anxiety and the danger of tests and treatments. These concepts are highly interrelated though the links between them are seldom made explicit.

Chapter 7

The concept of risk and measures of disease frequency
Incidence and prevalence

Objectives

On completion of the chapter you should understand:

+ that risk is the likelihood of an individual in a defined population developing a disease or risk factor;

+ that epidemiology measures who gets disease in what quantity (absolute or actual measure of risk) and how this quantity compares with other populations (relative measure of risk);

+ that a risk factor is a characteristic that is associated with disease or precursor of disease;

+ the meaning and application of the words rate, ratio and proportion in everyday and epidemiological language;

+ that the principal measures of disease frequency in epidemiology are the incidence and prevalence rates;

+ the differences and similarities between incidence rate estimated using a person-time denominator and using a population denominator;

+ that there are great challenges in accurately measuring the events (numerator) and populations at risk (denominator) needed to calculate incidence and prevalence;

+ the interrelationship between incidence and prevalence;

+ the advantages of using subgroup specific as opposed to overall rates.

7.1 Introduction: risks, risk factors, and causes

In everyday language, risk is the possibility of suffering harm or loss or danger, while a person at risk from an environmental or behavioural factor is someone endangered. This everyday concept of risk factors is clearly a causal one, that is, a risk increases a person's chances of harm, loss, or danger, or indeed, of contracting a disease. Risk in epidemiology also usually refers to the likelihood (probability) of dying or developing a disease, or its precursors, so the word is used similarly to everyday language. In epidemiology our prime interest is in the interaction between the probability of disease, or risk, and those environmental, individual, and social characteristics which influence the risk. Where there is an association with an increased probability of disease in those with such characteristics, the characteristics are called risk factors. Reflect on the question in Box 7.1 before reading on.

> Box 7.1 **Risk factors and causes**
>
> Reflect on the phrases 'risk factor' and 'causes of diseases'. What is the difference between them?

In epidemiology the phrase 'risk factor' does not necessarily imply that the characteristic has a causal effect (association is not causation). The phrase 'risk marker' is sometimes used in preference to risk factor, simply to emphasize that no causal relationship is presumed. It has no logical advantages to counter the disadvantage of its unfamiliarity and it wrongly implies that a risk factor (rather than marker) is causal. When a causal relationship is agreed between disease and risk factor the phrase causal factor, or simply cause, is used. For example, we say smoking is a cause of coronary heart disease (CHD), but for most CHD 'risk factors' (e.g. hyperhomocystinaemia, low levels of high density lipoprotein cholesterol (HDL), high C-reactive protein, job strain) we may imply, but rarely claim, a causal role.

In contemporary epidemiology there is imprecision in the interpretation and use of these vital phrases. The confusion leads to attribution of cause where it is merely association, and alternatively the failure to speak of an association as causal when it is. Such confusion has led to much criticism of epidemiology. Chapters 3, 4 and 5 explain the difficulties involved in achieving causal understanding, and the reader will appreciate that a cautious approach is usually to be applauded rather than criticized. As already discussed, associations rarely turn out to be causal, but their analysis is the starting point of causal understanding in epidemiology. Seeking causal understanding from analysis of associations is like panning for gold, for it usually yields nothing but grit and mud (error and bias), sometimes gold flakes and specks (risk factors, relating to the causal pathway but not demonstrably in a causal way), sometimes a nugget (causal factor) and rarely a gold mine (understanding of the entire basis of a disease). Like panning for gold, a great deal of hard work is required to find a gold mine, and when it is discovered, panning alone will not be enough, and much intensive and sophisticated equipment and skills will be needed to take full advantage of the discovery. In epidemiology, this implies working with other laboratory and population-based scientific disciplines (including social sciences) to gain understanding of the mechanisms by which the cause operates. This chapter and the next two consider the basic epidemiological tools needed for this task.

7.2 **Quantifying disease frequency, risk factors, and their relationships**

Epidemiological studies measure, present, and interpret frequency of disease and of factors that influence this. In its methods epidemiology is a quantitative science, though in its theory and applications, the ideas of qualitative sciences are vital. The epidemiological question is, who gets the disease in what quantity (absolute measures) and how does this compare with other populations (relative measures)? Table 7.1 lists the main measures that answer these questions and are to be discussed in this and the next chapter.

While there are many measures, two underpin virtually all epidemiology: incidence and prevalence rates. These are discussed in detail in this chapter. Table 7.2 gives brief

Table 7.1 Some epidemiological measures in relation to whether they provide actual (absolute) or relative frequency

Numbers of cases	Actual
Proportional mortality	Actual
Proportional mortality ratio	Relative
Overall (crude) prevalence and incidence rates	Actual
Specific prevalence and incidence rates	Actual
Standardized rates	Actual/relative mix
Standardized ratios	Relative
Relative risk	Relative
Odds ratio	Relative
Attributable risks	Actual
Numbers needed to treat and prevent	Actual
Life years lost	Actual
Disability adjusted life year (DALY)	Actual
Quality adjusted life year (QALY)	Actual

Table 7.2 Introduction to incidence and prevalence rates

Measure	Key features	Type of study	Formulae
Incidence	Count of new cases over a period of time in a population of known size defined by characteristics (age, sex, etc.), and place and time boundaries	Disease register Cohort Trial	New cases ÷ population-at-risk or New cases ÷ time spent by the study population at risk
Prevalence	Count of cases (new and old) at a point in time in a population of known size defined by characteristics (age, sex, etc.) and place	Cross-sectional Disease register	All cases ÷ Population at risk

definitions of incidence and prevalence rates and indicates the type of studies (discussed in Chapter 9) from which data are derived to make the calculation. The epidemiological strategy for working out causes of disease works best by using the comparative (relative) approach, while that for assessing a population's health needs works best by examining that population's health pattern (absolute approach).

Epidemiology needs accurate information on the timing and locations of observations, and number and characteristics of disease cases, of people with risk factors, and of the population from which they derive. Numbers of cases, or people with the risk factors, comprise the numerator, the population from which they come is commonly the denominator. Epidemiology has developed a terminology based on, but not corresponding exactly to, everyday and mathematical words for similar ideas. This is a potential cause of difficulty, for which there is no easy remedy. The fraction, numerator divided by the denominator, is in practice called the rate in epidemiology, in public health and medicine. The dictionary meaning of the word rate, which corresponds best to its use in epidemiology, is a quantity (in epidemiology usually a disease or risk factor for disease) measured with respect to another quantity (in epidemiology usually a population). Some writers, basing their views on sciences such as physics and chemistry, which are distant in concepts, methods, and applications from epidemiology, advise that all rates must have a time dimension, but this has caused a rift between theoretical definitions and practice, a confusion in terminology, and quarrels about semantics. Some flexibility, and awareness of the issues, are recommended.

A ratio is any number in relation to another, and a rate comprising the numerator in relation to the denominator is, therefore, a type of ratio. The word ratio is commonly used in epidemiology, but is usually reserved for summarizing the division of one ratio by another, as explained in Chapter 8 in the discussion of the proportional mortality and morbidity ratios, standardized mortality ratio, and odds ratio. In epidemiology the word rate is usually, but not always, used for a ratio where the numerator and denominator have different qualities, for example, deaths/population time. A proportion in epidemiology is usually a ratio where the numerator is a part of the denominator, so both must have the same qualities, for example, deaths due to one cause/deaths due to all causes. To avoid the controversy around the word rate some writers say, for example, incidence instead of incidence rate. I have done this sometimes. Strictly, however, the incidence of a disease is a count of new cases unrelated to a denominator, and therefore not a rate by any definition (and similarly for the word prevalence).

Disease frequency is usually measured by the incidence rate and/or the prevalence rate. From basic data on disease, death, risk factors, and population counts many summary measures of health status and risk, some of which are listed in Table 7.1, can be calculated as shown in this and the next chapter. Different ways of presenting the same data have a major impact on the perception of risk and, in particular, relative and actual (or, absolute) measures of frequency portray dramatically different priorities. Epidemiological data should be presented, wherever possible, to indicate both relative and actual frequency as discussed in Chapter 8.

The prevalence and incidence of diseases (and of their risk factors) are constantly changing, mainly because the environment within which populations live is changing. Frequency data must, therefore, be described in the context of the population, the place, and the time of the study. Readers should search for these crucial contextual details, which are too often missing in reports of investigations (Chapter 10).

The following principles in the analysis of differences and changes in disease frequency apply to all epidemiological measures but are explained and emphasized for incidence rates. However, the likelihood of artefacts explaining differences and changes in disease frequency is greater with prevalence measures than with incidence rates simply because prevalence rates are more complex, being influenced not only by disease occurrence but also by death and recovery.

7.3 **Incidence and incidence rate: the concepts of incidence density, person-time incidence, and cumulative incidence**

The meanings of the word incidence in epidemiology that correspond to its dictionary definition are: the act of happening and the occurrence or the extent or frequency of occurrence. The meaning of incidence in everyday English is broad, which explains why this word is so commonly used to mean different things even in epidemiological writing. In epidemiology incidence rate is the frequency of *new* occurrences of an event in a population at risk of the disease in a period of time (Table 7.2). The word new is the key defining feature. The meaningful interpretation of disease incidence requires the number of new cases (the numerator), the population at risk (denominator), the time period, and the place of study.

The incidence rate is a fundamental measure in epidemiology and yet the concept underlying it has evolved in recent decades and it is difficult to grasp and convey. Presently there are two main variants, sometimes, but often not, differentiated as the person-time incidence and cumulative incidence, which are easily confused with each other (Table 7.3 summarizes some of their qualities). Person-time incidence is also known as incidence rate, and estimates incidence density, instantaneous incidence rate, hazard rate, and force of morbidity or mortality. Person-time incidence rate ranges from zero to infinity, as a number of deaths might occur over a short period of time. Cumulative incidence is also most usually simply referred to as incidence rate (or incidence proportion, or cumulative incidence or proportion), so causing confusion with person-time incidence rate. Cumulative incidence rate is also often used synonymously with risk. The cumulative incidence rate varies from 0 to 1 (or 0–100 per cent). Readers will need to become accustomed, and alert to, these two related concepts underlying incidence rates.

The need for these two approaches can be best understood by an example. If the cumulative incidence rate of a disease is 20 per cent per year and we follow up 100 people, after six months, on average, 10 people will develop the disease. For diseases that occur only once these 10 people are no longer at risk. This would certainly be true for

Table 7.3 Qualities of the incidence rate obtained using the person and person-time denominator (numerator is identical)

Person denominator (cumulative incidence rate)	Person-time denominator (estimate of incidence density)
Ranges from 0 to 1*	Ranges from zero to infinity
Measures absolute risk (probability) of new disease e.g. cases/10 000 people = 5%	Not clearly interpreted as a measure of absolute risk e.g. 50 cases per 1000 person-years
Can be used to construct relative risks	Can be used to construct relative risks
Incidence rates can be calculated with population estimates, e.g. from a census, and disease from a register	Person-time cannot be calculated in population estimates
Can only be used directly in cohort studies where study participants are enrolled at about the same time	Can be used either when enrolment is at about the same time *or* when enrolment is spread over time

*When the denominator is the population at the beginning of the study. When the denominator is adjusted for those no longer at risk cumulative incidence and incidence density converge.

many infectious diseases that are followed by life-long immunity. This would also apply to those chronic diseases that only occur once. When the outcome of interest is death, then these 10 are no longer at risk. The denominator is 100 only at the beginning of the population at risk study. In theory, for first event only studies, as each case occurs it should be subtracted from the denominator. So, in our example, the denominator would be approximately 95 at the three-month stage, 90.25 (not 90) at six months, 85.7 (not 85) at nine months and 81.5 (not 80) at twelve months. In a large population, and a common disease, the denominator would be diminishing almost continuously. To take this fully into account we would need to measure incidence rate in very small increments of time. There are theoretical measures of the occurrence of disease over a period of time approaching zero. Figure 7.1 illustrates this point. The formula for one, force of morbidity (adapted from the 1st edition of the Dictionary of Epidemiology by Last), is (change in t, time, approaching zero, or Δt).

$$\frac{\text{Probability that a person well at time } t \text{ will develop the disease in the interval from } t \text{ to } t \text{ plus change in } t \, (\Delta t)}{\text{Time from } t \text{ to } t \text{ plus change in } t \, (\Delta t)} \tag{7.1}$$

This is not a formula that most readers of this book will need but they will come across these ideas.

A number of closely linked concepts relating to the incidence rate at a point in time are described by these effectively synonymous phrases – forces of morbidity and mortality, hazard rate, instantaneous incidence density, instantaneous incidence rate, disease intensity, and person-time incidence rate. In practice epidemiologists mainly work with the last of these. The person-time denominator is simply the amount of time that the study population as a whole has spent at risk (disease-free, or alive, in the case of mortality studies).

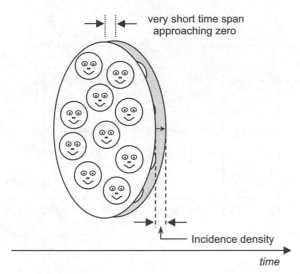

Fig. 7.1 Incidence density, forces of mortality/morbidity, hazard rates, disease intensity: a pictorial representation.

The formula for this is:

$$\frac{\text{Person-time}}{\text{incidence rate}} = \frac{\text{New occurrences over a period of time}}{\text{Time spent by the study population at risk over this period}} \quad (7.2)$$
$$\text{of time (person-years of observations)}$$

$$\text{Or more simply (after Rothman)} = \frac{\text{Disease occurrences}}{\text{Sum of time periods}} \quad (7.3)$$

Figure 7.2 illustrates the idea behind this way of measuring incidence rate. This formula provides investigators with great flexibility, particularly in cohort studies where investigators know, for each person, the exact date of entry into the study and the date of onset of disease or death. Its flexibility also allows study subjects to enter the study at different times, and it makes handling losses to follow-up and death easy (for these simply contribute less time to the denominator). It does have some disadvantages. Firstly, it does not give an easily interpreted direct measure of risk; the incidence rate will be expressed, for example, as 102/10 000 years. Secondly, there is an assumption underlying this estimate, which needs checking, that the incidence rate in those entering the study at different times, and those lost to follow-up, is the same as in others in the study population. Thirdly, the formula assumes that the disease occurs evenly over time, for the time periods contributed by those in the study for a short time are given the same weight as those contributed by people in the study for a long time. This definition gives the outcome for a person contributing 50 years to a study five times the weight of a person contributing 10 years, and 50 times the weight of those contributing one year. The number of people in the person-time denominator can be judged only from a knowledge of the average time period of observation, which is only a reasonable

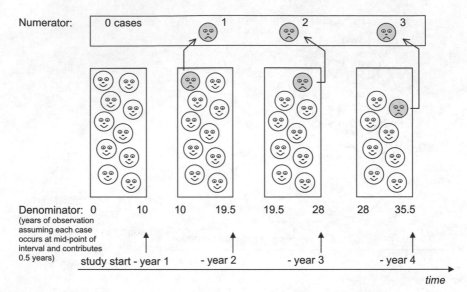

Fig. 7.2 Incidence rate—3 cases per 35.5 person-years—estimated using the person-time denominator: a pictorial representation.

estimate if there is no skew in the distribution (so investigators need to ensure this information is provided). The person-time denominator assumes that the rate is constant over the varying time periods each individual is observed. Most diseases, however, present different risk at different ages and calendar periods. A study with a large number of people with small time contributions may, therefore, come to a conclusion different from that of a study comprising mostly people with large time contributions.

In historical and much current epidemiological practice, this problem of the diminishing denominator has been sidestepped. The standard, and time honoured, formula for incidence rate is

$$\frac{\text{New occurrences over a period of time}}{\text{Population at risk over that period of time}} \tag{7.4}$$

The resulting fraction is usually multiplied by an appropriate number; for example, by 100 to give a percentage, or by 1000 to give a rate per thousand. When the baseline population is the denominator this measure is referred to as cumulative incidence rate. It is a direct measure of the probability of a new event occurring in a population, and hence the risk of that event. In this formula the person-based denominator is fixed at one point in time, usually at the beginning or middle of the time period; for example, if the study is 1-year long, the denominator might be the baseline population. If the disease is recurrent, and the investigator is interested in all and not just new occurrences, then using a baseline denominator is correct, for the whole population remains at risk of the event of interest. Deaths should, however, be subtracted from the denominator if possible. When the person denominator is so adjusted, person and person-time rates converge.

Investigators, particularly in studies of the initiating causes of disease, often choose to study only first occurrences. If so, when the disease is common, adjusting the denominator is advised. If the incidence of the disease or death was only 0.5 per cent per year then on practical (but not theoretical) grounds the investigator might argue that adjusting the denominator is unnecessary, for it would only decrease from 100 to about 99.75 at the six months stage, and have no important effect on the calculation.

In most studies the denominator is not adjusted because the information is not available to do this, the investigators have not thought to do so, the outcome is too rare for it to matter, or because investigators are interested in all events.

Do the exercise in Box 7.2 before reading on. To prepare you may wish to read the relevant sections on cohort studies in Chapter 9 (Section 9.6) first.

Box 7.2 **Two approaches for measuring Incidence**

(a) Imagine a cohort study with follow-up over 5 years to answer the question: What is the incidence of coronary heart disease in 45–74 year old people? Consider the advantages and disadvantages of the two approaches for measuring incidence.

(b) Imagine a study of the incidence of coronary heart disease or mortality based on a register of diseases (or deaths) compiled for 5 years. Again, consider the advantages and disadvantages of the two approaches for measuring incidence.

In the cohort study ((a) in Box 7.2) the decision on which formula to use will, in theory, depend on the design of the study. If the cohort is assembled at one point of time—say all people born on one day, or army personnel retiring in a particular month of the year—then there is an open choice. In the case of CHD in 45–74 year olds, we could enrol all people of this age from a general practice or other population registers providing age. The participants would then be followed up over time to observe the outcome. The denominator could be the study population at the beginning or the midpoint of the interval of time in question. Alternatively the person-time denominator could be used. If the study sample in the cohort is recruited over a prolonged period of time, say over years, then a person denominator is not appropriate. The elegant choice is the person-time denominator.

Mostly, incidence rates are calculated by setting up registers of deaths or disease (as in (b) in Box 7.2), and using census or other estimates of the size of the population from which the cases arose. Information on migration, and other means by which a person is effectively lost from the system capturing data for the register, is not usually available on all the individuals making up the denominator. The assumption is made that the population is fairly stable and usually the mid-point of the time period is used. If the disease is uncommon, as is usually the case, adjusting the denominator to remove the new cases would make little difference to the incidence rate. If the disease is common, the denominator could be adjusted by assuming that the cases occur evenly through the year so reducing the denominator by 50 per cent of the number of cases. In this kind of study, with no information on each of the individuals in the denominator, there is no added value to a person-time based denominator. Table 7.4 summarizes the advantages and disadvantages of the two types of denominator.

The concepts and algebraic formulae for incidence require reflection, but putting the concepts into practice in measuring the incidence of disease accurately is a still greater challenge. The following discussion of measuring events (numerators) and population (denominators) is applicable to all rates in epidemiology.

Table 7.4 Main advantages and disadvantages of person and person-time denominators in the context of (a) cohort and (b) register-based studies of incidence rates

	Advantages	Disadvantages
(a) Cohort study		
Person denominator	Measures risk directly	Requires everyone in the study to be enrolled at about the same time
	Choices of time periods to present incidence data on e.g. 1 year, 5 years	Not easy to account for losses to follow-up
		Baseline population is an inaccurate estimate of the population at risk for common diseases
Person-time denominator	Very flexible in coping with people entering and leaving study at different times	No easily interpreted direct measure of risk
	Study population can be enrolled over long periods of time	Assumes disease occurrence is even across time
		Requires information on date of onset of disease (year of onset is not enough)
(b) Register based study		
Person denominator	Can use population size data from census and other sources if necessary	Accurate census based estimates of denominator are required
	Can use population at mid-point of interval as estimate	Routine population data may give inexact denominator size
	Otherwise as for cohort studies	Otherwise as for cohort studies
Person-time denominator	Not usually applicable, but if it were, then as for cohort studies	Information to calculate person-years is not usually available

7.4 **Numerator**

In contemporary epidemiology the greatest need is for accurate data collection. The difficulties start with the numerator, that is, the number of events (numerator is the mathematical term for the upper number in a vulgar fraction as in the formula for incidence rate). Epidemiological studies are usually based on diagnoses made by someone else, not the investigator. There have been some notable exceptions, mainly work by single clinical investigators such as the general practitioner William Pickles who described the pattern of occurrence and natural history of several diseases in his own patients (Pickles 1939). With the advent of the multidisciplinary, team-based approach of modern health care, the specialization of medical practice, and the need for large studies, epidemiologists rarely make their own diagnoses. Herein lies a difficulty. How can epidemiologists ensure that the diagnoses are accurate? Clearly, they cannot be sure, but their confidence will be increased by a valid case definition, information on symptoms, signs and tests relevant to the case definition, and healthcare staff who have been trained well and in comparable ways in diagnosis.

An information system is needed to hold the clinical data to which the case definition can be applied and from which a list of cases can be extracted. Since neither the basic clinical information, nor the diagnosis, is likely to be recorded in unambiguous and consistent words, a means of judging the evidence to make or affirm a diagnosis is needed. A patient may have several diseases in the course of one illness. Imagine, for example, a person who has a feverish illness diagnosed on laboratory tests as influenza, who develops cough and shortness of breath shown to be pneumonia, followed by a deep venous thrombosis. The doctors suspect that pulmonary embolus has occurred but before it can be confirmed by tests, the patient collapses and dies unexpectedly. Assume that there is no postmortem because the relatives refuse permission. These diagnoses will need to be extracted from a complex set of medical records. Difficult decisions need to be made. Which diagnoses will go on the death certificate (and ultimately our research database) and in what order? Do the exercise in Box 7.3 now.

Box 7.3 **Entering diagnosis on a death certificate**

Complete the specimen death certificate in Table 7.5 for the above person. Take care to order the causes as instructed.

Imagine that you are an epidemiologist who acquires 600 000 such death certificates on all causes of death and that you wish to study the incidence of mortality from pulmonary embolus. The task of extracting a list of cases of death due to pulmonary

Table 7.5 Specimen death certificate

CAUSE OF DEATH

The condition thought to be the 'Underlying Cause of Death' should appear in the lowest completed line of Part 1.

I (a) Disease or condition directly leading to death

  (b) Other disease or condition, if any, leading to I(a)...

  (c) Other disease or condition, if any, leading to I(b)...

II Other significant conditions CONTRIBUTING TO THE DEATH but not related to the disease or condition causing

it ....

  ....

embolus is not a trivial one, not least because some differences in writing style and words is inevitable, with some doctors using pulmonary thrombosis, some lung embolus, some omitting it altogether from the death certificate. Compare your completed certificate with mine below.

1a Pulmonary embolus

 b Pneumonia

 c Influenza

11 Deep venous thrombosis

One solution, which makes both the choosing of diagnosis and the handling of data easier, is a list of codes for disease. There are several such sets of codes but the most important one is the International Classification of Diseases (ICD) of the WHO.

The order in which the causes of death are listed on the certificate of death is important, for there is a long tradition that only the underlying cause of death is coded, analysed and published. This tradition has been overturned recently in the UK, and all the causes are now coded and available for analysis. Before reading on do the exercise in Box 7.4.

In studies of incidence there is the additional complication, which does not apply to death as here, that a decision needs to be made on whether the case is a new case

Box 7.4 **Coding of diagnosis**

◆ Based on your completed death certificate code the causes of death (see Table 7.6).

◆ Reconsider your choice of order of causes of death after reading the coding rule from the ICD (see Table 7.6).

Table 7.6 Selected codes from ICD-10, with brief notes on coding rules

Chapter IX	**Diseases of circulatory system**	I00–I99	
	Hypertension	I10–I5	
	Ischaemic heart disease	I20–25	
	Cerebrovascular	I60–69	
	Phlebitis and thrombophlebitis	I80	I80.0 of superficial vessels of lower extremities
			I80.1 of femoral vein of other lower extremities (Deep vein thrombosis)
	Other venous embolism and thrombosis	I82	
	Varicose veins of lower extremities	I83	
	Pulmonary embolism	I26	
Chapter X:	**Disease of respiratory system**	J00–J99	
	Influenza due to influenza virus	J10	(J10 with pneumonia)
	Influenza, virus not identified	J11	(J11 with pneumonia)
	Viral pneumonia, not elsewhere classified	J12	
	Bacterial pneumonia, not elsewhere classified	J15	
	Pneumonia, organism unspecified	J18	
	Respiratory failure, not elsewhere classified	J96	
Chapter XVII: Symptoms, signs, etc not elsewhere classified		R00–R99	
	Respiratory arrest (cardiorespiratory failure)	RO9.2	

Note: The causes of death to be recorded are all those that resulted in or contributed to death, and the circumstances of accident or violence which produced injury.

The underlying cause of death is (a) the disease or injury which initiated the train of events leading directly to death or (b) the circumstances of the accident or violence which produced the fatal injury.

Adapted from the international classification of diseases tenth edition (see Permissions).

or an old one and whether the person is in the at risk group under study. The investigator with 600 000 death certificates (or hospital records) has much work to do to turn these into useful epidemiological information, including the accurate count of cases. (My codes are I26, J18, J10, I80.1.)

Two examples, lower limb amputation and Legionnaires' disease, provide contrasting perspectives on the problem of achieving accuracy in the numerator. The words 'lower limb amputation' convey the essence of the case definition of the problem and it is a small step to define it in terms of anatomy, that is, what part of the limb is amputated. Further, there is no need for the diagnosis to be confirmed by a doctor or by checking medical records. With such a problem the patient will almost certainly have been treated by the health service. The main obstacle to obtaining an accurate numerator is maintaining a case register. Since nearly all cases are likely to be hospitalized, the problem is simply one of collating and extracting the information from the information systems of the relevant hospitals. The obvious place to look for data is the hospital admissions or discharges information system, or the operating theatre records or the limb-fitting centre. Figure 7.3 shows the result of a study. Of the 291 cases identified, only 17 were recorded in all three information systems. If the authors had relied on operation records alone, which seems a reasonable strategy, 192/291 (66 per cent) of cases would have been identified. In this example, even for such a straightforward diagnosis, the difficulty in defining the numerator is extreme.

There is a strong movement for health care to be planned rationally based on data from routine sources and rigorous healthcare needs assessment. Figure 7.3 illustrates the perils of such an approach, even for such a clearly defined condition. The resources for a 'needs' based service planned using 'routine' information from the discharge data would have been depleted rapidly. Until we have accurate systems for measuring need,

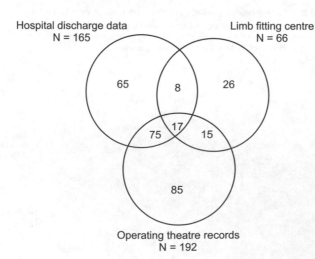

Hospital discharge data
N = 165

Limb fitting centre
N = 66

65 8 26

75 17 15

85

Operating theatre records
N = 192

Fig. 7.3 Use of routine information to measure the number of people with limb amputation: ascertainment based on three data sources. Data from Leeds Health Authority (England), July 1992 to December 1993. Total number of cases of LEA = 291 (source of data, Bodansky, 1997; unpublished figure from Williams, see Permissions).

it is best to incorporate information on past resource requirement in planning the health service. When information is available from several independent sources, the capture-recapture technique, originally designed for measuring the size of animal populations, can sometimes be used. Discussion of this technique is beyond the scope of this book (see references).

In contrast with lower limb amputation the nature and case definition of Legionnaires' disease is complex. This pneumonia cannot be differentiated from other forms of pneumonia clinically and has a wide spectrum of presentation (see Chapter 6); some patients have minimal illness and others a wide variety of signs and symptoms. Most patients are likely to be cared for in the community (as a flu-like illness or pneumonia) rather than be admitted to hospital. The first challenge is for the physician to consider this diagnosis. The second is to order the necessary laboratory tests. The tests are often difficult to interpret, especially as culture of the organism is only successful in a minority of cases. There was, until the publication of ICD 10 very recently, no specific ICD code for this pneumonia so information about cases could not be extracted by searching in routine information systems, including those for hospital inpatients. This meant that for epidemiological studies a specific register of cases had to be created and maintained. Since the diagnosis requires both clinical and laboratory information the register cannot be maintained from laboratory records alone. As it is a rare disease, incidence studies require the participation of a large number of physicians in supplying information to a registry. Add to this the need to comply with the rules on protecting the confidentiality of clinical information and it is not surprising that there is a huge 'iceberg' effect for this (and similar) diseases. Fewer than 10 per cent of all cases are counted in most registers. The reader should ponder on the difficulties of measuring the incidence of this and similar diseases.

To calculate the incidence of disease the procedures for registration of cases will need to include rules to judge whether a case is new or old and decide whether to include recurrences. For example, in a study of the incidence of bronchiolitis, the common cold or acute myocardial infarction, the investigator needs to decide whether only the first occurrence is included as a new case or whether each occurrence is to be included. As there is no general rule each study will need to make this decision in the light of its aims. These decisions are not always easy except for the incidence of mortality, diseases which are irreversible (e.g. amputation of a limb), diseases which usually occur only once (e.g. measles), or diseases agreed by definition or convention to be lifelong diseases (e.g. diabetes). Where the prime purpose of the study is to measure the frequency of disease to assess its importance or need for services all cases must be included. Where the aim is to make comparisons between populations to develop or test causal hypotheses there is a choice. In measuring the incidence of stroke, for example, all new and recurrent cases will probably be included if we are doing the study to measure the need for services or evaluating interventions. In a study of whether cholesterol is a causal risk factor for stroke, possibly based on studying groups of subjects with low and high cholesterol, there is a choice. Interpretation of the findings of such a study is usually easier if first occurrences only are included.

There is a truism that epidemiology is the science of denominators; but that is simplistic. The accurate collection of numerator data is an enormous, underestimated problem in epidemiology.

7.5 **Denominator**

The quality of the data on the denominator (the lower number in a vulgar fraction) is crucial. Our need is to know the number of people at risk of disease. As a simple rule, if people are at risk of being in the numerator, the population from which they came should be in the denominator. Clearly, women are not endangered from testicular cancer, or men from cancer of the cervix. In these cases the denominator would be sex-specific. It is common and good practice in epidemiology to consider men and women separately for most analysis, for their disease patterns are often different. If their patterns are demonstrably not different, data can be combined. Often, the choice of denominator is common sense but sometimes it is not. Try the exercise in Box 7.5 now.

Box 7.5 **Defining the denominator**

◆ What might be your denominator for a study defining the incidence rate of
    (a) infant mortality;
    (b) the sudden infant death syndrome ('cot' death); and
    (c) myocardial infarction?
◆ What information would you need to make a rational choice?

The key step is to understand the definition of the health problem under study. The infant mortality rate is by definition the number of deaths within the first year of life. The word infant, actually meaning a very young child, has been given a more precise meaning here. The logical denominator would be the population of 0–1 year olds, or the person-years of observation of a cohort of newborns (which is less because of deaths, migrations and losses to follow-up). By definition, however, the denominator for infant mortality rate is the number of live births. The reason is a practical one, this information is easy to obtain, is accurate and up-to-date. Effectively, this defines a cohort for which outcomes are obtained from mortality data. In contrast, to know the size of the population of 0–1 year olds would require a more regular census or only occasional data analysis (the population census is done every 10 years). To measure person-years of observation would need follow-up of members of our cohort individually. Since infant mortality rates are less than 1 per cent in industrialized countries, to follow up individuals to collect 100 deaths would need a study of more than 10 000 infants. The formula for infant mortality rate in a particular year can now be seen as a pragmatic compromise, and is:

$$\frac{\text{Number of deaths in infants under one year in year x}}{\text{Number of liveborn in year x}} \qquad (7.5)$$

To choose a denominator for sudden infant death syndrome (SIDS) we need to know the definition of the disease, which is:

> sudden death of an infant under one year of age, which remains unexplained after a thorough case investigation, including performance of a complete autopsy, examination of the death scene, and review of the clinical history.
>
> (US National Institute of Child Health 1991)

The denominator is infants less than 1-year old. The denominator choice here is driven by the definition of the disease, for identical deaths after the first year would not be called SIDS or 'cot' deaths.

For the incidence rate of myocardial infarction the denominator would be those at risk. It would be reasonable, in designing a study of incidence rates, to exclude children and adolescents, for myocardial infarction is extremely rare in these groups. There is no scientific rationale for excluding the elderly, one sex (usually women are excluded), or particular ethnic groups. If the numerator comprises selected cases based on age, sex, or ethnic group then the denominator will need to reflect this. In research focusing on the causes of disease those who have already had a heart attack before and are therefore no longer at risk of having a *first* attack, might reasonably be excluded.

The cause of a recurrent myocardial infarction may be different from a first one, hence deserves separate study. If the information is to be used for priority setting or health needs assessment the study should measure the incidence of first, recurrent and total infarcts.

The principles in terms of establishing the numerator and the denominator, discussed in the context of disease incidence studies, are similar but more complex in relation to prevalence, as discussed next.

7.6 **Prevalence and prevalence rate**

Prevalence is, in plain English, the extent to which something exists. In epidemiology (Table 7.2) prevalence is the count of all instances of the factor of interest in the study population. For simplicity, the remainder of this section assumes the factor of interest is a disease, but it could be something else, such as a behaviour or an abnormal value in a blood test. As with incidence, prevalence is usually expressed in relation to a population at risk, but sometimes another type of denominator may be chosen; for example, prevalence of congenital abnormalities is usually expressed in relation to the number of live births.

The key features of prevalence are given in Table 7.2. The term prevalence rate reflects its widespread usage but, as discussed earlier, some authorities contend that a rate must have a time dimension. The argument has led to confusion. *Last's Dictionary of*

Epidemiology (2001) states that prevalence is a number, not a rate and prevalence 'rate' (Last's quotations) is a proportion, not a rate. All rates (and incidence figures) are numbers, so this property does not exclude prevalence from being a rate. Proportions and rates are both a subset of ratios. Readers are advised to consider these arguments and adopt the usage they feel comfortable with – I use either the traditional, widespread, and continuing approach of expressing prevalence as a rate or the emergent (but, strictly speaking, inaccurate) trend simply to call this measure prevalence.

There are three types of prevalence rates. The point prevalence rate comprises all the cases of a disease that exist in a place at a point in time. In practice not all cases are either diagnosed or discovered (false negatives), and some cases are misdiagnosed (false positives). The denominator is chosen to represent those at risk. The population at risk is often specifically recruited into the study. In studies where the investigators have not recruited the population at risk, the denominator is usually derived from population estimates. It is unlikely that such estimates will exist for a point in time (e.g. they are usually mid-year estimates, from the census). Inaccuracy in estimating prevalence is, therefore, likely. In a study of the prevalence of, say, menstrual irregularity, the denominator would be women who are menstruating, and a choice of the age group 15–45 years of age might be reasonable. For prevalence, unlike incidence, there is no requirement to exclude from the denominator those people who already have the disease. As the denominator includes the numerator the prevalence is, mathematically, a proportion and ranges from 0 to 1 (or, 0–100 per cent). The formula is simple:

$$\text{Point prevalence rate} = \frac{\text{All cases of the factor of interest at time x}}{\text{Population at risk at time x}} \quad (7.6)$$

Point prevalence rate does not always gauge the burden of disease in a way that is helpful to health organizations that plan their work over periods of time.

Period prevalence is a way of recognizing and overcoming the limitations of prevalence studies done at a point in time. All cases whether old, new, or recurrent, arising over a defined period, say a year or two, are counted. The denominator is the average population over the period (or mid-point estimate). Period prevalence, which combines the concept of incidence and point prevalence, is particularly useful in gauging the burden of episodic, recurrent diseases such as depression, anxiety, or migraine. Both point prevalence and incidence, alone, tend to underestimate the size of such problems so a combination is desirable. The formula is:

$$\text{Period prevalence rate} = \frac{\text{All cases (old and new) of the factor of interest during time period}}{\text{Average population at risk during time period}} \quad (7.7)$$

Lifetime prevalence is the ultimate extension of the idea of period prevalence, and is the proportion of the population who have ever had the disease. This can be derived systematically from a birth cohort study (where people are followed up from birth); we can derive the proportion of the population who have ever had asthma by the age of 5, 10, 15, 30, 45 years or more until all are dead. Lifetime prevalence has value for drawing attention to how common some disorders are. For example, over a lifetime mental health problems are extremely common. The formula is:

$$\text{Lifetime prevalence} = \frac{\text{No. who ever had the factor of interest during lifetime}}{\text{Population at risk (at the beginning of the time period)}} \quad (7.8)$$

The algebraic formulae for prevalence rates are simple but, as with incidence, their measurement is problematic. Most of the principles discussed in relation to incidence apply to prevalence; for example, the need for a valid case definition and information to judge whether a case qualifies, a system for collection of information on the numerator, and defining and measuring an appropriate denominator. Imagine we are interested in measuring the prevalence of type 2 diabetes. Now try the exercise in Box 7.6 before reading on.

Box 7.6 **Defining the numerator and denominator for the prevalence of diabetes**

In general terms consider the steps you will need to take to count the numerator and denominator to measure the population prevalence of type 2 diabetes.

The first and crucial step is to decide on the definition. The usual choices are:

- The WHO definition of a plasma glucose of more than 11.1 mmol/litre two hours after a standard oral glucose tolerance test. To meet this definition your study population will need to undergo this test which involves fasting overnight, then drinking the standard glucose drink and having blood taken 120 minutes later. This will require a special study, for such information does not exist in routine information systems. Since such a test is potentially dangerous or inadvisable in those with diabetes, not everyone will be able to do it.

- The definition of the American Diabetes Association of a fasting plasma blood glucose level of ≥ 7 mmol/l. Again this information does not exist in records so a special study will be needed. This test is simpler than the glucose tolerance test but will lead to a different list of people diagnosed and a different prevalence than the WHO definition above. In both of these definitions, the denominator will be the people who undergo the test.

- Definitions based on clinical diagnoses made on the basis of a mixture of symptoms, signs, and of a variety of diagnostic strategies used in normal clinical practice. This approach is relatively easy, for the cases can be identified from medical records or registers, but is likely to underestimate the prevalence greatly, and perhaps pick up half of all cases. Sometimes access to medical records will not be possible, leaving the investigators to rely on self-report of doctors' diagnosis by the study participants at interview or by questionnaire. This will underestimate the prevalence even more, for some participants will fail to report such a diagnosis.

The second step is to select an appropriate population at risk. Identifying unbiased sample populations, and enlisting their cooperation in prevalence studies is a formidable task as discussed more fully in Chapter 9. Unlike incidence, which is concerned with events including death, point prevalence studies are usually of survivors. With the exception of autopsy-based prevalence studies, for example, measuring the prevalence of congenital heart disease in sudden infant death syndrome, deaths are not included. The duration of the prevalence study depends on what it measures: point, period, or lifetime prevalence. Point prevalence studies should take place on a particular day or narrow time interval. In practice, observations on hundreds, sometimes thousands, of people cannot be made in this way and measurements take place over months or even years. Figures 7.4 and 7.5 are simple illustrations of the effects this can have. Figure 7.4 is a study of a common permanent condition in 20 people, divided into four groups to make fieldwork easier, and spread over the year. The lines show the onset of the disease. The shading in the figure, which shows the fieldwork periods, is simply to help the counting. Do the exercise in Box 7.7 before reading on.

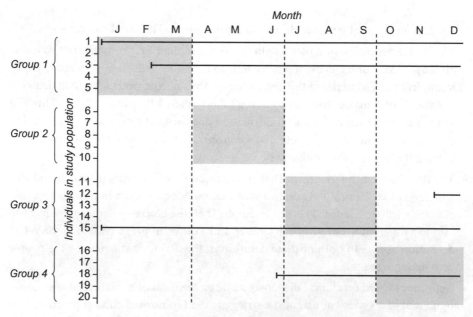

Fig. 7.4 Study of a common permanent problem. Each horizontal line denotes a case and shading the fieldwork order.

Box 7.7 **Measuring prevalence and incidence rates in a permanent condition**

In Fig. 7.4 what is the point prevalence rate in January, July, and December? What is the cumulative annual incidence rate? What is the period prevalence rate? What is the lifetime prevalence rate? Have the fieldwork team identified all cases? What would be the effect of doing the study in a different order, say group 4 went first, group 3 followed, etc.

The point prevalence is 10 per cent in January (two cases exist, nos. 1 and 15), 20 per cent in July (four cases, nos. 1, 3, 15, 18), and 25 per cent in December (nos. 1, 3, 12, 15, 18). The (cumulative) incidence is 12.5 per cent (3 new cases/18 at risk; two already had the disease). The period prevalence is the initial prevalence plus incidence, 25 per cent. Here the denominator is 20, the entire population under study. We cannot calculate lifetime prevalence on these data; we need to know what will happen to our study population until they die. Of these cases only one (no.12) will be missed by the fieldwork team; the fieldwork is before the date of onset. If the fieldwork order was changed, for example, group 4 first (January–March), group 3 second (April–June), group 2 third (January–September), and group 1 last (October–December), case no. 18 would also be missed (in addition to case 12). In the study, as actually conducted, cases are missed and the prevalence is underestimated.

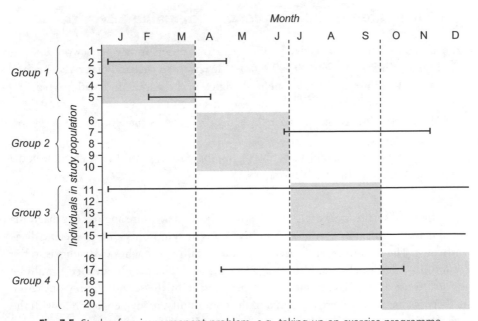

Fig. 7.5 Study of an impermanent problem, e.g. taking up an exercise programme.

Figure 7.5 represents a study of a changeable condition, say, taking up an exercise programme. Do the exercise in Box 7.8 before reading on.

Box 7.8 **Measuring incidence and prevalence rates in a changeable condition**

- What is the point prevalence of exercise uptake in January, July, and December?
- What is the cumulative incidence rate and period prevalence of exercise uptake by end-December?
- Have the fieldwork teams identified all the cases?
- What would be the effect of a different order of field work , say group 4 went first, group 3 second, etc

---

The point prevalence is 15 per cent in January (3/20, nos. 2, 11, 15), 20 per cent in July (nos. 7, 11, 15, 17), and 10 per cent in December (nos. 11 and 15). The cumulative incidence of exercise uptake is 3/17 which is 17.6 per cent (nos. 5, 7, 17). The period prevalence is 30 per cent. On this occasion our fieldwork team misses no cases. If the fieldwork order had been group 4 (January–March), 3, 2, 1 then cases 2, 5 and 17 would have been missed. Now try the exercise in Box 7.9 before reading on.

Box 7.9 **Incidence and prevalence in planning a service**

A health authority (or an equivalent body such as an insurance agency or a managed care organization) serving 500 000 people wishes to cost and plan a service for the medical and surgical management of angina in the population, with particular emphasis on the numbers of cases requiring surgery.

You are invited to assist. Consider the general principles that you would apply to the task.

Consider the relative merits of measuring incidence, point prevalence, period prevalence, and lifetime prevalence rates.

The first and surprisingly difficult task is to define and measure angina. The diagnosis of angina is a clinical one with no definitive signs or symptoms and no specific diagnostic test. The sensitivity and specificity of the main approaches to diagnosis in the community, that is, clinical history or ECG, are low. The health authority could be advised to use data based on numbers of people seen by the service in previous years. As there is a massive iceberg of angina in the community, many people, often with the severest disease and destined for sudden death or MI, will be missed.

The second difficult task is to differentiate those people with angina who would benefit from surgery from those who would do as well on medical therapy. The usual way to do this is coronary angiogram, an invasive procedure whereby the narrowing of the coronary arteries is displayed using X-ray techniques. The dangers of this procedure are sufficient to preclude its use in epidemiological surveys of apparently healthy populations. For this reason a preliminary test—the exercise ECG—is done, and those positive get the angiogram, which is the key test in helping to decide whether surgical treatment is appropriate.

The investigator needs to define angina for the purpose of this task and design a study to estimate the fraction of cases that will require surgery. Since angina is rarely a problem in the young, it could be reasonable to limit the investigation to adults, perhaps 35 years or more. The incidence rate is not helpful for planning here because it hugely underestimates the burden of the problem. The point prevalence estimate is the number of people with angina in the community. Period prevalence (say over a year) is probably the most useful measure, for it informs the planner of the number of people in the community that will require service in that year. Lifetime prevalence is of no immediate value here. The period prevalence could be measured by a combination of clinical examinations and tests, and a register of cases. Once the population of angina patients has been identified, further tests, including exercise ECGs and angiography will help to identify the need for surgery or medical management. Incidence and prevalence are clearly related. This is discussed below.

7.7 Relationship of incidence and prevalence

There is a close relationship between incidence and prevalence. The relationship is shown in simple form in Fig. 7.6, as the bath model. The inflow is the incidence, the bath water the prevalence (pool of cases). The prevalence pool is changed by death, recovery, or migration (the outflow). Figure 7.7 develops this simple idea in relation to a population. The population is enhanced by births and immigration, and diminished by deaths and emigration. This is the water supply to the bath. Some incident cases die before reaching the prevalence pool, such as sudden infant death syndrome cases. The recovered cases may rejoin the main population.

There is a mathematical relationship between incidence and prevalence, which only works in fixed populations. Imagine a fixed population of newborn infants all of whom survive for the duration of the study, say five years. The number of new cases over five years (5-year cumulative incidence) of a chronic, lifelong but non-fatal disease, let us say amputation of a limb, and the total number of cases at the end of the study (5-year period prevalence) are identical. If the duration of the disease is less than lifelong or death occurs, then the period prevalence will be smaller than the 5-year cumulative incidence. In fixed populations, when the prevalence is low, the prevalence is approximately equal to the incidence rate × average duration of disease among those observed. It follows that incidence rate is approximately = point prevalence rate ÷ duration; and duration is

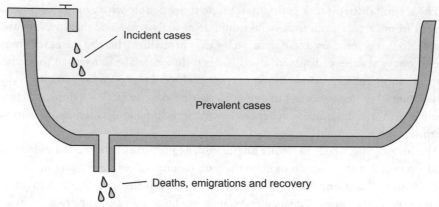

Fig. 7.6 Incidence, prevalence, and the bath model of disease (Adapted from a figure provided by Howel, see Permissions).

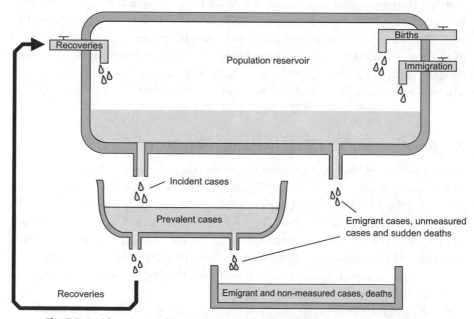

Fig. 7.7 Incidence, prevalence in a natural population: the population reservoir.

approximately = point prevalence rate ÷ incidence rate. In a dynamic population, however, the prevalence of a disease cannot be predicted from knowledge of the incidence (or vice versa) because of migration into and out of the population, deaths, changing disease rates, changes in prognosis, and error in measuring the incidence (or prevalence) accurately. In practice, either both the prevalence and incidence are measured or a choice of one is made. The formula can be used, at best, as an approximation. The exercise in Box 7.10 provides a simple example to permit you to develop your understanding. Do this exercise before reading on.

Box 7.10 **Incidence and prevalence of gunshot wounds**

Imagine a population of 10 000 new army recruits. Your interest is in the incidence and prevalence of gunshot wounds on war duty. Assume all gunshot wounds lead to permanent visible damage. You follow the recruits for one year. All of the study population survive, all medical records are available, and all are available for interview and examination. Assume that the occurrence of gunshot wounds is spread evenly through the year, and that at recruitment none had such a wound. Over the year you find that 20 recruits had a gunshot wound.

- What is the cumulative incidence rate of gunshot wounds? What is the incidence rate based on the person-time denominator?
- What is the point prevalence rate of having had a gunshot wound at the beginning, middle and end of the year?
- What is the period prevalence rate over the year?
- If the incidence rate remains the same over time, what is the prevalence rate of ever being scarred by the end of five years?
- What is the average duration of a gunshot wound, among those scarred, by the end of the first year?
- What is the estimate of the point prevalence over the five-year period?
- What is the average duration of scarring over the five years?

The incidence rate (cumulative) of first scarring wounds, based on the denominator at the beginning of the study, is 20/10 000 per year = 2/1000 or 0.2 per cent. The alternative is to take the population at risk at the midpoint of the time interval, at 6 months. By then 10 people will have been scarred and hence are no longer at risk. The incidence rate then is 20/9990 = 2.002/1000 = 0.2002 per cent. The incidence rate estimated by the person-time denominator of first gunshot wounds is identical. The total person-years of observation is 9990 (9980 given by those unwounded, and 10 by those 20 people who were wounded for they give, on average, 0.5 years). The result is 20/9990 person years, that is, 0.002002 per person-year, or 2.002 per 1000 person-years, identical to the incidence rate based on the mid-interval denominator.

The point prevalence at the beginning is zero, and at 6 months, on average, half of all cases will have occurred, so it is 10/10000 and by the end of the year it is 20/10 000. The period prevalence at one year is also 20/10 000. The actual duration of scarring among cases is, on average, half of the time of follow-up. The prevalence is low and the population is fixed so our simple formula on p. 185 will give a good estimate. The average duration of a scarring wound at one year, is point prevalence at the midpoint of the interval ÷ incidence = 1 ÷ 2 = 0.5 year. The predicted approximate point prevalence at five years = annual incidence rate × average duration × years of observation.

$$= 2 \text{ per thousand} \times 0.5 \text{ years} \times 5 = 5 \text{ per } 1000.$$

The approximate average duration of scarring over the 5 years is $5/1000 \div 2/1000 = 2.5$ years.

The prevalence above slightly overestimates because there will be a decreasing number of cases in each successive year, as those who have already had a scarring wound cannot contribute twice to the prevalence of ever having had a gunshot wound, even though they can continue to contribute to the incidence of new scarring wounds (first and subsequent).

A better estimate of the period prevalence at 5 years is $99.6/10\,000$ (or $9.96/1000$) as follows:

- 1st year incident cases = 20, leaving 9980 at risk
- 2nd year incident cases = 0.2 per cent of 9980 = 19.96, leaving 9960
- 3rd year incident cases = 0.2 per cent of 9960 = 19.92, leaving 9940
- 4th year incident cases = 0.2 per cent of 9940 = 19.88, leaving 9920
- 5th year incident cases = 0.2 per cent of 9920 = 19.84, a total of 99.6 cases

The reader may wish to calculate the 5-year cumulative incidence based on the baseline and mid-point denominators, and the person-years of observation. For advanced understanding of the concepts of incidence and prevalence, readers may wish to consult Rothman (1988).

7.8 Choice of incidence or prevalence

As a general principle, for studies of the causes of disease, the incidence rate is preferred because it is not affected by variation in treatment and case-fatality, so differences between populations are easier to interpret. For studies of the burden of diseases of short duration (e.g. measles, influenza, diarrhoea, transient ischaemic attacks, ankle sprains, acute low backache), incidence is also preferred because point prevalence would underestimate the problem. The point prevalence figure would miss the recovered or dead cases. The period prevalence adds little to understanding here. As medical records tend to capture data on such diseases poorly, special studies will usually be required.

The prevalence rate is generally preferred as the measure of burden for long-lasting diseases even when these are rare (e.g. multiple sclerosis, renal failure). For health behaviours and other disease risk factors prevalence is the preferred measure (even in studies of disease causation). Prevalence is sometimes perceived in epidemiology as inferior to incidence. It is not. Both measures have inherent weaknesses and strengths, and different value in various circumstances.

7.9 Presenting rates

Rates can be presented for the whole population under study or for subgroups of that population. For example, the population of Scotland in 1999 was 5.195 million, and there were 60 277 deaths, giving an overall mortality rate of $60\,277/5\,195\,000 = 0.0116 = 11.6$ per 1000. Such an overall rate is commonly referred to as the crude mortality rate.

As the word crude has negative connotations a better term is actual overall rate. The actual rate can be subdivided by any characteristic of the population of epidemiological interest (e.g. age, sex) and calculated for different places and times. Such rates are called specific rates (e.g. age or sex specific rates) and this is called stratified analysis. Commonly used variables for subdivision of rates include age group, sex, ethnic group or race, social class, educational status, and marital status. Such variables are commonly referred to as epidemiological variables. The characteristics of a sound epidemiological variable were discussed in Chapter 1. Obviously, to calculate specific rates we need to be able to subdivide the population counts by these variables; we need to know the number of people in each ethnic group in the underlying population before we can calculate ethnic group specific rates. Such information may not be available, especially in small areas and in years other than the census year.

Specific rates permit rational and easy comparison of disease patterns in different places and times for they can be directly compared with each other, and questions asked about why differences occur. The answers are usually complex and elusive. Simple observations of difference in disease rates may lead to inspiration, as in the example of Semmelweiss's hypothesis of a transmissable cadaverous particle, arising from his reflection on mortality in two clinics (discussed in Chapter 5). More often the observations are merely noted or give rise to untested (sometimes untestable) hypotheses. For example, longstanding observations of greater lifespan (and lower mortality rates) in women compared with men are largely unexplained in specific biological or social terms as are differences in chronic diseases at different ages. Explaining differences in disease rates is exceptionally difficult science.

Although there are still intriguing differences in disease by sex and age, these variables are usually treated as confounding variables. Imagine that we observe that a seaside resort town such as Bournemouth has a higher actual overall (or crude) mortality rate from stroke than, say, a city such as Bristol. The likely explanation is one of low scientific interest; the seaside resort has more elderly people, for it is a place people move to after retirement. The overall higher rate, though true, is usually adjusted to take account of these differences in age structure of the population of the two cities using methods discussed in the next chapter. We would not usually investigate the role of age in causing differences in stroke between these cities.

7.10 **Conclusion**

Epidemiology is a practical and pragmatic science that is focused on measuring and explaining risk of disease in populations. This requires three distinct types of data in context of time and place: on diseases, on the factors that potentially cause disease, and the size and characteristics of the populations under study. Obtaining these data is a serious obstacle to epidemiology, even in the most advanced populations. The art of epidemiology lies in making judgements on the appropriate interpretation of, inevitably, inaccurate data. Epidemiological and other theories of health and disease are vital to guide such judgements and interpretations. Theoretical considerations around measurements and presentation of risk, and mathematical and statistical ideas on measurement of disease occurrence, underpin the practice of data collection. These are the factors that have driven change and advancement in an aspect of epidemiology that is based on mathematics, and prevent epidemiology being more than the toolbox of disease measurement.

The rate of disease, where a measure of the quantity of disease (the numerator) is considered in relation to a measure of the quantity of population (the denominator), lies at the core of epidemiological method. Two types of rates are dominant in epidemiology, incidence and prevalence. The two are clearly distinguished by being concerned with either new events (incidence) or events old and new (prevalence). These two measures are manipulated in epidemiology to produce a multiplicity of perspectives on population patterns of health and disease—and that is the subject of the next chapter.

Summary

Risk is the possibility of harm. In epidemiology risk refers to the likelihood of an individual in a defined population developing a disease or other adverse health problem. In epidemiology the association between risk of disease and both individual and social characteristics (risk factors) is often the starting point for causal analysis. Epidemiological studies measure, present and interpret disease frequency, usually by comparing the patterns in one population relative to another. Measures of disease frequency include incidence and prevalence rates.

The incidence rate is the number of new cases in relation to a population, time, and place. Two forms of incidence rates are in common use, cumulative incidence and person-time incidence rate. In cumulative incidence the denominator is the population, in person-time incidence the denominator is the sum of the time periods for which the individuals in the population have been observed. Prevalence rate measures all disease in a population either at a particular time (point prevalence) or over a time period (period prevalence, lifetime prevalence). There is a theoretical mathematical relation between the two measures, such that in a fixed population prevalence rate is approximately equal to the incidence rate multiplied by the duration of the disease. Rates are most accurately presented by age and sex groups ('specific' rates), but for ease of interpretation they may be grouped as overall (crude) rates, which can be adjusted for age and sex differences between compared populations. The collection of both disease and population data to achieve accurate figures of incidence and prevalence is problematic.

Chapter 8

Presentation and interpretation of epidemiological data on risk

Objectives

On completion of the chapter you should understand:

- that the aim of manipulating epidemiological data is to sharpen understanding of actual and relative risk of disease, but distortions occur easily;

- that epidemiological studies measure, present and interpret risk, often comparing one population with another, using relative measures;

- the idea behind, definition of, strengths and limitations of, and means of calculation of proportional mortality, proportional mortality ratio, actual overall (crude) rates, directly and indirectly standardized rates (and the standardized mortality ratio), relative risk, odds ratio, attributable risk, population attributable risk, years of life lost, numbers needed to treat, the quality adjusted life year, the disability adjusted life year;

- that the principal relative measure is the relative risk while the odds ratio can approximate it in particular circumstances;

- that attributable risk and population attributable risk are measures that help us to assess the proportion of the burden of disease that is caused by a particular risk factor;

- that the term avoidable mortality refers to the potential to avoid death or disability from the specified causes if the best possible healthcare actions were taken;

- that the number of years of avoidable life lost measures the impact of avoidable mortality and helps us to assess the effectiveness of health care;

- how epidemiological data contributes to assessing the health needs and health status of populations;

- the process of constructing summary measures of health status;

- that different ways of presenting the same data have a major impact on the perception of risk, so epidemiological studies should provide both relative and actual risk.

8.1 Introduction

Epidemiological data can be manipulated easily, with the purpose of extracting additional insights. Usually, but not always, the objective is to permit or sharpen up comparisons, whether over time or between places and population groups. This chapter introduces the main ways in which data are manipulated, with a warning that the end results are often artificial measures that change (and sometimes distort) the perception and interpretation of risk, a matter of utmost concern to a science where communication between researchers, health professionals, and the public is critically important.

8.2 Proportional morbidity or mortality ratio (PMR)

Sometimes the only reliable data we have are on cases. Comparisons between populations are difficult without population denominators to construct rates but these may not be available or they may be inaccurate. For example, there are usually no accurate population denominators for comparing disease and mortality outcomes by hospital. Studies of ethnicity and health in the UK are thwarted by the fact that ethnic code has been collected only at two censuses (1991 and 2001) and that records providing information on disease do not record ethnicity accurately (e.g. the death certificate has no ethnic code and in hospital admission records the code is often missing). Furthermore, some record systems and studies that do provide an ethnic code use a different classification from that in the census. The PMR is commonly used to study disease patterns by cause in settings where population denominators are not available, as illustrated here using mortality.

In the first step, the total number of deaths (not the population) is used as the denominator, and the deaths from each specific cause as the numerator. The proportional mortality (PM) is the resulting fraction, usually expressed as a percentage. The formula is:

$$PM = \frac{\text{Number of deaths due to cause x}}{\text{Total number of deaths}} \qquad (8.1)$$

Multiplying by 100 provides the PM as a percentage. The proportional mortality can be calculated by sex, age group or any other appropriate subdivision of the population. These figures can be compared between populations, places or time periods by calculating the proportional mortality ratio (PMR) which is simply the ratio of PMs in the two comparison populations, that is,

$$PMR = \frac{\text{PM in population A}}{\text{PM in population B}} \qquad (8.2)$$

In this formula population A is called the study population, population B the standard or comparison population, and the latter supplies the information on the expected proportion.

The PMR answers the question, is there a difference in the proportion of deaths attributable to disease x in one population compared with a second population? (Obviously, there can be no all-cause PM or PMR because it is always 100 per cent.) The PMR (formula above) can then be re-considered as:

$$PMR = \frac{\text{Observed proportion of deaths from a specific cause (study population)}}{\substack{\text{Expected proportion of deaths from a specific cause} \\ \text{(from the standard population)}}} \qquad (8.3)$$

Either the overall proportion in the standard population can be applied to obtain the expected proportion in all ages (the actual or crude PMR), or the age-specific proportions can be applied. If the latter is adopted the expected proportion is calculated for each specific age group, with the specific figures being summed (in effect standardizing for age, as explained in Section 8.3). The denominator may also be cause-specific. For example, we could look at deaths from coronary heart disease (CHD) as a proportion of deaths from stroke, or cancer, or accidents, rather than all causes.

Marmot and colleagues (1984), for example, were interested in the question, do people of Indian, Pakistani, Bangladeshi, and Sri Lankan ethnic origin (South Asians) living in England and Wales have a higher rate of mortality from coronary heart disease than the population as a whole? They studied mortality rates around the years of the 1971 census. The preliminary answer on the basis of mortality rates by country of birth was—possibly so. The problem was that some people born on the Indian Subcontinent were of European ethnic origin. Further, some South Asians were born in England and Wales. Neither the 1971 census nor the death certificate recorded ethnic group, only country of birth. The solution Marmot *et al.* adopted was to calculate the age-adjusted PMR (see Table 8.1). They tested the hypothesis that the proportional mortality in those with South Asian names (an indicator of ethnic group, not just birthplace), was different from that in those born in the Indian Subcontinent without such names, from African New Commonwealth born, and from the whole population of England and Wales. The proportional mortality of the whole population of England and Wales provided the standard. A PMR of 100 per cent would, therefore, reflect no difference between the ethnic groups and the standard population. Before reading on do the exercise in Box 8.1.

Box 8.1 **Assumption behind PMR**

Examine Table 8.1. How do the PMRs in the Indian ethnic group compare?

◆ What is the fundamental assumption that underpins valid comparisons between populations using PMRs?

◆ Were Marmot *et al.* correct in inferring that ischaemic heart disease was comparatively more common in the South Asian populations?

The magnitude of the PM depends not only on the number of deaths from the cause under study but also the number of deaths from other causes. In comparing PM between populations, therefore, differences might arise from either differences in the disease under study, or differences in other diseases. In South Asians, for example, cancers are less common than in the population as a whole, so the high PMR could be due to either a higher level of CHD or a lower rate of cancer. While the data in Table 8.1 favour the view that ischaemic heart disease is comparatively common in South Asians, the result is not conclusive (at least, on its own).

Table 8.1 PMR for ischaemic heart disease in male immigrants born in the Indian Subcontintent and the African New Commonwealth

	Observed deaths	PMR
Indian Subcontinent born		
Standard population		100
With Indian names, Indian ethnic origin	605	119
Without Indian names, 'British' ethnic origin	535	121
African New Commonwealth born		
With African names, African ethnic origin	28	56
With Indian names, Indian ethnic origin	23	120
With British names, British ethnic origin	39	84

Table developed from data in Marmot *et al.* (1984), p. 51—see Permissions.

The PMR can be considered as a preliminary, or corroborative, analysis tool. This is because its fundamental assumption, that the distribution of deaths from causes other than the one under study is the same in the two populations, is unlikely to hold. When it does the SMR (standardized mortality ratio) and the PMR are related, according to the formula given by Roman *et al.* (1984):

$$\text{SMR (for a specific cause)} = \frac{\text{All cause SMR} \times \text{PMR (for a specific cause)}}{100} \quad (8.4)$$

Clearly, proportional mortality is a simple and potentially useful way of portraying the burden of a specific disease within a population, and the PMR provides a way to compare populations. PMRs can be used to examine the association between an exposure and a cause of death. In our example of Marmot *et al.*'s study (Table 8.1), the exposure is South Asian ethnicity and cause of death CHD. The PMR then is one measure of the strength of the association, but for reasons already discussed in relation to the exercise in Box 8.1, a potentially flawed one.

8.3 Adjusted overall rates: standardization and the calculation of the SMR (Standardized mortality ratio)

When sound numerator and population denominator data are available, age and sex specific rates can be calculated and compared between times, places, and sub-populations (Chapter 7). These rates provide an undistorted view of the disease patterns in a population. Wherever possible, these rates should be presented.

Sometimes the numbers of study participants or study outcomes is small and age and sex specific rates are imprecise. The resulting data set may pose difficulties in interpretation. Age and sex specific tables are usually large and difficult to assimilate (e.g. Table 8.17). The obvious answer is to calculate a summary figure such as the overall (crude) rate.

For making comparisons of populations in comparative research, however, overall actual (crude) rates may mislead. The usual problem is that the age and sex structure of the compared populations differ, in other words age and sex are confounding variables. The simplest way to take this into account is to adjust (or standardize) the rates for age, sex or both, as discussed below. This is usual and good epidemiological practice. There are exceptions to this principle. Where the comparison populations are virtually identical in age and sex structure, age and sex adjustment will not alter the results. When age and sex differences in populations are potentially interesting or important explanatory factors for population disease patterns, rates should not be adjusted and age-specific and sex-specific data should be shown.

Adjusted rates have become the norm, but a warning is appropriate. The disadvantages of adjusted rates are substantial. As they are not true population based rates, they do not accurately measure the health status of a population, and resulting estimates of healthcare needs are wrong. For example, the age-adjusted rate for stroke in seaside resorts which attract the recently retired (such as Bournemouth), may be lower than in major commercial cities such as London but this is quite misleading. London's need for stroke services per unit of population is actually less than a place like Bournemouth's.

Summarizing a set of age-specific rates into one age-adjusted figure loses information, which is particularly important when differences are not consistent across age group or sex. For example, Table 8.2 shows that the overall SMR for lung cancer for women living near industry (zones ABC) was higher than in the control area (S). (Study details are in box 4.6.) The summary figure (SMR all ages) disguises the fact that mortality rates in the under 65 year olds were much higher in zones ABC while rates in over 75 year olds were actually lower in zones ABC than in zone S.

Where there are major differences in age and sex structure between populations, when adjustment is most needed, the method is least effective. These limitations also apply to the same population being compared at different time periods; for example, CHD in the USA in 1994 compared with 1940. Until recently USA CHD mortality data

Table 8.2 Standardized mortality ratios for lung cancer in women at all ages and by age group in larger zones[1] (ABC) compared with an area in Sunderland (S)

Population women (census 1991)	ABC 40332		S 22321	
	SMR	N	SMR	N
All ages	217	288	173	152
0–64	287	136	170	55
65–74	190	98	165	56
75+	161	54	192	41

[1] Standardized to England Wales population with 5 year age groupings, N = observed number of deaths; SMR = standardized mortality ratios. Adapted from Pless-Mulloli et al. (1998), Environmental Health Perspectives **106**, 189–96—see Permissions.

were adjusted using the 1940 age structure, but for the 1996 analysis the population structure of the year 2000 was used. The calculation based on the 1940 structure gave a rate of 86.7/100 000, compared with 187.1/100 000 using the 2000 structure (the explanation for this extraordinary result is given below).

Before reading on do the exercise in Box 8.2, based on Table 8.3.

Box 8.2 **Interpreting age-specific and actual overall (crude) rates**

Consider the age-specific and actual overall rates in Table 8.3. Comment on the age structure, and the effect this has on the overall rate, which varies in populations A, B and C. Why does this effect occur?

Table 8.3 shows three populations with radically different age structures. Population A is not untypical of industrialized countries, with similar numbers of people in the three decades. Population B is clearly an unnatural age structure. This could be the age structure of hospital specialist doctors, or university academic staff. This could also be the age structure in the aftermath of war, decimation by a disease such as AIDS or the result of the major industry closing down, for example, in a mining town, leading to

Table 8.3 Age-specific and overall (crude) rates in three populations of varying size

Age group	Population size	Cases	Rate (as %)
Population A			
21–30	1000	50	5
31–40	1000	100	10
41–50	1000	150	15
Actual overall rate	3000	300	10
Population B			
21–30	500	25	5
31–40	1500	150	10
41–50	3000	450	15
Actual overall rate	5000	625	12.5
Population C			
21–30	5000	250	5
31–40	1000	100	10
41–50	200	30	15
Actual overall rate	6200	380	6.1

emigration of the young. Population C is also unnatural in structure. It could be the population of soldiers, university students, doctors in the training grades, or the population in a new suburb with low cost homes for families.

The age-specific rates show that the disease rates are identical in the three populations and that they rise with age. The actual overall (crude) rates differ markedly. Why? Population B has high overall rates because it has a comparatively older population. The larger number of older people is weighting (exerting influence upon) the summary figure. In effect, the size of the population in each age group provides a set of weights that are applied to the overall rates. While the actual overall rates are accurately describing the disease experience in each of the three populations, the comparison of the overall rates is misleading us into thinking there are differences, because the weights exerted by the population structure differ. These differential weights cause confounding. Age is, here, the confounding factor.

There are two main techniques for standardizing the rates to nullify the effects of the differing age structures and make overall comparisons possible—direct and indirect. In the direct method the age-specific rates from the study population are applied to a standard population structure. Table 8.4 shows the results of doing this with a relatively young (a) and relatively old (b) population as the standard. Before reading on, reflect on the exercise in Box 8.3.

Table 8.4 Standardize with the direct method: effect of young and old standard populations

Standard population	Population size	Applying age-specific rates from Table 8.3 to standard population: cases expected		
		Population A	Population B	Population C
(a) A young population (age group)				
21–30	3000	150*	150	150
31–40	1500	150	150	150
41–50	500	75	75	75
Overall	5000	375	375	375
Overall standard rate = 375/5000 = 7.5%				
(b) An older population (age group)				
21–30	200	10	10	10
31–40	1000	100	100	100
41–50	5000	750	750	750
Overall	6200	860	860	860
Overall standardized adjusted rate = 860/6200 = 139/1000 = 13.9%				

* Example: from Table 8.3 we see that the rate in the age group 21–30 in populations A, B, and C is 5%. In the young standard population (a) there are 3000 people. We expect, therefore, that 5% of them will develop the disease, i.e. 150 people.

Box 8.3 **Effect of directly standardizing on overall rates**

Consider the age structures of the standard populations, and the age-specific and overall rates in Table 8.4. What is the relationship between the overall standardized rates in Table 8.4 and those in Table 8.3? Why are the overall rates now the same in populations A, B and C? What is the influence of a relatively young and relatively old standard population?

Whichever standard population is used, young (a) or old (b), the identical age-specific rates in populations A, B and C obtained from Table 8.3 lead to the same number of cases expected in Table 8.4 and, therefore, an identical overall (standardized) rate. Here the standard population structure supplies the weights and these are, therefore, the same in all comparison groups. The use of a young standard leads to a low standardized rate (7.5 per cent), and an old standard to a high rate (13.9 per cent). (This explains why the standardized rate of CHD in the USA rose greatly when a modern, older age structure replaced the younger, 1940 age structure.) The problem is that the overall result of 7.5 per cent in Table 8.4 is not real, and differs from all the overall rates in Table 8.3.

The second approach is called indirect standardization. Here, the standard population supplies disease rates, not population structure. These rates are applied to the study population structure to answer the question: how many cases would have occurred if the study population had the same rates as the standard population? The observed figure is divided by the expected cases. This resulting figure is the standardized morbidity (or mortality) ratio and is usually expressed as a percentage. Table 8.5(a) shows a set of rates in the standard population, and these are high, while those in 8.5(b) are low. The overall rates (Table 8.3) and standardized rates in the three populations A, B and C differ. Why? Because the standard rates are weighted differentially by the different population structures. Here the population structures from populations A, B and C are weighting the standard rates.

Rates adjusted by the indirect method are weighted (or biased) in relation to the age and sex structure of the population under study. The summary output from such adjustment is the SMR. This means that SMRs from several study populations cannot be compared with each other. Only SMR comparisons between the study population and the chosen standard population are valid. This principle is usually breached. Where comparisons are to be made between several populations, strictly, either specific rates, or those adjusted by the direct method should be examined.

8.4 **Relative measure: relative risk**

The incidence rate (cumulative) is the prime measure of risk in epidemiology. To see how the risk varies between populations (say, those with and without a particular risk factor) the incidence rates (age-specific, overall, or standardized) can simply be compared. Alternatively, we can calculate the relative risk (Table 8.6) which is the ratio of

Table 8.5(a) Standardization with the indirect method

Standard population (high rates)

Age group	Population	Cases	Rate (%)
21–30	40 000	4000	10
31–40	50 000	7500	15
41–50	60 000	12 000	20
Total	150 000	23 500	15.7

	Population A		Population B		Population C	
	Population	Cases expected	Population	Cases expected	Population	Cases expected
21–30	1000	100	500	50	5000	500
31–40	1000	150	1500	225	1000	150
41–50	1000	200	3000	600	200	40
Total	3000	450	5000	875	6200	690
Overall rate (standardized)	15%		17.5%		11.1%	
Observed*/expected (standardized morbidity/ mortality ratio, SMR)	$\frac{300}{450} = 66\%$		$\frac{625}{875} = 71\%$		$\frac{380}{690} = 55.1\%$	

* Observed from Table 8.3—no. of cases in total

Table 8.5(b) Standardization with the indirect method

Standard population (low rates)

Age group	Population	Cases	Rate (%)
21–30	40 000	2000	5
31–40	50 000	3750	7.5
41–50	60 000	6000	10
Total	150 000	11 500	7.7

	Population A		Population B		Population C	
	Population	Cases expected	Population	Cases expected	Population	Cases expected
21–30	1000	50	500	25	5000	250
31–40	1000	75	1500	113	1000	75
41–50	1000	100	3000	300	200	20
Total	3000	225	5000	438	6200	345
Overall rate (standardized)	7.5%		8.8%		5.6%	
Observed*/expected (standardized morbidity/ mortality ratio, SMR)	$\frac{300}{225} = 133\%$		$\frac{625}{438} = 143\%$		$\frac{380}{345} = 110\%$	

* observed from Table 8.3—no. of cases in total

Table 8.6 Incidence rate, relative risk (RR), odds ratio (OR), and 2 × 2 tables

Risk factor/exposure	Clinical outcome		Total
	Diseased	**Not diseased**	
Present (exposed)	a	b	a + b
Absent (not exposed)	c	d	c + d
Total	a + c	b + d	a + b + c + d

(a) Incidence in those with the risk factor = a/a+b. (With the baseline population as the denominator.)

Incidence in those without the risk factor = c/c+d.

(b) $RR = \dfrac{\text{incidence in those with risk factor}}{\text{incidence in those without risk factor}} = (a/a + b)/(c/c + d)$.

(c) $OR = \text{cross product ratio} = \dfrac{a \times d}{c \times b}$.

two incidence rates: that in the population of interest divided by the rate in a comparison (or control or reference) population. (When the incidence rates are based on the person-time denominator the ratio is sometimes named the rate ratio.) The term is derived from the fact that we are relating the risk of disease in those with the risk factor to those without. The relative risk is the most important summary measure of the size of the effect of the risk factor on disease rates and, hence, the strength of the association in epidemiology. The formula for relative risk based on cumulative incidence rates is simple (see Table 8.6), but the interpretation is not.

The relative risk (RR) can be calculated from all studies providing incidence data: cohort studies, disease register studies with valid estimates of the denominator, trials and (most exceptionally) cross-sectional surveys (see Chapter 9). The RR can never be calculated from case-control studies which do not give incidence data, though, as discussed in Section 8.5, in some circumstances the odds ratio calculated from such a study provides an acceptable estimate of the relative risk. Before interpreting any relative risk always critically review the underlying data to judge the likelihood and extent of error and bias. Before reading on do the exercise in Box 8.4.

Box 8.4 **False estimates of relative risk**

Consider why the relative risk might provide a false picture of the effect of the risk factor on disease and hence strength of the association.

The problems lie in the measurement of disease incidence (Chapter 7). Differences between populations may reflect differences in the accuracy with which the diagnosis is made (numerator inaccuracy) or the population counted (denominator inaccuracy). For example, young people are less likely to consult for medical care, are more likely to be undercounted at census, and most likely to be lost to follow-up or be a non-responder in surveys. A different incidence of a disease in 15–24 year olds, compared to 25–34 year olds, may reflect such factors, rather than, say, effect of age. The time periods for the measurements of incidence need to be comparable to avoid spurious differences arising from time trends. Data are often collected for large areas and presented for small areas. This process may create errors by incorrectly attributing cases and population at risk to the smaller areas. These and other factors need to be checked before calculating and interpreting relative risk. Now do the exercise in Box 8.5 before reading on.

Box 8.5 **Calculating and interpreting relative risk**

Imagine that the incidence of lung cancer is compared in two cities, one with polluted air (A), the other not (B). In the polluted city there were 20 cases in a population of 100 000; in the other city 10 cases in a population of 100 000. Assume accuracy in the numerators and denominators.

◆ What is the relative risk of lung cancer in the polluted city (A)?

◆ What is the relative risk of lung cancer in the less polluted city (B)?

◆ Do we know the precision of this estimate of relative risk?

◆ What explanations are there for the higher relative risk in the polluted city?

◆ What questions will you consider before concluding that there is a real association between pollution and lung cancer?

The relative risk of lung cancer in the polluted city is:

$$\frac{\text{incidence in A}}{\text{incidence in B}} = \frac{20/100\ 000}{10/100\ 000} = \frac{20}{10} = 2 \tag{8.5}$$

The relative risk of lung cancer in city B compared with A is:

$$\frac{\text{incidence in B}}{\text{incidence in A}} = \frac{10/100\ 000}{20/100\ 000} = \frac{10}{20} = 0.50 \tag{8.6}$$

We do not know the precision of the estimate but it can be assessed by calculating confidence intervals around the point estimate (the student should consult a statistics textbook on how to do this).

The obvious explanation is that the pollution in town A causes lung cancer, and doubles the risk. Before reaching this conclusion, however, the investigator needs to ask questions such as these:

◆ Is the age distribution of the populations being compared similar? As lung cancer is more common in older people it may be that town A has more older people. The solutions to this potential problem are to base relative risk calculations on age-specific rates or use age standardized rates (Section 8.3).

◆ Are the prevalences of the known causal and protective factors for lung cancer different in town A from those in town B? If town A has a higher prevalence of smoking or other causal factors (or less exposure to protective factors such as antioxidants) then the increased relative risk may not be attributable to pollution. The solution is to do prevalence studies in cities A and B on the major causal factors.

◆ Were the risk exposure patterns several decades ago, when the disease was induced, similar to those in the present? (Data on exposure patterns in the distant past may not be available.)

◆ Were there differences in health care in the two cities?

Healthcare differences between towns A and B are unlikely to explain the differences in lung cancer incidence, though tobacco and pollution control campaigns in town B may have been more effective than in town A. If the study had been of lung cancer mortality, however, differences in diagnostic acumen leading to earlier detection of disease in town B, or better and more effective treatment in town B, are potential explanations. Equally, if the cancer under study were breast cancer or cervical cancer, then a higher quality of the screening programme in town B would be a potential explanation for differences in both incidence and mortality.

Once these explanations are considered and due adjustments to the RR made, the investigator can consider the relative risk as a fair measure of the strength of the association and can apply frameworks for causal thinking to judge whether pollution is the probable cause of the higher relative risk in town A (see Chapter 5). The methods by which adjustments to the RR are made, except for age and sex by standardization of the incidence rates as already discussed, are beyond the scope of this book.

8.5 **The odds ratio (OR)**

The odds ratio is a popular measure of association in current epidemiological practice. The term odds ratio is an apt description for it is simply one set of odds divided by another. The odds are the chances in favour of one side in relation to the second side. In the epidemiological context, the odds are the chances of being exposed (or diseased) as opposed to not being exposed (or diseased). In a standard 2×2 table (Table 8.6) the odds of exposure to the risk factor for the group with the disease are then $a \div c$ and for the group without disease, $b \div d$. The odds ratio for exposure is simply the odds $a \div c$ divided by the odds $b \div d$. Similarly, the odds of disease in those exposed to the risk factor are $a \div b$, and for those not exposed, $c \div d$.

These formulae can be expressed as:

$$\text{Exposure odds ratio} = \frac{a}{c} \div \frac{b}{d} \quad \text{and,} \quad \text{disease odds ratio} = \frac{a}{b} \div \frac{c}{d} \quad (8.7)$$

Arithmetically, it is usually easier to multiply than divide, so to simplify this formula we use the arithmetical rule that division by a fraction is equivalent to multiplication by the inverse of the fraction; for example, division by 1/3 equals multiplication by 3/1. So, the odds ratio can be expressed as:

$$\text{Exposure odds ratio} \frac{a}{c} \times \frac{d}{b} \quad \text{and} \quad \text{for disease odds ratio} = \frac{a}{b} \times \frac{d}{c} \quad (8.8)$$

This eqn (8.8), usually expressed as '$\frac{a \times d}{b \times c}$' is known as the cross-product ratio. It is exactly the same for exposure and disease. As it is so easy it has become the standard way of calculating the odds ratio. Product is another word for multiplication, so the phrase cross-product ratio is descriptive of the diagonal direction of the multiplication in a 2×2 table (table 8.6).

The drawback of the cross-product ratio is that the epidemiological idea behind the use of the odds ratio is lost. The epidemiological idea is a simple one: if a disease is causally associated with an exposure, then the odds of exposure in the diseased group will be higher than the corresponding odds in the non-diseased group. If there is no association, the odds ratio will be one. If the exposure is protective against disease, the odds ratio will be less than one. This idea fits in with the basic question behind a case-control study (Chapter 9). For a cohort study (see Chapter 9) the corresponding idea is that if an exposure is associated with a disease then the odds of disease in the exposed group will be higher than in the non-exposed group.

The odds ratio is a means of summarizing and quantifying these differences, just as a relative risk provided a way of summarizing differences in incidence rates. Before reading on, do the exercise in Box 8.6.

Box 8.6 **Disease, relative risk, and odds ratios**

Imagine that a disease is caused by lack of exercise (called exposure). You compare the exercise habits of 1000 cases of this disease with 1000 similar people who are disease free. You set out your data as in Table 8.6. Which group will have the higher odds of not taking exercise? Will the odds ratio be more or less than one? Can you calculate the relative risk in this example?

Now, imagine you follow up 1000 people over time who do take exercise and 1000 who do not and count the number of cases over time. Which group will have the higher odds of becoming diseased? Can you calculate the relative risk in this example? In these two examples in what circumstances will the OR approximate the RR? Why? Based on Table 8.6, try to figure this out for yourself before reading on.

If a disease is caused by an exposure the cases of the disease will have more exposure than controls, so in the first study in Box 8.6 (a case-control study) the odds of exposure to the risk factor, lack of exercise, will be higher in cases and the odds ratio will exceed 1. In the first study the relative risk cannot be calculated because we have no incidence data. In the second study, which is a cohort study, the exercise group will have the lower odds of disease. This study will provide incidence data, so relative risk can be calculated.

In the second study, for both the odds ratio and the relative risk the numerators (a, and c, as in Table 8.6) are identical. The denominators are different, that is, b and d, respectively, in the odds ratio, and $a + b$ and $c + d$, respectively, in the relative risk. When b is similar to $a + b$, and d is similar to $c + d$, the odds ratio and relative risk will be similar. This happens when the disease is rare, that is, when a and c are small in relation to b and d. Before reading on do the exercise in Box 8.7.

Box 8.7 **Calculating odds ratios**

A study of a disease compared cases with non-cases, and found that 25/100 cases took no exercise compared with 10/100 of the non-cases.

+ Develop a 2 × 2 table to display the data.

+ Calculate the odds of exposure in cases and non-cases.

+ Calculate the odds ratio using eqns (8.7) and (8.8) given earlier.

+ How does the difference between the two prevalences of exercise (25 per cent vs. 10 per cent) compare with the odds ratio?

+ Which is the more accurate way of assessing the differences between the two groups, the odds ratio or the comparison of prevalences?

+ Which gives the better feel for the degree of association between the disease and exposure, prevalence rate ratio or odds ratio?

Table 8.7 shows the data and the results for the calculation of odds ratios for the exercise in Box 8.7. The first calculation (exposure odds) follows the epidemiological logic, but it gives the same answer as the alternative formula which is easier to calculate.

Table 8.7 Odds ratio relating to Box 8.7

Risk factor/exposure	Disease group	
	Case	**Control**
No exercise	25(a)	10(b)
Exercise	75(c)	90(d)

The odds of exposure in:
case group: $a \div c = 25 \div 75 = 1/3$;
control group: $b \div d = 10 \div 90 = 1/9$.
The odds ratio:

$$OR = \frac{a \div c}{b \div d} = \frac{25 \div 75}{10 \div 90} = \frac{1/3}{1/9} = 3.0 \ (= \text{exposure odds}).$$

$$OR = \frac{a \div c}{b \div d} = (a \div b) \times (d \div c) = \frac{a \times d}{b \times c} = \frac{25 \times 90}{10 \times 75} = \frac{2250}{750} = 3.0$$

(=cross-product ratio).

In epidemiology one of the key goals is to compare the health experience of one group with another, so our measures should give a feel for the degree of difference between groups. Here we see a 2.5 fold difference in the prevalence rate (25 per cent vs. 10 per cent) change to a threefold difference in odds ratio. Clearly, the two approaches are giving different results. Before reading on, try the exercise in Box 8.8.

Box 8.8 **Varying prevalence of exposure: impact on odds ratio and its validity as an indicator of differences between populations**

- What happens to the difference between the picture provided by the prevalence rate ratio and the odds ratio if the percentages exposed in the disease group were 15 per cent and in the control group 6 per cent (scenario 1)?

- What happens if the percentages were 50 per cent in the diseased group and 20 per cent in the control group (scenario 2)? In both these scenarios, as in Box 8.7, the prevalence in the disease group is 2.5 times that in the control group.

Table 8.8 Odds ratios in relation to exercise in Box 8.8: effect of changing prevalence

	Case	Control
Scenario 1		
No exercise	15	6
Exercise	85	94

$$OR = \frac{15 \times 94}{85 \times 6} = \frac{1410}{510} = 2.76$$

	Case	Control
Scenario 2		
No exercise	50	20
Exercise	50	80

$$OR = \frac{50 \times 80}{50 \times 20} = \frac{4000}{1000} = 4.0$$

The odds ratio approximates the prevalence rate ratio when the exposure is infrequent, but not when it is common as shown in Table 8.8. When $a:c$ is similar to $a/a+c$ (prevalence) and $c:d$ is similar to $c/d+c$ (prevalence) the odds ratio and prevalence rate ratio approximate each other. This happens when the prevalence is low. Before reading on do the exercise in Box 8.9 which concerns incidence.

The results are given in Table 8.9. The odds ratio is higher than the relative risk in both instances, and is greater when the disease incidence is higher (in people with diabetes). In cohort studies, the odds ratio best corresponds to relative risk when the disease incidence is low (which is often the case over short-term follow-up).

The odds ratio is an extremely popular summary measure in epidemiology despite its disadvantages, for three main reasons. First, in several study designs it approximates well to the relative measures of prevalence rate ratio and relative risk in some circumstances so provides an alternative measure of association. Second, in case-control studies where relative risk cannot be calculated, it provides an estimate of this. Third, the odds have desirable mathematical properties permitting easy manipulation

Box 8.9 **Effect of changing incidence on OR**

Imagine that an exposure to a causal factor triples the incidence of a disease, that is, the relative risk is three. This disease has a baseline incidence of 1 per cent per year (in the non-exposed group). Imagine also that the baseline incidence is double in people with diabetes, that is, 2 per cent, and that the relative risk associated with exposure is the same, 3. You follow up 100 non-diabetic and 100 diabetic subjects with the exposure, and an equivalent number without the exposure. The study lasts 5 years. Work with 5-year cumulative incidence and a denominator of 100.

Create two 2 × 2 tables to show the data for diabetics and non-diabetics and calculate the OR of disease in the exposed group in relation to those not exposed. Compare the odds ratio with the RR of 3.

Table 8.9 Relative risk and odds ratios associated with an exposure in people with and without diabetes: annual disease incidence at baseline = 1% and RR = 3 (5-year follow-up)

	Not diabetic		People with diabetes	
	Diseased	**Not diseased**	**Diseased**	**Not diseased**
Exposed	15	85	30	70
Not exposed	5	95	10	90
	$RR = \dfrac{15/100}{5/100} = 3.00$		$RR = \dfrac{30/100}{10/100} = 3.00$	
	$OR = \dfrac{15/85}{5/95} = \dfrac{15 \times 95}{5 \times 85} = 3.35$		$OR = \dfrac{30/70}{10/90} = \dfrac{30 \times 90}{10 \times 70} = 3.86$	

in mathematical models and statistical computations, as, for example, in multiple logistic regression. For example, in epidemiology we are usually focused on the disease or other adverse outcome. If, however, non-occurrence of disease is of equal interest the OR provides a symmetrical result while the RR does not as shown below.

From the preceding data on people without diabetes in Table 8.9 the RR for being diseased is:

$$\frac{a}{a+b} \div \frac{c}{c+d} = 3.00 \tag{8.9}$$

The RR for not being diseased is:

$$\frac{b}{a+b} \div \frac{d}{c+d} = \frac{85/100}{95/100} = 0.89 \tag{8.10}$$

The relative risk of not being diseased (0.89) is not reciprocal of 3, which is 1/3.

The OR for being diseased is 3.35 and the OR for not being diseased is:

$$\frac{85 \times 5}{95 \times 15} = \frac{425}{1425} = 0.298 \tag{8.11}$$

This odds ratio (0.298) is the reciprocal of 3.35. The OR has this arithmetical advantage. The odds ratio, of course, is also an independent measure of association.

There is a vigorous debate on the merits and problems with odds ratios. Epidemiologists need to be aware that misinterpretation of the odds ratio is common, so care is needed when reading papers reporting it. Many writers, wrongly, treat the odds ratio as if it were a true measure of risk. Statistical packages may label the output of odds ratio analysis as relative risk, creating a trap for the unwary investigator and reader. Some researchers, wrongly, use relative risk as a general term for any summary measure of comparison between groups.

Odds ratios give a fair estimate of the following:

♦ The prevalence rate ratio when the prevalence of exposure is low.

♦ Relative risk in a cohort study when the disease incidence is low in the control group, usually taken as less than 10–20 per cent, which is usually true for specific causes, except in long-term studies.

♦ The relative risk in a case-control study when the exposure in the control group represents the population from which cases derive (and, in some designs, when the disease is care). (See also p. 250).

As with relative risk the OR only makes sense if the study is well executed and can be related to a population.

These conditions are sometimes not met. The odds ratio must be interpreted with care.

Odds ratios are not comparable across times, populations and between places if the exposure levels and incidence rates differ substantially. If we are interested, for example, in the dimension of the association between smoking and lung cancer in men and women, the odds ratios are not comparable across sexes if the underlying smoking prevalence differs in men and women. The odds ratio from a study done in London is likely to differ from one in Tokyo simply because the exposure status in the control group differs even when the relative risk is identical (the point is illustrated in table 8.9).

Prevalence rate ratio and RR are stable and independent of either exposure or incidence levels but the odds are not. While it is true that the incidence of most diseases is rare, it does not apply to long-term cohort studies, especially in people with concomitant disease that increases the risk. The implications of this are often ignored. While the relative risk is virtually never calculated in cross-sectional studies for its association with incidence data (rarely available from cross-sectional studies) is strong, the odds ratio often is (in preference to the prevalence rate ratio). In these circumstances its interpretation as an estimate of relative risk is erroneous. As a measure of association, and an alternative to the prevalence rate ratio, it has the disadvantages demonstrated above. In cross-sectional studies the prevalence of exposures is usually high (and the prevalence of disease is sometimes so) and the odds ratio may be a poor estimator of prevalence rate ratio. The error in interpretation is often important. Ease of calculation of the odds ratio should not override its limitations.

8.6 Measurements to assess the impact of a risk factor in groups and populations

As discussed in Chapter 5 knowledge of the causes of diseases is the surest route to their prevention and control. In a few diseases there is a unique, known causal factor, for example, nutritional disorders such as scurvy, infections such as measles, and environmental diseases such as asbestosis. All cases of such diseases are attributable, by definition, to one cause. By removing asbestos from the environment we can eliminate asbestosis, and by removing the measles virus we eliminate all measles. Cases of diseases that clinically mimic scurvy, asbestosis, and measles will, by definition, be a result of different causes and be different diseases. Often, however, removal of the causes is impossible because we do not know what they are, or removing them is too difficult or costly or the causes are multiple and complex.

Indirect methods to estimate the effect of reducing the causal factor may therefore be needed. For example, the organisms causing Legionnaires' disease cannot be eliminated so we may attack them by methods such as maintaining hot water supplies at temperatures that prevent bacterial growth, disinfecting water systems, cleaning equipment and plant, re-engineering water systems, and even by encouraging the population not to smoke. For some chronic diseases there are several risk factors, for example, stroke, ischaemic heart disease, and cancers such as those of the breast and the colorectal tract. The problem that now arises is choosing between alternative actions for there is limited time, money, energy, and expertise. There is also uncertainty about the benefits and costs of alternative actions. We need ways of helping to make choices by predicting the possible consequences. Attributable risk provides a way of developing the epidemiological basis for such decisions. An extension of the concept—population attributable risk—is discussed in Section 8.6.2. Attributable fraction/proportion and population attributable fraction/population are among several synonyms for this concept.

Before reading on reflect on the exercise in Box 8.10.

Box 8.10 **Epidemiological information to choose between priorities**

Several hundred factors have been associated with coronary heart disease. That said, the following modifiable risk factors have been established as important:

- high levels of some lipids in the blood, particularly low density lipoprotein (LDL) cholesterol;
- high blood pressure;
- smoking;
- low levels of physical activity;
- obesity;
- diabetes.

Imagine that there are insufficient resources to tackle all six of these risk factors. What epidemiological information would help us to choose between them to reduce coronary heart disease in a population?

Some of our information needs are as follows:

♦ Solid evidence that each of these risk factors is a component of the causal pathway and not merely artefactually or statistically associated with the disease. Such data usually comes from case-control studies, cohort studies, and trials (Chapter 9), together with supporting information from the laboratory and clinical sciences, to provide understanding of the biological basis of the disease. We need to specify the causal model we are using to judge the evidence (Chapter 5).

♦ Knowledge of the frequency of each risk factor in the population (Chapter 7). If a risk factor is rare then action to reduce it will have little effect on the incidence of the disease in the population. In devising a strategy for controlling coronary heart disease, for example, diabetes will be a more important risk-factor in South Asian and Afro-Caribbean populations than in European origin populations, simply because diabetes is about three to four times more common in these populations.

♦ A precise estimate of the additional risk that each risk factor imposes on our population. If the relative risk of CHD among those with diabetes was 1.1 (a 10 per cent increase) the impact of controlling diabetes would be much smaller than if the RR was 3 (a 200 per cent increase).

♦ An understanding of the actions that are (or might be) effective in reducing the prevalence of the risk factor and their costs (this latter subject, health economics, is beyond the scope of this book).

♦ Assuming success in reducing the prevalence of the risk factor, the reduction in disease outcome (attributable risk). The formulae to calculate attributable risks are shown in Tables 8.10 and 8.11 and are discussed in Sections 8.6.1 and 8.6.2.

Table 8.10 Formulae for attributable risk (synonym: attributable fraction)

Attributable risk (AR) answers the question: What proportion of the risk in those *exposed* is attributable to risk factor X?

$$AR = \frac{\text{Risk in exposed} - \text{background risk}}{\text{Risk in exposed}} \qquad \text{(eqn 1)}$$

$$= \frac{\text{Incidence in exposed } (I_e) - \text{Incidence in unexposed } (I_u)}{\text{Incidence in exposed } (I_e)} = \frac{I_e - I_u}{I_e} \qquad \text{(eqn 2)}$$

$$= \frac{RR_e - RR_u}{RR_e} \qquad \text{(eqn 3)}$$

$$= \frac{RR - 1}{RR} \qquad \text{(eqn 4)}$$

RR can sometimes be estimated by $OR = \dfrac{OR - 1}{OR}$ $\qquad$ (eqn 5)

To express AR as a percentage we multiple by 100

Abbreviations: AR = attributable risk; RR = relative risk; I = incidence; e = exposed; u = unexposed; OR = odds ratio.

Table 8.11 Formulae for population attributable risk (PAR) (Synonym: population attributable fraction)

PAR answers the question: What proportion of the incidence in the population as a whole is attributable to risk factor X?

$$PAR = \frac{\text{Risk in total population} - \text{Risk in unexposed population}}{\text{Risk in total population}} \qquad \text{(eqn 1)}$$

$$= \frac{\text{Incidence in total population} - \text{Incidence in unexposed population}}{\text{Incidence in total population}} = \frac{I_p - I_u}{I_p} \qquad \text{(eqn 2)}$$

or an alternative formula based on relative risk and prevalence data

$$PAR = \frac{P_e(RR - 1)}{1 + P_e(RR - 1)} \qquad \text{(eqn 3)}$$

or an alternative formula based on odds ratio and prevalence data $= \dfrac{P_e(OR - 1)}{1 + P_e(OR - 1)}$ (eqn 4)

Abbreviations: I = incidence; p = population; u = unexposed population; e = exposed; P = Prevalence of risk factor (P_e = proportion of population exposed); RR = Relative risk; OR = odds ratio.

8.6.1 Attributable risk/exposed group

The question being answered by attributable risk is—how many cases would not have occurred if a particular risk factor had not been present? Another way of framing the same question is, what proportion of disease incidence in those exposed to the risk factor is attributable to that particular risk factor? Finally, in shorthand, what is the attributable risk associated with a risk factor? The answer is conceptually simple: from the total number of cases, subtract the number that would have occurred anyway, even if the cases had not had the risk factor. This number can never be known as a fact, but it can be estimated from the control, or unexposed, group. These 'excess' cases represent those attributable to the risk factor. It is more elegant to express this excess risk as a percentage. Table 8.10 shows five formulae (these are easy to understand when applied to a practical example, as will be done below). In eqn 1 the background risk (estimated from the control group) is subtracted from the risk in the exposed (study) group and expressed as a fraction of the risk in the exposed group. The difference in the two risks is the excess risk. Equation 2 simply substitutes incidence rates for risk.

Attributable risk (AR) is, therefore, the excess risk expressed as a fraction of total risk in the exposed group. The excess risk can also be derived as the relative risk in the exposed group minus the relative risk in the unexposed group which is, by definition, 1 (eqn 3 and 4). The total risk in this exposed group is simply the relative risk. The benefit of this formula is that when the odds ratio is an accurate estimate of RR, it can be used to provide AR even without incidence data (eqn 5).

Before reading on do the exercise in Box 8.11.

Box 8.11 Calculating attributable risk

From Table 8.12, calculate the attributable risk associated with smoking based on eqn (2) and (4) given in Table 8.10. Now do the same for smoking and coronary heart disease.

Table 8.12 Relative, excess, and attributable: study of lung cancer and coronary heart disease in heavy smokers and non-smokers. See base of page for calculation

	Annual death rates per 100 000	
	Lung cancer	**Coronary heart disease**
Heavy smokers	166	599
Non-smokers	7	422

Adapted from Mausner and Bahn (p. 170); original data from Doll and Hill 1956. *British Medical Journal* (1956), pp. 1071–1081, with permission from the BMJ Publishing Group.

So, from the cohort study data in Table 8.12, among heavy smokers the excess risk of lung cancer associated with smoking is $166-7 = 159/100\,000$ persons annually. We can express this as attributable risk by using eqn 2 in Table 8.10 with the total rate as the denominator, and the excess risk in the exposed group as the numerator, as shown in the table ($159/166 \times 100 = 95.8$ per cent). This percentage is identical to that obtained using relative risk (eqn 4 in Table 8.10).

We are claiming, therefore, that among heavy smokers 95.8 per cent of the lung cancer cases were attributable to smoking. By implication, if the cause could be removed, in heavy smokers the disease would be reduced by up to 95.8 per cent and 159 lives would be saved per 100 000 of the population of heavy smokers. The attributable risk for CHD was 29.5 per cent.

It is worth noting that the excess risk is dependent on the actual incidence rate. Table 8.12 shows that even though the relative risk of coronary heart disease in heavy smokers was 1.4, the excess risk of deaths (177) was greater than that for lung cancer (159), where the relative risk was 23.7. The public health impact of stopping smoking is potentially even greater via CHD prevention than with lung cancer prevention.

Since the removal of the cause may arise from preventive health programmes, attributable risk is an indication of their potential benefits. The concept of attributable risk is, potentially, a powerful tool in public health practice but we should critically appraise the underlying assumptions.

The first and foremost assumption is that the risk factor is a causal one. If not, the calculation of attributable risk is merely an arithmetical exercise, which makes false

Table 8.12 (*continued*)

	Annual death rates per 100 000	
	Lung cancer	**Coronary heart disease**
Relative risk (RR)	23.7	1.4
Excess risk for smoking based on incidence formula	$166 - 7 = 159$	$599 - 422 = 177$
Attributable risk given as a percentage of all risk; based on incidence	$\dfrac{159}{166} = 95.8\%$	$\dfrac{177}{599} = 29.5\%$
Attributable risk based on relative risk formula given as a percentage; based on RR	$\dfrac{23.7 - 1}{23.7} = 95.8\%$	$\dfrac{1.42 - 1}{1.42} = 29.5\%$

promises. (At best, the calculation then answers the question: if the associations turn out to be causal, what will be the attributable risk?) The second assumption is that the incidence data apply elsewhere to other populations. It may be that in other populations the relative risk is the same, but the incidence in the unexposed population is lower, say 3.5 per 100 000. Then, the incidence in the exposed populations would be 83 per 100 000 (3.5 × 23. 7, i.e. baseline incidence times relative risk), and the excess risk 79.5 per 100 000. When expressed as a percentage, the attributable risk would remain at 95.8 per cent, but the potential for lives saved by the intervention is substantially less at 79.5 lives per 100 000 of the population.

The third assumption is that the study is valid and accurate. The true incidence rates and relative risk may not be the same as the point estimates, so allowance needs to be made in calculating attributable risk. The precision of these estimates can be reflected in confidence intervals. So it may behove planners to use various incidence rates and relative risks within the range given by the confidence intervals.

There is also a need to understand the underlying natural history of disease and causal model. How does smoking operate as a carcinogen? What are the causal mechanisms? Is there a threshold effect? Will smokers personally benefit from stopping or has the carcinogenic damage been done already? Without this understanding we cannot properly interpret the attributable risk or offer rational advice to smokers. If the damage is irreversible, the potential lives saved according to the attributable risk may not be achievable and public health efforts might concentrate on preventing children taking up smoking. If the damaging effects are reversible then smoking cessation is a higher priority. (The latter is the case.)

Another important consideration is whether smoking interacts with other factors to cause lung cancer or whether it acts alone. If it acts alone then an intervention to reduce smoking will achieve the promise indicated by the attributable risk. If, however, there are other interacting factors the effect may be greater or less than predicted. To take a well-known example, smoking and asbestos interact in the causation of lung cancer and increase the incidence rate greatly. Stopping smoking in a community of shipbuilders previously exposed to asbestos may yield benefits far greater than predicted from a study based on British doctors.

8.6.2 **Population attributable risk**

From a public health perspective we are interested in the benefits of an intervention both to the exposed group and to the whole community. The question of interest to the whole community is, what proportion of the disease experience in the population (not just the exposed population) is attributable to a particular exposure? This clearly depends on how common the exposure is. If a community had no or very little exposure to smoking, as in Sikh women living in the Punjab, India, then cases of lung cancer in that population must be caused mainly, if not wholly, by other factors.

The measure that answers this question is known as the population attributable risk (or fraction or proportion). The formulae are in Table 8.11 on p. 210. Essentially, eqns (1) and (2) are similar to that for attributable risk except that the risk or incidence is not in the exposed group but in the entire population (or a random sample of the population). As such studies are rare, population attributable risk is often calculated by combining data from representative cross-sectional studies providing prevalence of exposures and relative risks from cohort studies usually from selected populations as in eqn (3) and its equivalent for odds ratios (eqn (4)). The attributable risk is, effectively, being weighted by the prevalence of the exposure in eqns (3) and (4).

Population attributable risk can overturn perceptions and conclusions derived from studying relative risks. The population attributable risk rises as the excess risk, the relative risk, and the prevalence of exposure rise. In contrast, relative risk is unaffected by change in prevalence of exposure.

The population attributable risk can help to answer questions such as: if a choice needs to be made on which exposure to reduce, which will have the bigger impact on disease incidence? Try the exercise in Box 8.12.

Box 8.12 **Choosing between options for public health campaigns**

Let us say that a sum of £100 000 is available for a health promotion programme to reduce coronary heart disease mortality. We can spend it on either reducing smoking *or* increasing the level of exercise. Assuming that the relative risk associated with both risk factors is 2, that changes of prevalence are equally permanent, and that the cardioprotective effect occurs quickly; which choice will give a better return in lives saved?

First make a judgement on which of the two preventive programmes you prefer.

Now consider which is more common, smoking or lack of exercise?

Calculate population attributable risk with prevalence of smoking of 20 per cent, 30 per cent, 40 per cent and 50 per cent and prevalence of lack of exercise 60 per cent, 70 per cent and 80 per cent. (These are realistic prevalences in the context of industrialized countries.) Has the result altered or substantiated your earlier judgement?

Table 8.13 shows the result. Given the assumptions, the population attributable risk calculation supports a programme to increase exercise uptake. Clearly, this is a simplistic example. Nonetheless, the calculation makes the expectation of risk to be averted explicit.

Both population attributable risk and attributable risk are theoretical exercises which provide estimates to help pose and debate options. To assess the benefits in

Table 8.13 PAR* for smoking and not taking exercise

	PAR (%)
Prevalence of smoking (%)	
20	16.7
30	23.1
40	28.6
50	33.3
Prevalence of not taking exercise(%)	
60	37.5
70	41.2
80	44.4

* Formula: $\dfrac{P_e \times (RR - 1)}{1 + P_e \times (RR - 1)} \times 100$

e.g. for first row

$PAR = \dfrac{0.20 \times (2 - 1)}{1 + 0.20 \times (2 - 1)} \times 100 = \dfrac{0.2}{1.2} \times 100 = 16.7\%.$

practice, trials need to be done (Chapter 9). In the absence of such trials the validity of population attributable risk/attributable risk estimates remains questionable.

8.7 Presentation and interpretation of epidemiological data in applied settings

The interpretation of epidemiological findings, and of the picture or pattern that arises, is greatly influenced by the mode of presentation of data. If practical decisions are to be made, then providing data in several formats is essential. Two principles nearly always hold: give the actual figures in addition to the summaries arising from statistical manipulation and present absolute and relative rates. Pressures of space and time acting against following these principles should be resisted. Table 8.14 summarizes some of the requirements in presenting disease data. Before reading on do the exercise in Box 8.13.

> ## Box 8.13 **Need for data in Table 8.14**
>
> - What unique information or interpretation does each column supply?
> - What difficulty would the absence of the information cause to the user of the information?
> - What harm could arise from the misinterpretation arising from such omissions?

Table 8.14 A standard table for organizing information for the assessment of the pattern of disease in applied settings

		Absolute measures		**Relative measures**	
Disease or condition	Number of cases	Rate (incidence or prevalence)	Rank position on number of cases or rate	PMR/SMR/relative risk/odds ratio	Rank on SMR

The first column gives the disease or condition. The value of this is self-evident. What is not self-evident is that a label for a disease may differ across times and places and even between diagnosticians working in the same health service. As discussed earlier, standardized definitions applied by trained observers are necessary. The simplest way to provide a definition is to give the standard name of the disease or condition and give its ICD code (or use other standardized coding systems). Without written definitions, the data have little lasting value, especially in terms of comparison.

Worse, the data may be misinterpreted. For example, the label heart disease is not enough, and is open to erroneous interpretation, particularly in places where ischaemic heart disease arising from atherosclerosis is not dominant (e.g. where rheumatic heart disease is common).

The second column states the number of cases for each specific cause. (The less satisfactory alternative is to give the total number of cases for all causes as the denominator and the percentage relating to each disease/condition.) This information has unique value to the health service planner and professional delivering care, in deciding the staffing, accommodation, and supplies needed or used. The numbers also give the best idea of the scale of the health problem and hence help to develop a sense of priority. The numbers are also needed to assess whether the sample size is adequate, to permit alternative presentations and analyses of data and to check for errors which are hidden by all summaries.

The rate is the primary epidemiological tool to permit comparisons over time, and between places and populations but it does not have the immediacy of case numbers. That there were 5000 deaths from a particular disease in a community of 500 000 people last year gives a different impression from knowing the death rate was 10 per 1000 per year, though one can be calculated from the other. Age-specific and overall (crude) rates have the advantage that they can be easily understood and applied to different populations. When the rates are adjusted for confounding factors the resulting rates have no reality and cannot be used directly for healthcare planning. This is the penalty paid for increased comparability. Depending on the context, there may be a need for both overall (crude) and adjusted rates. The source of the population denominators used to construct rates needs to be recorded, preferably as a footnote to the table, or space permitting, somewhere in the paper or report. Unlike case numbers, population denominators are usually easily accessible.

The directly adjusted rate is, to some extent, a relative measure of disease frequency and not, as at first sight, an absolute one. It is the disease experience adjusted in relation to the standard population. (The standard population used in adjustment needs to be described.) This and other relative measures, such as the SMR (indirectly adjusted rates), RR, and OR, can be used to refine the picture using the power of analysis of similarities and differences. Finally, the diseases/conditions can be ranked on these relative measures. Rankings aid interpretation and evaluation of the importance of different diseases/conditions.

Relative measures unleash the potential to generate hypotheses to explain differences. The problem is that attention tends to be focused on differences at the expense of similarities, and more attention is given to diseases which are relatively common even although they may be less important as a cause of illness and death than those which are relatively less common. These points are illustrated in Table 8.15. The list of diseases/conditions highlighted by an analysis focused on absolute (actual) frequency

Table 8.15 Deaths and SMRs* in male immigrants from the Indian Subcontinent (aged 20 and over; total deaths = 4352)

Cause	Number of deaths	% of Total	SMR
By rank order of number of deaths— actual/absolute approach			
Ischaemic heart disease	1533	35.2	115
Cerebrovascular disease	438	10.1	108
Bronchitis, emphysema and asthma	223	5.1	77
Neoplasm of the trachea, bronchus and lung	218	5.0	53
Other non-viral pneumonia	214	4.9	100
Total	2626	60.3	–
By rank order of SMR— relative approach			
Homicide	21	0.5	341
Liver and intrahepatic bile duct neoplasm	19	0.4	338
Tuberculosis	64	1.5	315
Diabetes mellitus	55	1.3	188
Neoplasm of buccal cavity and pharynx	28	0.6	178
Total	187	4.3	–

* Standardized mortality ratios, compared with the male population of England and Wales, which was by definition 100.

Source of original data for the construction of this table: Marmot *et al.* (1984).

This table is adapted from that published by Senior and Bhopal, *BMJ* 1994; **309**, 327–30. Published with permission of the BMJ Publishing Group.

Table 8.16 Actual, adjusted, and relative measures

Actual/absolute measures	Adjusted measures, relative but not explicitly so	Relative measures
Numbers	Weighted/adjusted numbers	Proportional mortality ratio
– Overall		Standardized morbidity or mortality ratio
– Specific to age, sex, class, etc		Prevalence rate ratio
Percentages	Weighted/adjusted percentages	Relative risk
Proportional mortality		
Age specific and actual overall rates (crude)	Weighted/adjusted rates	Odds ratio
Attributable and population attributable risks		
Life years lost		
Numbers needed to treat		

is quite different from that highlighted by the relative approach. Table 8.16 lists the main epidemiological measures of disease frequency as absolute, adjusted, or relative. Life-years lost are discussed in the next section and numbers needed to treat thereafter.

8.8 **Avoidable morbidity and mortality**

Death and much sickness, disability, and disease is unavoidable so the idea of avoidable mortality or morbidity can be confusing. Avoidable mortality (or morbidity) is the idea that there is potential to avoid death (or morbidity) from specified causes if the best possible public health and healthcare actions were taken. For example, death from appendicitis is avoidable given early diagnosis and treatment and some morbidity ought to be (e.g. rupturing of the appendix). The causes of avoidable mortality and morbidity are chosen on the potential for prevention or cure so they change with advances in knowledge.

The avoidable causes of death tend to be those where a preventive and therapeutic intervention has been developed, and the causal chain understood sufficiently to break the link through intervention. The research challenge for these conditions is to implement (and evaluate) effective services. For non-avoidable conditions the challenge is to develop new interventions and, usually, this will need aetiological understanding.

Calculating how many years of life would potentially be saved if all avoidable deaths were averted (years of life lost) measures the impact of avoidable mortality in a population, assesses the potential benefits of actions to reduce avoidable mortality, and is a test of the healthcare system. The age at which death would have occurred naturally if the avoidable cause of death had not occurred, the key data item, is of course unknown so it is estimated. Usually, the expected age at death is set at the average life expectancy in the population. For example, assuming the life expectancy was 75 years, a 74 year old woman dying of lung cancer would have one year of life lost. In fact, life expectancy at the age of 74 is about 10 years, so in truth about 10 years of life were potentially lost. It would be more accurate, though not so simple, to calculate the anticipated life expectancy of the dead individual based on the population average at that age. Sometimes a lower age cut-off (65 years usually) is taken as a measure of premature mortality. Clearly, the idea of premature death is arbitrary and refers simply to chronological age. Deaths over this age, however, may be premature if the health status of the deceased was good, while some persons below 65 years may be riddled with disease and their deaths may be timely.

The years of lost life approach gives emphasis to death in the relatively young. Given an expectation of life of 75, a death at the age of 10 would yield a years of life lost figure of 65, the same as 13 deaths at the age of 70. Clearly, there is no moral, social, legal, or religious set of values to justify equivalence of these yields. Yet, here is a rationale for, and echo of, the fact that societies usually hold the prevention and treatment of death in childhood as a higher priority than death in older ages.

Years of life lost can change the perceived importance of problems, which seem relatively unimportant in the light of disease rates. For example, injury has emerged from the shadows partly because of the powerful impact of years of life lost analysis (see Chapter 10, Section 2, on priority setting). The years of life lost approach provides a common denominator for judging the priority to be given to each cause of mortality. The concept provides a means of comparing the performance of the healthcare system with the best possible and can be used to set targets. For example, it would be reasonable to say that the organization of the healthcare system as a whole should mean that patients with appendicitis are sufficiently well informed that they seek advice early, and that doctors are able to make the diagnosis and operate to prevent deaths. The setting of targets relating to avoidable mortality and evaluation of their achievement provides a powerful means of audit.

The years of life lost approach can be refined further by incorporating disability and quality of life as discussed below. Before doing so let us look at Lee's analysis of 10 health status measures.

8.9 Comparison of summary measures of health status

Lee explored age-specific mortality rates for pneumonia and suicide in Taiwan, 1995, using 10 summary measures, including years of life lost. Table 8.17 shows age-specific population size, number of deaths, and rates. Before reading on, readers may wish to summarize the results of the table, in terms of the pattern of deaths.

There were more deaths from pneumonia (3070) than from suicide (1618). Pneumonia deaths occurred mainly in the age groups over 55 years and the number of deaths rose with age, except in the 85 years plus group. By contrast most deaths from suicide were in the 20–74 age groups with the peak number in the 25–44 age groups. The age-specific rates generally confirm the picture derived from case numbers for pneumonia but show that the highest rates were in the 85 years plus group. For suicide

Table 8.17 Population size and mortality due to pneumonia and suicide in Taiwan, 1995

Age	Population	Pneumonia Death	Mortality[a]	Suicide Death	Mortality[a]
0–4	1 596 058	59	3.70	0	0.00
5–9	1 608 446	14	0.87	0	0.00
10–14	1 918 327	11	0.57	12	0.63
15–19	1 988 479	11	0.55	44	2.21
20–24	1 790 146	6	0.34	105	5.87
25–29	1 886 651	18	0.95	163	8.64
30–34	1 959 013	31	1.58	165	8.42
35–39	1 846 480	27	1.46	145	7.85
40–44	1 632 355	36	2.21	154	9.43
45–49	1 060 675	29	2.73	92	8.67
50–54	866 026	65	7.51	102	11.78
55–59	799 674	90	11.25	114	15.86
60–64	718 617	167	23.24	114	15.86
65–69	655 406	266	40.59	125	19.07
70–74	457 317	431	94.25	131	28.65
75–79	263 482	583	221.27	66	25.05
80–84	149 406	638	427.02	59	39.49
85+	71 094	588	827.07	27	37.98
Total*		3070		1618	

[a] Per 100 000 population.   * Added by the author.
Adapted from Lee, *Int J Epidemiol* 1998; **27**, 1053–6—see Permissions.

age-specific rates indicate an increasing problem with age, the greater number of deaths in the 25–44 age group simply being a function of larger population size. The differentials in the rates for pneumonia are huge; for example, the 80–84 year olds have a relative risk of pneumonia mortality about 1255 times that in the 20–24 age group. By contrast, the equivalent relative risk for suicide is 6.7.

What happens to this picture when summary measures are used? Lee used 10 summary measures, but for simplicity the number has been reduced to six here. Table 8.18 shows that both the crude rate and the age-standardized rate show pneumonia deaths to be about twice as common as suicide mortality. The cumulative rate and life-table risk are much greater for pneumonia. The measures of years of life lost (YPLL and CRPLL), however, show these to be much lower for pneumonia than for suicide. The point is that the perception of the relative burden of disease depends on the choice and mode of data presentation. Table 8.19 summarises the qualities of these measures, as a stepping stone to more advanced studies.

Table 8.18 Comparison of various health-status measures in quantifying the impacts of pneumonia death and suicide in Taiwan, 1995

Measure[a]	Pneumonia	Suicide	*Ratio of pneumonia/ suicide
Crude rate	14.44[b]	7.61[b]	1.9
ASR	14.55[b]	7.06[b]	2.1
CR	0.0834	0.0122	6.8
Life-table risk	0.0353	0.0080	4.4
YPLL	20 208	43 500	0.5
CRPLL	35.1[c]	55.0[c]	0.6

[a] ASR: age-standardized rate, CR: cumulative rate, YPLL: years of potential life lost, CRPLL: cumulative rate of potential life lost.
[b] Per 100 000 population.   [c] In days.   * Column added by the author.
Adapted from Lee, *Int J Epidemiol* 1998; **27**, 1053–6—see Permissions.

Table 8.19 The properties of some health-status measures as summarized by Lee

Measures[a]	Between-group comparison	Need for an external standard	Value judgement on death	Lifetime projected risk	Individual-level interpretation
Crude rate	No	No	No	No	No
ASR	Yes	Yes	No	No	No
CR	Yes	No	No	Yes	Yes
Life-table risk	Yes	No	No	Yes	Yes
YPLL	No	No	Yes	No	No
CRPLL	Yes	No	Yes	Yes	Yes

[a] ASR: age-standardized rate, CR: cumulative rate, YPLL: years of potential life lost, CRPLL: cumulative rate of potential life lost.
Adapted from Lee, *Int J Epidemiol* 1998; **27**, 1053–6—see Permissions.

8.10 **DALY, disability adjusted life years, and QALY, quality adjusted life years**

The underlying idea behind these measures is that life expectancy free of disability or impairment is of greater value than life expectancy with such problems. A year of life with a disability or illness such as stroke, diabetes, or multiple sclerosis is said to be worth less to an individual than a year of life without. This is an idea that is controversial. The logical but morally and ethically dubious extension of this idea is that a year of life of a disabled or sick person is worth less than that of another person free of such disability or sickness.

In population settings these measures provide a means of gauging the burden of disease. In contemporary life, unlike other eras, the equal worth of different populations is rarely questioned. In making choices between healthcare interventions, and by implication populations to be served, these concepts have provided a way of presenting information and spurring debate and, fortunately, not for discriminating between who gets services.

The key question is this: how much less is a year of life with a particular disability worth than a year free of that disability? In the quality adjusted life year approach the answer is derived by asking people, usually those with the disability and their relatives, and others without a disability. This type of questioning yields a so-called utility value for particular health states, usually expressed on a scale of 0 to 1. Such surveys show that some states, like irreversible coma, are commonly judged to be worse than death. A year of life in coma, for example, may have no value (or even a negative one). In contrast, a year of life with a minor disability, say correctable short sightedness, may have little or no negative impact on perceived quality of life and hence the quality adjusted life year. The quality adjusted life year provides a means of adjusting the value of life expectancy, and hence years of life lost, by disability. Clearly, however, the adjustments are based on subjective judgements which depend on who is asked, by whom, when, and how. The judgements are unlikely to be lasting, as social values change and advances in management of disease occur. The quality adjusted life year has proved to be particularly useful in health economics where it has provided an outcome against which costs can be considered (cost-utility studies).

Disability adjusted life years are similar in concept to quality adjusted life years. The main difference is that disability is used to value the life year lost or gained, and not the perceived effect on value of life as in the quality adjusted life year. The life years lost for each individual are, as usual, based on potential life expectancy minus years actually lived. To this value is added the loss caused by disability, after weighting. The weights vary for each diagnosis, for example, for angina the weight used in the Global Burden of Disease Project (see Murray *et al.* 1997) was 0.095, for congestive heart failure it was 0.171 and for acute myocardial infarction it was 0.395. Assuming that cases of acute myocardial infarction are disabled for 3 months (0.25 of a year), on average, then 100 cases would contribute 9.8 years of disability adjusted life years (100 cases $\times$ 0.25 years $\times$ 0.395 (weight) = 9.8). Some will go on to develop angina (9.5 disability adjusted life years per 100 cases of angina per year) and heart failure (17.1 disability adjusted life years per 100 cases per year). The value of these morbidity weights is critical. The weights were changed in the Global Burden of Disease (GBD) Project between 1994 and 1996. Mental disorders moved from 3rd to 1st ranking cause of disability adjusted life years after the change.

The disability adjusted life year calculations can be refined by including a discount rate, age weighting, sensitivity testing using different disability weightings, and restriction of analysis to avoidable causes of death and disease. The discounting argument hinges on the view that a health benefit now is worth more than a health benefit in the future. The argument is as for money, for a pound (or dollar) now is worth more than a pound made available in 5 years time. So, a disability adjusted life year lost or gained is weighted in accord with the discount rate (3 per cent in the Global Burden of Disease Project). Saving one life at age 0 would result in 80 life years saved using the World Bank standard life table (which uses a life expectancy of 80 at birth, and about 85.17 once 75 years are achieved), and saving the life of a 75 year old saves 10.17 years. Without discounting, however, the infant life is worth about 8 lives at 75 years. With discounting this is not the case because the short-term benefits gained by 10 people aged 75 years exceed very long term benefits to be gained by the one infant.

In the Global Burden of Disease Project disability adjusted life years at age 25 were valued highest. A year of life at age 2 was valued at 20 per cent of the value at 25, and at 70 years the value was 46 per cent of that at 25 years. Age weighting is a controversial matter that openly accepts a stance that is ageist. The quality adjusted life years and disability adjusted life years are summary measures suitable for policy analysis. A summary measure useful for clinicians and patients is the number needed to treat or prevent.

8.11 Numbers needed to treat (NNT) or to prevent (NNP)

The accurate perception of risk is vital to making decisions, particularly where the patient must give informed consent and understand the risks and potential benefits. The numbers needed to treat (NNT) is a measure that combines directness with simplicity. It simply states the number of people who need to be treated for one patient to benefit. Conceptually, the same measure could be applied to preventive measures (numbers needed to prevent, or NNP) but this is done less often.

The calculation of accurate NNT needs incidence rates for outcomes, from a well-conducted trial (Chapter 9). So if in a reliable trial we found:

- incidence of outcome in the untreated group = 30/1000 and
- incidence of outcome in the treated group = 25/1000 then

- the reduction in risk $= \dfrac{30-25}{1000} = 5/1000$ and

- NNT = 1000/5 = 200

In this trial five people in every thousand benefit, 0.5 per cent. In other words 1 in 200 benefit, or alternatively, 200 need to be treated for one to benefit. The reduction in risk is known as the absolute risk reduction (and it is similar in concept to excess risk). The NNT is the reciprocal of the absolute risk reduction. Before reading on, reflect on the exercise in Box 8.14.

Box 8.14 NNT in relation to other summary measures

Compare the directness and value of this information with alternatives e.g. stating the two incidences possibly as percentages, the excess risk, the attributable risk, the relative risk, or the odds ratio.

The physician can explain to the patient that the risk (incidence) of disease will decline from 30/1000, or 3 per cent, to 25/1000, or 2.5 per cent. While the rates may not be easily understood, the percentages will be. The absolute risk reduction can simply be stated as 5/1000 or 0.5 per cent (the excess risk is 5/1000). These all suggest modest benefits. These are all measures of absolute risk.

The relative risk here (the treated group is exposed) is

$$\frac{25/1000}{30/1000} = 0.83$$

or a 17 per cent decline (and the odds ratio is, essentially the same here).

The relative risk (and OR) imply a 17 per cent reduction in risk, a seemingly large benefit. Essentially, there is a substantial benefit on a very low baseline, for the risk of the adverse outcome is very low even in the absence of treatment. This is another example of relative and absolute measures leading to very different perceptions. The NNT tells the patient simply that for every 200 people treated one will benefit. By comparison with the other measures, this one requires no technical knowledge or sophistication in mathematics.

The NNT based on results in a trial, of course, may not apply to real healthcare settings, simply because trials enrol highly selected patients. The NNT, nonetheless, usually provides a more sobering assessment of benefits than the relative risk or the odds ratio. Policy makers and clinicians have been quick to apply NNTs to therapies but not to preventive actions. This may reflect a fear that public support may be lost by this approach for the NNP tends to be large. The NNP and NNT can be calculated from cohort and case register studies providing incidence data, but such figures might not be reliable (Chapter 9).

8.12 Describing the health status of a population

One of the vital contributions of epidemiology is the measurement of the health status of a population. The first challenge is to define health. Based on the WHO definition, health is not merely the absence of disease or infirmity but a state of physical, mental, and social well-being. To be healthy it is necessary to be alive, functioning, and to have a sense of well-being. Before reading on do the exercise in Box 8.15.

Box 8.15 Describing health status: choice of measures

Imagine you are asked to describe the health status of your population to a new minister of health. The minister has no previous background in the health field. What kinds of measures would you choose to portray the health of your community?

Consider not only the specific types of data, but also the qualities of the data you would seek out.

Obviously, your data set will be a mix of health and disease measures, but less obviously, it ought to include both qualitative and quantitive information. Qualitative information may include the public's and professionals' values, beliefs, and attitudes in relation to health and disease. Quantitative measures will be both self-reported such as on smoking, alcohol, and exercise habits, and directly measured such as height, weight, visual acuity, blood pressure, and cholesterol. There may be information on actual health-related events, such as recent mortality and morbidity rates and life expectancy, and future anticipated trends. The portrait of health would be incomplete without an indication of the healthcare facilities and services and the effects of such services. These might be described as structures (number of doctors, nurses, hospitals, etc.), processes (consultation and hospitalization rates, etc.), and outcomes (effect on morbidity, mortality, and well-being). These points are captured in Tables 8.20, 8.21 and 8.22.

The next step, beyond description, lies in explanation. This requires relating the determinants of health status such as age, sex, social and economic status, ethnicity, and health-related behaviours, to the measures of health status, and through study of

Table 8.20 Creating a health portrait: some qualities of required health status data

Health and disease
Qualitative and quantitative
Self-reported and measured (e.g. weight)
Actual death rates and anticipated disease trends
Health service structure, number of doctors, processes (e.g. consultation), and outcomes (e.g. death)

Table 8.21 General classification of some indices of health status

Socio-economic
Demographic
Behavioural
Physiological/Biochemical/Anatomical/ Pathological/Microbiological
Genetic
Psychological
Morbidity
Mortality
Health care

Table 8.22 Specific examples of some health status measurements

Biological function	Social function	Well-being	Disease and death	Health service utilization
Physical measures such as, Height Weight Body shape and obesity	Reproductive status of the population e.g. fertility rates	Mental well-being e.g. General Health Questionnaire	Mortality and morbidity rates overall and by cause	Consultation activity
Physiological function e.g. blood pressure, heart rate	Activities of daily living	Well-being e.g. as self-reported	Life expectancy, as measured from current mortality rates	Effectiveness of services
Biochemical status, e.g cholesterol level, plasma glucose, antioxidant levels	Social networks	Attitudes to health and health-related behaviours	Predicted disease and life expectancy patterns	Equity of health service use
Genetic profiles e.g. prevalence of sickle cell trait or cystic fibrosis gene	Health-related behaviours		Disability: prevalence and severity	

the relationships deriving conclusions about cause and effect. To complete the description of health status, therefore, the minister should be informed on these matters too.

Population-based data tend to be rich in information on death rates, and poor on function and well-being. As comparing health status between time periods and between populations and places is likely to be important in developing and interpreting the profile the minister will need to be reassured that the validity and quality of measurement is high.

In summary, the health minister might reasonably expect your presentation to include specific information on:

- the population and its characteristics, generally;
- life expectancy, disease states, and causes of disability and infirmity;
- measures of physical well-being;
- measures of mental and social well-being;
- measures of functioning;
- measures relating to health services;
- explanation of variations.

The next section discusses how these measures can be expressed in a consistent and easily understood way.

8.13 **The construction and development of health status indicators**

Having chosen an aspect of health—whether life expectancy, death rates, or fertility—we need to define how the indicator is to be constructed and calculated. The general principles are those underlying the calculation of incidence and prevalence rates, but the practice varies for each indicator, usually being reflected by the availability of data, as illustrated with life expectancy and maternal mortality. Table 8.23 exemplifies the construction of some key health indicators. Life expectancy at birth, or at a specified age, is not based on a theoretical expectation for the individual or the actual living population but the years of life lived calculated from the most recently available mortality rates in the population. Life expectancy is calculated from life tables (discussion of these is beyond the scope of this book). In most societies, therefore, life expectancy estimates are underestimates, because mortality rates will drop in future. This, however, is not a certainty as the experience in some Eastern European countries and Russia (due to economic difficulties) and some African countries (due to AIDS) has shown. Knowing the life expectancy permits us to estimate the potential years of life lost by an individual (as discussed previously). The point is that a workable solution is found to estimate that which cannot be known.

The maternal mortality rate is an excellent example of how pragmatic decisions are made. We are actually interested in deaths in women associated with any aspect of

Table 8.23 Examples of the construction of some indices

Indices	Defining and operationalizing the index
Life expectancy	Years of life in a population expected on basis of current mortality rates ÷ population
Maternal mortality rate	Deaths from puerperal causes during pregnancy or within 42 days ÷ live births
Stillbirth (synonym, fetal death) rate	Stillbirths per 1000 total births
Neonatal mortality rate	Deaths in 28 days per 1000 live births
Perinatal mortality rate	Stillbirths + 1st week deaths ÷ total births
Postneonatal rate	Post 28 days to first year deaths ÷ live births
Infant mortality rate	Deaths at <1 year ÷ live births
Birth rate	Live births ÷ population
Fertility rate	Live births ÷ women 15–44 years
Abortion rate	Number of abortions ÷ women 15–44 years
Consultation rate	Number of consultations ÷ registered population
Hospitalization rate	Discharges and deaths ÷ population
(Death rates)	As discussed earlier in Chapter 7

childbirth. The first challenge is to define those causes of death that are associated with childbirth. Rather than create a long list of specific causes, the definition is a general one: any cause related to or aggravated by the pregnancy or its management but not from accidental or incidental causes. This leaves a judgement that is made by the health professional and the coder. The next question is whether there is to be a time limit. According to the WHO definition a maternal death needs to occur during pregnancy or within 42 days of the termination of pregnancy. The denominator for this rate ought to be all pregnancies. This figure cannot be estimated accurately so the definition, pragmatically, uses live births. The principles illustrated here are that definitions need to work in widely varying circumstances, to permit comparable data, say from rural China and from inner London. This requires absolute clarity (e.g. as in the time limit of 42 days) and the use of readily available data; for example, number of live births rather than, say, pregnancies or the number of women registered at antenatal clinics. The resulting fraction is multiplied to create a whole number, and is calculated for an appropriate time period. Most rates are expressed as rate per 1000, 10 000 or 100 000 and per year.

In most rates relating to health events around birth the number of births is used rather than population size. Sometimes the denominator is all births, sometimes live births. The reader has no option but to learn the definitions, though there is some logic behind the choices. The rate of stillbirth and of perinatal mortality includes live and stillborn in the denominator, the rate of neonatal mortality does not, for good reason. The numerator of stillbirth and perinatal mortality includes stillborn, so the denominator does too. The numerator for neonatal mortality excludes the stillborn, so the denominator excludes them too.

Sometimes definitions cannot be agreed internationally, either for national legal reasons or because the availability of data differs too greatly. The WHO definition of perinatal mortality uses live births in the denominator whereas most industrialized nations use all births, dead or alive. Clearly, live births are easier to count accurately than all births.

Definitions are subject to periodic review and revision. There are, as the reader can see, intricacies and controversies behind apparently simple definitions of commonly used rates.

8.14 **Conclusion**

Clearly, epidemiological purposes, theories and study design underpin measurement, presentation, and interpretation of data. To a surprising extent, however, the capacity to measure and analyse data also alters our theories and study designs. Practical matters such as ease of analysis, and the availability of computers and computer software, also alter our choice of measures and mode of presentation. This, in turn, has a dramatic effect on the interpretation of data and the conclusions and recommendations arising. The interpretation of data, more than most aspects of epidemiology, is influenced by investigators' philosophy on the nature of knowledge (epistemology) and by the theories they hold.

Most epidemiologists adhere consciously or subconsciously to the doctrine of positivism, that is, the philosophic system that is based on facts, acquired by empirical observations, and logic. Anecdote, opinion, intuition, experience, and even observations made informally are not easily admitted as evidence. In this book and in Chapters 3, 4, 7 and 8 specifically I have emphasized that facts do not exist in a vacuum, but are extracted by analysis and interpretation from data that are invariably flawed. These 'facts' are contestable, and not surprisingly epidemiologists are known for their capacity for critique (see Chapter 10, Sections 10.10 and 10.11).

These general points could be illustrated with many examples but let us consider just two, one reflecting a measure (the odds ratio), the other an approach (relative and absolute risk).

The odds ratio has had a profound impact on epidemiology. Its use can be traced to a paper by J. Cornfield in 1951 entitled, 'A method of estimating comparative rates from clinical data. Applications to cancer of the lung, breast and cervix' (see References). The appeal of the odds ratio at that time was its capacity to yield an estimate of the relative risk from case-control studies (Chapter 9). With increasing understanding of when the estimate was a good one, came a change in the design of case-control studies with an emphasis on studying incident cases and on ensuring controls were representative of non-cases. The mode of analysis, therefore, altered the theoretical understanding and design of case-control studies. Yet, there is no imperative to analyse a case-control study using an odds ratio. Landmark case-control studies on adenocarcinoma of the vagina (Herbst *et al.*) published in 1971, and on smoking and carcinoma of the lung (Doll and Hill) published in 1950 and 1952 do not, for example, report odds ratios. Presently, the case-control study and the odds ratio are inextricably intertwined. The odds ratio has now become a dominant summary measure in a range of studies, despite its drawbacks, because its mathematical properties make analysis easy (e.g. in a logistic regression model).

Different ways of presenting the same data have a major impact on the perception of risk, and in particular relative and actual risks portray dramatically different priorities giving different perspectives on the health needs of populations. Usually, relative measures of risk are more useful in aetiologic enquiry while actual measures are better in health planning and policy.

The tensions inherent in the choice of whether to present data using a relative or absolute risk approach go to the core of epidemiology. What is epidemiology for? Is it a science aiming for causal understanding? If so, the 'compare and contrast' mode of analysis is the time-honoured way of generating hypothesis and the relative risk approach is right. If, however, epidemiology is equally (or even predominantly) concerned with feeding into health policy, needs assessment, and health planning, then the burden of disease as measured by absolute risk is of critical importance. In practice the relative risk approach tends to dominate. Ideally, investigators should report both relative and absolute risk, hence achieving a dual purpose. This simple advice is usually resisted because it creates extra work, makes the messages harder to convey, and takes up scarce publication space.

The example in Table 8.15 of the mortality of Indian Subcontinent born men illustrates the vastly different perspectives offered by relative and absolute risk. It also raises a question about how researchers see the world. Why did other investigators not report their data in this way? Why, so often in race and ethnicity research, is the reference or standard population a 'white' one? Why is the health of the 'white' population not compared with the minority ethnic groups using the latter as the reference population? The answers are not simply technical ones. One explanation is that there is an ethno-centric approach whereby the population that is dominant in status and numbers is automatically assigned as the standard because investigators (most of whom come from or are trained in such populations) see the world through the eyes of this population.

The measurement and portrayal of risk is a dynamic and creative aspect of epidemiology with much scope for innovation. Lee's (1998) work described in this chapter illustrates this well. The challenges of creating simple, understandable, and valid summary measures of health states are formidable. There is the task, at the interphase of epidemiology and public health, of putting measures together to create a profile of the community's health, and using this as a foundation to help improve it.

Epidemiological data on diseases can be combined with other information such as socio-economic circumstances, social values and attitudes to health, and behaviours relevant to health, to build up a community health profile. Combining data sets in this way helps to generate causal understanding of disease processes in populations and the means of developing interventions to improve public health. As epidemiology is a positivist discipline founded on empirical observation, mastery of data interpretation is vital to its proper practice.

Summary

Basic epidemiological data on disease occurrence and population structure can be manipulated and presented in many ways. The choice should be guided by the purposes of the research and the likely application of the findings. Data manipulation, inevitably, helps both to sharpen the findings and to distort them. Epidemiological summary measures, broadly, estimate absolute risks (e.g. numbers, rates, life years lost, numbers needed to treat) or relative ones (e.g. adjusted rates, relative risk, odds ratios).

Different ways of presenting the same data have a major impact on the perception of risk, and in particular relative and actual risks portray dramatically different perspectives on the health needs of populations. Usually, relative measures of risk are more useful in aetiologic enquiry while actual measures are better in health planning and policy. Epidemiological studies should indicate both relative and actual risk.

Avoidable mortality (and morbidity) refers to the potential to avoid death (or morbidity) from a number of specified causes if the best possible healthcare actions were taken. Years of life saved if such deaths were avoided help to measure the impact of avoidable mortality in the population. Avoidable mortality helps us to focus on priorities for new research, apply epidemiological knowledge in public health, guide healthcare actions, and assess effectiveness of health care.

Epidemiological data on diseases can be combined with other information such as socio-economic circumstances, social values and attitudes, and behaviours relevant to health, to build up a community health profile. Combining data sets in this way generates causal understanding of disease processes in populations and the means of developing rational interventions to improve public health.

Chapter 9

Study design

Objectives

On completion of the chapter you should understand that:

- understanding disease causation and measuring the burden of disease are the two key purposes underlying epidemiological studies;
- epidemiological studies are unified by their common purposes, by their utilization of the survey method and their dependency on the concept of a defined population;
- all study designs potentially contribute to questions of cause and effect, health policy and planning, and clinical practice;
- a clinical case-series is a coherent set of cases compiled by one or a few clinicians;
- a population case-series study, consisting of a set of cases in a defined population and time, lays the foundation for description of disease by place, time, and characteristics of population;
- if cases are compared with non-cases from the same population the design is that of a case-control study, which generates and tests causal hypotheses, through the analysis of associations;
- a cross-sectional study measures disease and risk factor prevalence in a sample of individuals in a population in a defined time period, mainly to explore the burden of disease but also to generate associations;
- a cohort study consists of a sample of individuals in a population followed up over time to observe changes in health status, to measure disease incidence, and to examine associations between risk factors and health outcomes;
- a trial is similar in design to a cohort study except that the investigators impose an intervention on one or more of the study populations;
- the ecological 'design' is a mode of analysis based on variables being studied in relation to places rather than individuals;
- there are conceptual and practical interrelationships between study designs.

9.1 Introduction: interdependence of study design

There is a growing number of apparently disparate study designs used in epidemiology and the labels used to describe them are numerous. There are five basic designs based on individual data as listed in Box 9.1 and summarized in Table 9.1, which outlines some of their characteristics and overlapping purposes. Confusion about these five designs is common, and is accentuated by the varying use of existing terms and continuous development and invention of new ones.

There are modifications of these study designs to suit different purposes. For example, there are retrospective and prospective cohort studies and there are case-series studies based on clinical records and population-based registers, and many forms of trial design. Most discussions tend to consider each design as being distinct but this is taxing, particularly when a study has atypical features, or comprises a mix of designs. It is important, therefore, to understand the ideas which underlie study design, particularly in terms of purpose, form, analysis, interpretation, and basis in the concept of population. Such understanding helps to define the common ground, and relative unity, of epidemiological study design.

The goal in common of epidemiological studies is understanding the frequency, pattern, and causes of disease in populations and they are usually analysed using a mix of the measures considered in Chapters 7 and 8. They are also united by their reliance on the survey method, defined by Last as an investigation in which information is systematically collected but in which the experimental method is not used (I assume, for the purposes of the discussion here, that the word experimental is used in the laboratory sense). Epidemiological studies are all rooted in the concept of population in that knowledge of the relation between the people studied and the population from which they originate is essential for interpretation, generalization, and application of data. Vital epidemiological questions, therefore, include these: Where and when was the study done? Of which population is the study group a subset? What are the characteristics of the study and wider populations? Are the findings generalizable to the whole of the population in the community, and to communities elsewhere? These questions will be reconsidered in the context of critical appraisal of epidemiological papers in Chapter 10. The underlying or base population, then, is the starting point.

All epidemiological studies permit comparisons of disease experience in terms of one or more of the triad of time, person, and place. They all contribute to measuring

---

Box 9.1 **Five basic epidemiological designs for studies based on individuals**

- ◆ case-series (clinical and population)
- ◆ cross-sectional
- ◆ case control
- ◆ cohort (prospective and retrospective)
- ◆ trial.

Table 9.1 Epidemiological designs and applications: an overview

Study design	Essential idea	Some research purposes
1. Case-series and population case-series	Count cases and relate to population data to produce rates and analyse patterns Look at characteristics of cases for causal hypotheses	Study signs and symptoms, and create disease definitions Surveillance of mortality/morbidity rates Seek associations Generate/test hypotheses Source of cases or foundation for other studies
2. Cross-sectional	Study health and disease states in a population, or populations, at a defined place and time	Measure prevalence of disease or related factors Seek associations between disease and related factors Generate/test hypotheses Repeat studies to measure change and evaluate interventions
3. Case-control	Look for differences and similarities between a series of cases and non-cases	Seek associations Generate/test hypotheses
4. Cohort	Follow up populations relating information on risk factor patterns and health states to the outcomes of interest	Study natural history of disease Measure incidence of disease Link disease outcomes to possible disease causes, i.e. seek associations Generate/test hypotheses
5. Trial	Intervene with some measure designed to improve health, then follow up people to see the effect*	Test understanding of causes Study how to influence natural history of disease Evaluate the benefits and costs of interventions

* Measures designed to worsen health or to make no difference would be ethically unacceptable.

the burden of disease or risk factors *and* study the relationship of disease and causal factors, though to a greatly varying extent. This unity and integration is not only theoretical but is also demonstrated by the way one study design leads to another, the relatively minor modifications needed to switch the study design, and the way they complement each other, particularly in adding to the weight of evidence in causal analysis (all discussed below). One of the epidemiological criteria for causality is consistency, which requires evidence from more than one study, preferably using different study designs (Chapter 5).

Most textbooks refer to an ecological study design but here this is considered as a mode of analysis. This issue is briefly discussed in the section after the basic five designs, the focus of this chapter, are explained. First we consider the value of several dichotomous classifications of study design.

9.2 **Classifications of study design: five dichotomies**

There are several classifications of study design, presumably developed to simplify the task of learning about them. Three major and commonly used dichotomies (division into two parts) distinguish between descriptive and analytic studies, retrospective and prospective studies, and observational and experimental studies (Table 9.2). The term descriptive, in these circumstances, implies a study which provides information about the pattern of disease or risk factors but not the underlying causes. The term analytic applies to studies exploring hypotheses about causes of disease but, by inference, not primarily concerned with patterns. This is a false dichotomy because insights about hypothesis on the causation of disease are inherent in the pattern of disease and risk factors in all epidemiological studies. The pattern is used both to generate and to test hypotheses. Equally, description is a necessary step in analysis. All epidemiological studies are simultaneously descriptive and analytic, in the sense of exploring hypotheses. One of the finest examples of causal thinking in epidemiology is the investigation by Semmelweiss of childbed fever, where so-called descriptive data were the foundation for a causal hypothesis (Chapter 5, Table 5.1). Table 9.2 shows the traditional view on whether the five study designs in Box 9.1 are descriptive or analytic. Readers will need to reflect on the value and limitations of this dichotomy.

Retrospective studies are said to be concerned with data in the past and prospective ones with data in the future (Table 9.2). The terms retrospective and prospective have been used synonymously with case-control and cohort studies, respectively. The distinction between retrospective and prospective studies is inaccurate, for case-control studies may enrol subjects prospectively and cohort studies may enrol subjects retrospectively (see later) and both do, of course, collect data on risk factors in the past. This classification has been largely abandoned except to describe two forms of cohort study,

Table 9.2 Fitting design to five dichotomous classifications

Design	Descriptive/ Analytic	Retrospective/ prospective	Observational/ Experimental	Beginning with disease/causes of disease	Specific comparison group/no such group
Case-series (clinical and population)	Descriptive	Retrospective	Observational	Disease	No
Cross-sectional	Descriptive	Retrospective	Observational	Both simultaneously	Usually not
Case-control	Analytic	Retrospective	Observational	Disease	Yes
Cohort (prospective and retrospective)	Analytic	Prospective and retrospective	Observational	Usually causes	Usually, yes (though it may be integral to the study poulation)
Trial	Analytic	Prospective	Experimental	Usually disease, but sometimes causes of disease	Yes, with exceptions

prospective and retrospective. Table 9.2 shows the results of applying this classification to the five study designs.

The observational study is one where the investigator observes the natural course of events. The experimental study is one where the course of events is deliberately altered. The investigation of a natural experiment is, strictly speaking, an observational study (Table 9.2). Most epidemiology is observational, for experiments are the exception. This classification is, therefore, of little practical help. These three dichotomous classifications may or may not be helpful to readers, but are needed to understand epidemiological writings which use them.

Some alternative dichotomous classifications may help readers. One important distinction lies with the presence or absence of disease at the beginning of a study (Table 9.2). Studies where the disease has already occurred focus on the risk factors which lead to it or influence its course. Studies where the risk factor is present but no disease has yet occurred focus on the occurrence of disease and other outcomes.

Another division in epidemiology is between studies which incorporate a specific comparison group and those which do not (Table 9.2). Those with comparison groups are generally better for testing hypotheses about disease causation than those without, and have usually been done with this as a primary goal. The scientific paradigm, strong in epidemiology, is to seek understanding through comparing and contrasting, comparing like-with-like, and ensuring that the principles derived can be repeated and generalized across geographical areas and time periods. The use of a comparison population helps to achieve this. The distinctions in Table 9.2 may help understanding but they cannot be used as the basis of definitive classification. The classification in Box 9.1 has simplicity as a merit.

The five study designs are explained using the concepts of population (Chapter 2) and the natural history of disease (Chapter 6).

9.3 **Case-series: clinical and population based**

Table 9.1 gives a brief summary and Table 9.2 indicates how case-series fit the dichotomous classifications. The clinical case-series is usually a coherent and consecutive set of cases of a disease (or similar problem) which derive from either the practice of one or more healthcare professionals or a defined healthcare setting such as a hospital or family practice. Clinical case-series are usually put together by clinicians on a topic of their interest. A case-series is, effectively, a register of cases. The cases can be analysed to aid clinical practice and research and explored in an epidemiological way by seeking commonalities and differences in characteristics within the set of cases.

Figure 9.1(a) illustrates the concept of a clinical case-series using coronary heart disease (CHD) deaths. Typically, a hospital clinician or group of clinicians would compile the case notes of all the cases seen, and analyse them to learn about the disease. As Fig. 9.1(a) illustrates, the cases may, indeed are likely to, live outside the defined geographical boundary and may include patients from overseas. People living in the area

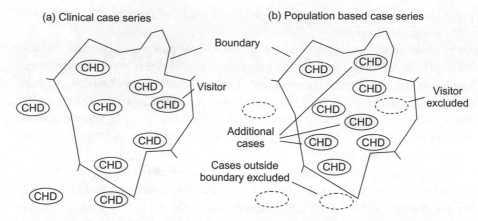

(a) Clinical case series

(b) Population based case series

Boundary

Visitor

Additional cases

Cases outside boundary excluded

Visitor excluded

- Identify cases seen by one or more clinicians
- Case series is unlikely to be a complete set of cases
- Assess characteristics of cases
- There is no accurately defined boundary so rates cannot be calculated

- Only cases within a defined boundary are included
- Note that there are extra deaths compared to the figure for the clinical case series
- The extra cases symbolize those not seen at the clinical facility e.g. street deaths

Fig. 9.1 Concept of clinical and population based case-series.

but not under the care of these particular clinicians would not be included, and usually rates cannot be calculated because the population corresponding to the list of cases cannot be defined well.

Clinical case-series are of value in epidemiology, especially for studying symptoms and signs and creating case definitions, and are important for clinical education, audit, and research. When a clinical case-series is complete for a defined geographical area for which the population is known, it is, effectively, a population-based case-series consisting of a population register of cases.

Figure 9.1(b) illustrates a population case-series. There are two main differences from Fig. 9.1(a). First, only cases within a defined geographical area are included and, second, extra cases (e.g. street deaths, coroners' cases, etc.) are included. Effectively, a population case-series is a collection of the cases seen by all clinicians serving a particular area, and attempts to include also people living in the area but seen by clinicians working in distant parts. In short, the list of cases is complete for a geographical area and particular time period. To achieve this usually requires a clear and well-administered system of data collection or a rigorous case finding study. Ideally, temporary migrants and visitors (and these may be overseas patients) should be excluded.

The biggest and epidemiologically most important case-series are registers of serious diseases or deaths, and of health service utilization (e.g. hospital admissions). These population case-series are usually compiled for administrative and legal reasons but are used by statisticians and epidemiologists for population surveillance of health. Reflect on the questions in Box 9.2 before reading on.

Box 9.2 **Differences and similarities in clinical and population case-series**

- Is there, conceptually, a difference between a clinical case-series and a population one?
- What are the differences? In what circumstances are clinical and population case-series identical?

The main difference between the clinical and the population case-series is that in the former the list of cases is likely to be incomplete. The cases will come from an undefined area and the population from which they come from may not be known. The exception to this occurs when the clinician(s) compiling the series provides all the care to the population in a defined catchment area or has collected information on all cases diagnosed by other clinicians (including pathologists doing postmortems) within that area. This is unlikely to occur except for rare and distinctive diseases or for rural areas, with small populations and a single healthcare provider. The difficulties of compiling a complete case-series were discussed in Chapter 7 (Section 4) in relation to counting the numerator for calculating incidence. Reflect on the question in Box 9.3 before reading on.

Box 9.3 **Case-series and the natural history of disease**

How does the case-series (clinical and population) contribute to our understanding of the natural history of disease?

Figure 9.2 shows a case-series of patients with suspected, and overt coronary heart disease. Clinical case-series may also include the dead. The cases are, therefore, at a variety of stages in their natural history and the spectrum of symptoms, signs, and severity is likely to be broad. By delving into the past circumstances of these patients, including examination of past medical records, and by continuing to observe them to death (and necropsy as appropriate) clinicians can build up a picture of the natural history of a disease. The population case-series is a systematic extension of this series but which includes additional cases, such as those dying without being seen by the clinicians. Such cases will add breadth to the understanding of the spectrum and natural history of disease; for example, sudden death in the home setting from a first myocardial infarction will not appear in the hospital doctor's case-series but will in the population-based case-series of deaths and will be particularly valuable if linked to postmortem data.

Making full epidemiological use of case-series data needs information on the population to permit calculation of rates, and to develop an understanding of the context in

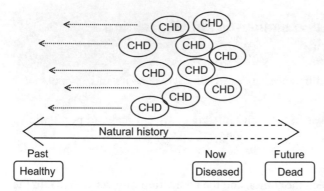

Fig. 9.2 Natural history of disease in case-series.

which the population develops disease. The choice of the population at risk needs an understanding of the biology of the disease and the purpose of the analysis. For example, for cervical cancer only the adult female population need be considered and for Alzheimer's disease the population at risk might be restricted to those over 65 years of age.

The epidemiological challenge is to develop a complete case-series and to collect additional data to make sense of the resulting analyses. The case-series is the key to understanding the distribution of disease in populations and to the study of variations over time, between places, and by population characteristics. Furthermore, the case-series can provide the key to sound case control and cohort studies and trials.

The design of a case-series is conceptually simple. The investigator defines a disease or health problem to be studied and sets up a system for capturing data on the health status and related factors in consecutive cases. In practice, however, the difficulties of developing population case-series are so great that many countries have no valid case-series even for mortality. For example, India has a well-developed health service and service infrastructure with an established decennial census but does not have national mortality data.

To make sense of case-series data the key requirements are:

1   the diagnosis or, for mortality, the cause of death

2   the date when the disease or death occurred (time)

3   the place where the person lived, worked, etc. (place)

4   the characteristics of the person (person)

5   the opportunity to collect additional data from medical records (possibly by electronic data linkage) or the person directly

6   the size and characteristics of the population at risk.

The date and time of death, for example, is recorded on the UK death certificate. The death data can thereby be analysed in relation to the time of day, day of week, month, season and, over the long term by year, decade, or even century. When the death is not witnessed forensic methods can be used to judge the time of death. Information on the main residence is also usually available on the death certificate. This can be used to find the postcode, map grid reference number, enumeration district (census tract in the USA), ward, local government area, health authority area, region or state, and country. The home address is also vital to exclude deaths of visitors (a procedure which may not be routinely applied). Workplace address is important for many diseases but is not usually recorded in population case-series.

In geographic epidemiology, particularly in small area comparisons, the address is critical information in deciding whether the case is within the geographical area of interest. Computerized information systems usually record postcode, not address. Except in national studies, there are difficult decisions to be made on people living near the boundaries of the study area. Decisions on which enumeration district or ward a person lives in can be critically important. Population denominator data are usually only available on a grouped basis, that is, the number of people living in a particular area (in the UK the smallest such area is the enumeration district). In small area studies, the geographical boundary required for a study may not match that for which the denominator data are available. In this case, grid references based on the full postcode address may be used to assign location but even then errors are inevitable, depending on the precision of the method of conversion.

In compiling a case-series, data on some characteristics are easily obtained, such as sex and date of birth. For most other characteristics, obtaining reliable and valid information is a problem, for example, on race, ethnicity, religion, income, or socio-economic position. The problem of inaccurate information on the diagnosis was discussed in Chapter 7 (Section 4).

The population case-series register is unlikely to hold information on the natural history of disease. However, case-series data can be linked to other health data either in the past or in the future; for example, mortality data can be linked to hospital admissions including at birth and childhood, cancer registrations and other records to obtain information on exposures and disease. The cases may also be contacted for additional information on their lifestyles, socio-economic circumstances, family history, and so on. In effect, this type of action may turn a case-series design into a cohort design (described below).

Usually, case-series data are analysed using rates. There are at least three circumstances, in particular, where rates are not used. First, in the study of spatial clustering of disease using techniques of point pattern analysis based on the grid reference. The level of expected clustering may be assessed using a second case-series as a control. Clearly, the chosen control disease will be one not expected to show spatial clustering. The second circumstance is when the population is stable as is usually the case for studies of short time periods, as in an examination of the number of deaths by hour of the day or day of the week. The analysis here is on the count of cases. Even if denominator data were available for such short time periods it would be unwise to use them for the errors in measurement of the denominator would outweigh any advantage. The third case is when there is no suitable denominator, for example, in case-series derived in occupational settings where accurate information on the population at risk is unavailable or the study is of an ethnic group which has not been identified in a census. The partial solution usually adopted is to use proportional ratios, as explained in Chapter 8 (Section 2).

Rates from population case-series pose problems of interpretation. Many clinicians are likely to be contributing to the data set. In the case of national statistics, perhaps tens of thousands of them. Even for a register of a common disease in a single city there may be several dozen clinicians involved. The investigator, therefore, may have little control over the quality of numerator data, particularly in the case definitions applied and the variations in diagnostic methods. The case-series may cross time periods when accurate denominator data are not available, and this is usually so, except in the census year. Awareness of the problem, training of clinicians and coders, use of agreed disease classifications such as the International Classification of Disease (ICD) and basing studies around the census year are partial solutions.

Population based case-series have great advantages to counter their disadvantages, for example, data sets may be complete over long periods of time, there may be huge numbers of cases, and there are likely to be comparable case-series in different regions in one country and internationally. Much important epidemiology centres around such data, which are the key to health service strategy and planning, and the spur to both hypothesis generation and testing.

Studies based on population case-series permit two arguably unique forms of epidemiological analysis and insight. First, they can provide a truly national and even international population perspective on disease. Second, the disease patterns can be related to aspects of society or the environment that affect the population but have no sensible measure at the individual level (see also Chapter 2, Section 5). Some indicators of the social, economic, and physical environment are not calculable at an individual level (e.g. income equality); do not exhibit individual variation within a geographical area (e.g. ozone concentration at ground level and the thickness of the ozone layer in the Earth's atmosphere); or are not available in the required accuracy in large data sets (e.g. income). For example, studies have related international rates of multiple sclerosis to the latitude of the country, mortality rates to income inequality in a region or country, and infant mortality rates to the gross national product. Reflect on the question in Box 9.4 before reading on.

Box 9.4 **Making use of indicators with no valid individual measures**

How might epidemiology study the potential role in disease causation of factors which vary little between individuals within a region or nation; for example, fluoride content of the water, the hardness or softness of water supplies, or annual exposure to sunshine?

Sometimes health status or exposure data are available for an aggregate population but not for each individual separately. In these cases the relations between these aggregate measures are studied. For example, we may know the fluoride content of the water in the health authority areas of a country but not the fluoride intake of individuals. We may also know the amount of expenditure on oral health, and from that payments made for fillings, teeth extraction, and so on, but not the oral health status of each individual. These two data sets could be studied to seek associations. This type of study, based on aggregate data, is often referred to as an ecological or correlation design. This is, however, a mode of data analysis and not a design. Individual level data can be analysed in this way (but aggregated data often cannot be disaggregated). In this mode of analysis a unit of population has replaced the individual. The five study designs (Box 9.1) could, in theory, be analysed in this way. In practice, most ecological analyses are based on population case-series, though there is an increasing interest in trials based on units rather than individuals. This is discussed in more depth in Section 9.9.

Ecological analyses are subject to the ecological fallacy (see Pearce 2000). This fallacy states that the association found with aggregate data may not apply to individuals; for example, in aggregate a population with a higher risk of disease may have a higher exposure to the risk factors, but this association may not apply to individuals. Imagine a study of the rate of coronary heart disease in the capital cities of the world relating the rate to average income. It may be that within the cities studied, coronary heart disease is higher in the richer cities than in the poorer ones. This finding would fit the general view that coronary heart disease is a disease of affluence. We might predict from such a finding that rich people in the individual cities too have more risk of CHD than poor people. In fact, in contemporary times, in the industrialized world the opposite is the case: within cities such as London, Washington DC, and Stockholm, poor people have higher CHD rates than rich ones. The forces that cause high rates of disease at a population level are different from those at an individual level.

The ecological fallacy is usually interpreted as a major weakness of ecological analyses based on population case-series. The ecological analyses, however, inform us about forces which act on whole populations which may be in conflict with those that act on individuals (see also Chapter 2). Before reading on do the exercise in Box 9.5.

Box 9.5 **Applying individual data to populations**

- Reflect on whether observations on individuals are always applicable to populations. Can you think of an example of when this is so and when it is not?
- Why do you think this happens?

Studies of individuals are prone to the opposite of the ecological fallacy, the so-called atomistic fallacy. Here, the fallacy is to wrongly assume from observations on the causes of disease in individuals that the same forces apply to whole populations. For example, at an individual level a high income or a marker of material success, such as employment or access to a car, is associated with a lower rate of suicide. This does not mean that populations or societies which are rich have a lower rate of suicide or better mental health. The opposite seems to be true. As in the previous example of CHD and wealth, the forces that cause or prevent disease at the individual level, in the case of suicide factors such as family support, are different from those that work at societal level (e.g. social cohesion and expectations).

A third fallacy, which might aptly be called the fallacy of homogeneity, arises from the misinterpretation of population data from heterogeneous populations. This fallacy is most likely to arise in population case-series analyses because of limitations in the detail available on the study populations. For example, studies of ethnic groups often use broad labels such as white or Asian. European origin 'white' populations in England have a lower all-cause SMR than those born in the Indian Subcontinent (often called South Asians). While this is true, the highest mortality is actually within the Irish-born living in England, who are often included in the white population, whose SMR is much higher than that of the South Asian population. To take a second example, the South Asian population is often described as having lower smoking prevalence than white populations. Again, while this is true, the highest recorded prevalence of smoking is actually within the South Asian population, in Bangladeshi men, as is the lowest prevalence, in Indian men and women. These examples emphasize how extrapolating from one level to another (individuals to subgroups to whole populations) is not a straightforward matter.

The viewpoint that case-series studies (whether based on individuals or aggregate data) are descriptive, observational, and epidemiologically weak is inappropriate. The weakness lies in the quality of data, and is not inherent in the design. These studies offer some unique opportunities and perspectives on the pattern and causes of disease in populations, and provide a solid platform from which to explore the pathways to disease causation. Sometimes, they provide the only way to explore causality in human populations.

9.4 **Cross-sectional study**

Table 9.1 gives a brief summary and Table 9.2 shows how cross-sectional studies fit dichotomous classifications. A cross-section is the shape that results from cutting an object lengthwise. In doing so we expose and study a part of it. A cross-sectional study exposes and studies disease and risk factor patterns in a representative part of the population, in a narrowly defined time period. The rarely used synonym, prevalence study, captures the key role of cross-sectional studies in epidemiology. In addition, the cross-sectional study seeks associations, generates and tests hypotheses and, by repetition in different time periods, can be used to measure change, and hence evaluate interventions. Its focus is simultaneously on disease and population characteristics and risk factors. Comparisons between subgroups within the sample are invariably made, but the study can also be deliberately designed with comparison groups. The comparisons are usually based on differences in the prevalence of risk factors and diseases, and the association between risk factors and diseases.

An ideal cross-sectional study is of a geographically defined, representative sample of the population studied within a slice of time and space. Figures 9.3 and 9.4 illustrate the idea in relation to a study to measure the prevalence of CHD. A target population is defined (all ovals within the boundary in Fig. 9.3). A list is made or obtained of the target populations (called sampling frame), a sample of the population at a point in time is taken (shaded ovals), and measurements are made (preferably simultaneously) to

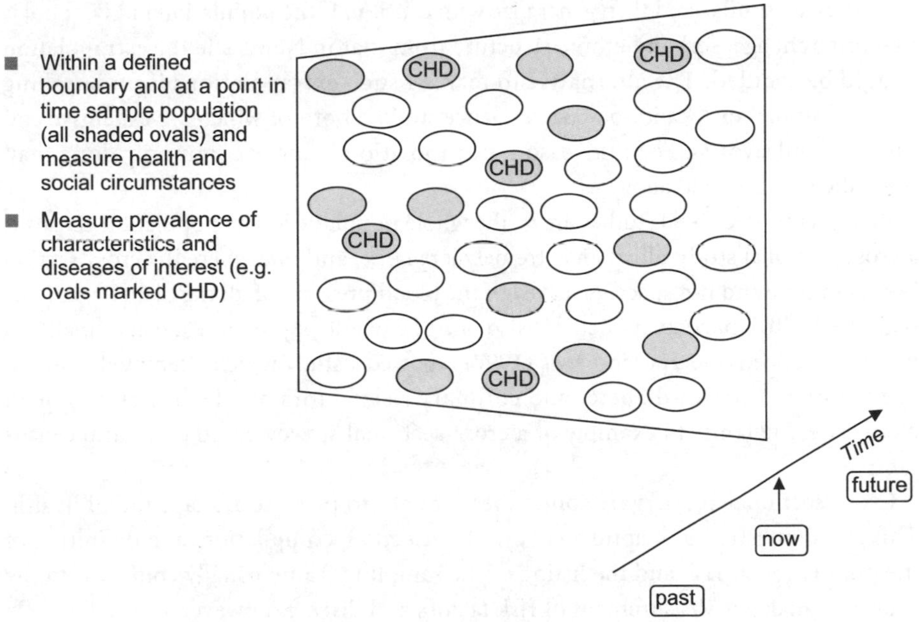

■ Within a defined
   boundary and at a point in
   time sample population
   (all shaded ovals) and
   measure health and
   social circumstances

■ Measure prevalence of
   characteristics and
   diseases of interest (e.g.
   ovals marked CHD)

Fig. 9.3 Concept of a cross-sectional study.

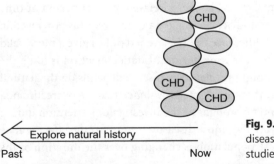

Explore natural history

Past

Now

Fig. 9.4 Natural history of disease in cross-sectional studies.

identify people with the characteristics of interest, here, coronary heart disease (marked as CHD). Assuming that the shaded ovals are representative of the population within the boundary, the findings on the sample are applicable to the whole target population. There are, of course, limitations of statistical variation and the method of selection, so generalization to the target population will need to be cautious.

Sometimes results are generalized to other distant populations too. For example, if the prevalence of CHD is 2 per cent in Liverpool, England, can this information be used in Newcastle, England? The answer is, probably, yes. This result is likely to be generalizable to Newcastle, England, but is unlikely to be valid in Newcastle, Australia. However, we would need to ensure that the characteristics of the populations of the two cities are similar and then generalize with caution. If the population in Liverpool is of a different age, sex, and ethnic structure from that in Newcastle the extrapolation should be avoided. The alternative to making such extrapolations is undertaking national studies or locality-based prevalence studies, both of which are expensive and difficult endeavours. For this reason, extrapolation is more commonly done than scientific rigour would allow.

Rarely, cross-sectional studies are of the whole population. The population census is a cross-sectional study, albeit an extremely large one, and one where the cross-section is only in time and not space. A survey of the blood pressure of all the diabetic patients registered with a particular doctor is also one of a whole population, albeit a small and narrowly defined one. Harland *et al.* (1997) reported a study which attempted to measure the prevalence of diabetes and coronary risk factors of all Chinese people in Newcastle, England; an example of a cross-sectional survey based on a mini census sample.

Cross-sectional surveys are sometimes thought to provide a 'snapshot' of health. This is a simplistic but helpful analogy. The selection, compilation, and definition of the population at risk and the listing of the sampling frame usually conforms to the snapshot analogy. Measurement of risk factors and disease, however, is usually made over a period of time which varies from as little as a day to several years. A rare example of a truly 'snapshot' study is the measurement of the prevalence of bedsores in Glasgow on 21 January 1976. (Ironically, the paper's title inaccurately describes this as a study of the incidence of pressure sores (Barbenel *et al.* 1977).)

In most studies the measurements are made over a relatively short period of time such as a year or two. The merit of a study collecting data over a year (as portrayed in Figs 7.1 and 7.2) is that any seasonal differences will be evened out to give a more valid annual measure of prevalence. When the time period of data collection is long, the degree of mis-measurement of the point prevalence of disease depends on the natural history. If the disease is permanent then the point prevalence may be overestimated because incident cases will occur and be brought to the investigator's attention during the duration of the fieldwork. Fortunately, most diseases are rare so the effect will be small. If the disease incidence or base population is changing over the duration of the study this too will affect the disease prevalence. If there is a dynamic but balanced state with new cases arising and old cases recovering in equal numbers then the mis-measure of the point prevalence is small. The mis-measurement of point prevalence is likely to be important for diseases which vary greatly by season or where the incidence of a disease is changing rapidly. The prevalence of a problem such as bedsores, for example, may be much higher in winter than summer. Here the date on which the study was done is important. It may be that to gauge the true picture repeat cross-sectional studies at different points of the year are advisable. Alternatively, the strategy of collecting data over a year (period prevalence) would also provide the better estimate. For the measurement of a rapidly changing phenomenon, such as the use of ecstasy in teenagers, the cross-sectional study would need to be conducted quickly and repeated to give useful results.

This cross-sectional study design is excellent for measuring the population burden of disease using prevalence rates, which are the most reliable summary measures obtained from such surveys. Data about the past medical history and other circumstances can be, and usually are, collected. This is illustrated in Fig. 9.4 in relation to the natural history of disease. In a cross-sectional study of a sample of the general ('well') population there will be people representing virtually all stages of health and disease, and the full range of exposures of interest. They will represent a wide spectrum of disease. Cross-sectional studies can only give indirect insights on the natural history.

People with severe disease, however, may be institutionalized and either not on the list from which the sample was drawn or not available for study. For example, in a study to measure the prevalence of heart failure, people with the most severe disease may be missed because they are hospitalized long term or have died since the sample list was prepared. While it is usual practice to exclude the recently dead from cross-sectional studies, there is no principle at stake. Data on dead people could be collected from clinical records or from acquaintances and family. For pragmatic reasons the recently deceased are usually excluded. This leads to survivor bias in cross-sectional studies; the portrait of diseases tends to exclude the most severe, possibly fatal, variants of disease. This imbalance can be partially corrected as discussed below.

The investigator may choose to restrict the sample, for example, by studying only people with disease. The sample may, for example, be taken from a register of people with diabetes, with the purpose of measuring the prevalence of smoking in relation to CHD. Such registers may include the recently dead and they can, in some circumstances, be studied.

In studies of the apparently well, cross-sectional studies discover people with previously unknown disease, that is, they uncover the iceberg of disease. The full spectrum of disease can be described only by a combination of cross-sectional surveys of the apparently well population and the diseased population, the latter more often obtained from clinical case-series than from cross-sectional studies. Reflect on the exercise in Box 9.6 before reading on.

Box 9.6 **Differentiating between a case-series and a cross-sectional study**

Reflect on the difference between a case-series study and a cross-sectional study of cases, basing your thinking on a particular problem such as heart failure or diabetes.

A case-series studies a coherent group of cases (or potential cases, i.e. those consulting) accrued over a period of time, sometimes over the entire career of a clinician or life of a clinic or service. By comparison, the cross-sectional survey of cases defines the geographical boundary for the study, and studies all or a sample of the patients under care at a specified and, usually, narrow period of time. For example, a study of all patients ever seen at a diabetic clinic, or those seen consecutively over a year, are case-series. The study of all or a sample of patients on the diabetes clinic's list compiled at a point in time is a cross-sectional study. The distinction is subtle, and emphasizes the interrelationships between study designs.

In theory, when the data on past diseases given by a cross-sectional study are accurate the disease incidence can be estimated (the problem of survivor bias needs to be considered). In practice, collecting accurate data on disease incidence using a cross-sectional design is a problem, mainly because subjects' memory of diseases is poor and medical records may be incomplete. The possibility of estimating incidence should not, however, be dismissed, particularly for populations and topics that do not easily permit follow-up studies, for example, young people joining the workforce (18–25 years), migrants from rural to urban areas in the developing world, or ethnic minority groups in the inner city. The mobility of these groups is high and cohort studies to collect incidence data may not be possible. Some topics, such as use of drugs, experience of sexually transmitted disease, or sexual behaviour, are so sensitive that the possibility of enrolling populations for follow-up cohort studies is small and information in medical records will be incomplete. For example, we may wish to study the incidence of gonorrhoea in young men of 18–25 years. In a cross-sectional study, information on whether and when in the last year the people in the sample had a diagnosis of gonorrhoea could be elicited to help estimate its true incidence. As clinic records are incomplete, population census denominator data unreliable, and the possibility of long-term follow-up of a representative sample of this population is small, the cross-sectional study offers a way of measuring incidence, albeit not an absolutely ideal one, which other studies cannot achieve.

An example is shown in Table 9.3 which is from the study summarized in Table 4.8 and Box 4.6. Here the incidence of consultation for asthma with a general practitioner (physician) has been calculated as well as the prevalence of asthma. A cross-section of people was identified from the register of the population registered with general practitioners

Table 9.3 Reasons for consultation by area in a cross-section of people registered with general practitioners in three areas of North-east England (shown here as zones CA, CB, CC)

	Zone CA	Zone CB	Zone CC
Number of people	734	724	734
Incidence rate of consultations per patient-year			
Total	3.97	4.45	3.86
Asthma diagnoses	0.04	0.05	0.06
Prevalence rate per thousand patients			
Asthma	74	97	113

Adapted from Bhopal *et al.*, *Occupational and Environmental Medicine* 1998; **55**, 812–22. With permission of the BMJ Publishing Group.

held by district health authorities. Medical case records were examined. The study illustrates that cross-sectional studies can do more than measure prevalence. Later, we will reflect on the similarity between this design and a retrospective cohort study (Section 9.6).

The cross-sectional study can be of populations in different places, so comparisons can be made (as in Table 9.3). Studies can also compare people with different characteristics, for example, there may be a sample of women and another of men, or one of people belonging to a Chinese origin population and another of the Indian population. Such studies are comparative cross-sectional studies. (But they are not case-control studies, which are discussed next.)

9.5 Case-control study

Table 9.1 provides a brief summary and Table 9.2 shows how case-control studies fit the dichotomous classifications. The case-control study is a comparative study where people with the disease (or problem) of interest are compared with people without that disease. The meaning of the word case is close to its medical use to describe the characteristics and medical history of a patient. The comparison, control or reference group supplies information about the expected risk factor profile in the population from which the case group is drawn.

The cases can be obtained from a number of sources: from a clinical case-series, a population register of cases, from the new cases identified in a cohort study, and from those identified in a cross-sectional survey. The ideal set of cases would be new (incident) and representative of all cases of the type of interest to the study question in the population under study. The cases from population registers and cohort studies usually meet this ideal the best. The cases identified in a clinical case-series are usually highly selected, while those from a cross-sectional study are usually prevalent ones, though there will be incident cases in a period prevalence study.

The cases are compared with controls, associations between the disease and potential risk factors are measured (usually by the odds ratio), and through analysis of similarities and dissimilarities hypotheses about disease causes are generated or tested.

Information is obtained on the social and medical history of cases and controls and on potential causal and confounding factors. As the causal factors have already had their effect in causing disease in the case group, and the information required is recalled from the past, the case-control study is sometimes referred to as a retrospective study, but this is not a particularly helpful term.

The basic idea is shown in Fig. 9.5. Ideally, the cases are related to a defined population (all ovals in Fig. 9.5). If the aim of the study is to explore the causes of coronary heart disease (marked on Fig. 9.5 as CHD), then new cases would be identified. From the same population are drawn a set of control subjects, marked with the letter C in Fig. 9.5. These control subjects should be chosen with no selection in relation to their pattern of exposure to the postulated causes, but should otherwise be alike to the cases. If, for example, the study was on the causes of CHD (say with a focus on exercise) in post-menopausal women of about 50–75 years, then the control group should also be of women in this age group. Obviously, recruitment of men or children into the control group would be inefficient, and if they were included in the analysis, highly misleading.

In some studies, controls are recruited to match each case; for example, if a woman of 53 years was recruited as a case, the investigator would seek a control of similar age (57 would be fine, but maybe not 72). This matching process is reducing the risk of confounding, here by age and sex. If a mix of ages is likely to arise anyway, the control group can be recruited without one-to-one matching. Matching cases and controls on several characteristics, such as sex, age, ethnicity, smoking status, and social class, is not advisable.

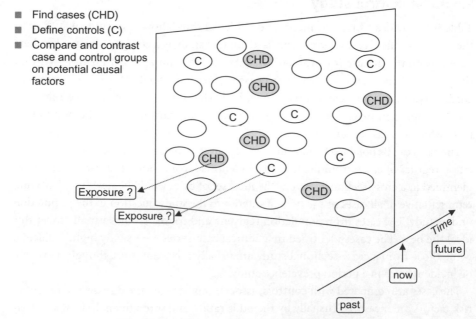

Fig. 9.5 Population concept of a case-control study.

Such matching procedures create difficulties in finding controls, require more complex statistical analysis, and run the risk of 'overmatching'. Overmatching leads to missed associations because the causal factors have been inadvertently matched for. For example, in the above study, if we matched women for smoking status, social class, and income, we may find no association between CHD occurrence and exercise habits, because exercise, smoking, social class, and income are linked. The matching process has created a selection bias, such that differences between cases and controls in exercise habits have been removed or reduced.

Information is collected to confirm (objectively) the presence of disease in cases and in some, but not all types of case-control study, the absence of disease in controls (though, of course, they may be at a prediagnostic phase of the disease's natural history), and on the past exposure to risk factors which may have caused the disease in both groups. This is shown in relation to the natural history of disease in Fig. 9.6. Since CHD develops over years or decades (and risk factors may operate even *in utero*, or be transmitted by previous generations) the collection of information on the causal exposures will need to delve deep into the past, and inevitably will be fraught with difficulty. The concept is clear: to find differences in exposure to the hypothesized causes in the past lives of cases as compared with controls.

These differences can be quantified and summarized either as differences in prevalence of exposure, or more usually as the odds ratio which in defined circumstances approximates to the relative risk (Chapter 8). An exposure that may have caused disease will be more common in cases than in controls giving an odds ratio greater than one, and one that may protect against disease will be less common, giving an odds ratio less than one.

The need for a population base for a case-control study is an especially interesting issue. Of the epidemiological designs, this one is most focused on establishing aetiology and least on measuring burden of disease or risk factors, which is a by-product. So why

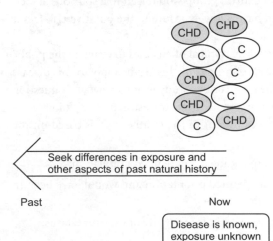

Fig. 9.6 Natural history of disease and case-control studies.

should it be population based? Surely, it may be argued, a finding of a difference between cases and controls is informing us about fundamental differences which apply irrespective of whether the population base is known or not. A classic study by Herbst *et al.* (1971) on the occurrence of the extremely rare disease adenocarcinoma of the vagina in girls and young women illustrates the issues. The study demonstrated an unequivocal association between the disease and use of diethylstilboestrol by mothers of cases in the first trimester of pregnancy; seven of eight cases were treated with the drug compared with none of the 32 controls. Might it be argued that the striking findings tell an underlying biological truth independent of the population base? Do the exercise in Box 9.7 before reading on.

Box 9.7 **Case control studies and the population base: example of the study by Herbst *et al.*.**

- Why do we need an understanding of the population base to execute the study and interpret the findings?
- In what way would the study be impaired if the population base were unknown?

There are both conceptual and pragmatic reasons why this unusually clear-cut study needs, and benefits from, a population base. We must know the geographical area and the time period when the cases occurred to draw an appropriate control group. If the cases are from all over the USA, and have been admitted to one or a few hospitals because of the reputations of the local surgeons, the control group also ought to be a USA wide sample. Taking a local control group may mislead. For example, if the local area physicians had a policy for not using diethylstilboestrol, while there was no such policy in the rest of the country, a local control group would lead to a spurious association; that is, the control group would have a low exposure to the putative risk factor because of a local policy.

We also need to know whether the cases are typical of all cases to evaluate the public health importance of the findings. Do the findings of this study apply to this disease generally? If the selection of cases in the case-control study is not known, this question cannot be answered satisfactorily. On a pragmatic note, the estimate of risk in a case-control study, the odds ratio, as a valid estimator of the relative risk, is based on the assumption that:

- the cases are incident cases drawn from a known and defined population;
- the controls are drawn from the same defined population and would have been in the case group if they had developed the disease;
- controls are selected in an unbiased way, e.g. independently of exposure status;
- and, in some types of study that the disease is rare.

Case-control studies are, for these reasons, best conducted within a population framework. One source of cases and controls that meet the above criteria is the population-based cohort study as discussed next. Some authorities (such as Rothman 1998) emphasize that all case-control studies ought to be conceptualized as part of a theoretical population cohort.

9.6 **Cohort study**

Table 9.1 provides a brief summary and Table 9.2 an analysis based on dichotomous classifications. It is common to hear people, particularly clinicians, speak of 'their cohort', simply meaning a group, irrespective of the study design. The word cohort is derived from the Latin cohors meaning an enclosure, company, or crowd. In Roman times a cohort was a body of 300–600 infantry. In epidemiological terms the cohort is a group of people with something in common, usually an exposure or involvement in a defined population group.

The cohort study involves tracking the study population over a period of time, a feature reflected in three synonyms for this design: follow-up, longitudinal, and prospective. As with the cross-sectional survey the cohort study population may be a general one, or one with characteristics of particular interest, for example, people with a defined lifestyle or even a disease. The hallmark of this design is that health outcome or health change data are obtained on the same individuals in a population at more than one time, not just once as in the cross-sectional study. The idea is to study part of the natural history of risk factors or diseases in individuals, and to relate one or more characteristics, exercise for example, to future outcomes such as coronary heart disease (Figs 9.7 and 9.8 illustrate this).

In Fig. 9.7 two groups are identified in the base population (all ovals), those who exercise (ovals marked E) and those who do not (NE). These two groups are followed up over time to ascertain the number of new cases of the outcome (CHD) in both groups, thereby calculating a disease incidence rate. Data are collected prospective to the construction of the sampling frame and assignment of exposure status, and this applies to retrospective cohorts too (see below). Figure 9.8 shows that cohort studies are future orientated in relation to the natural history of disease.

Comparison groups are usually identified within the cohort (e.g. people who smoke or do not smoke) but sometimes separate cohorts are set up at the outset. In the latter case, the cohort study is usually exploring a specific hypothesis, which dictates the nature of the comparison group. If a particular exposure or characteristic of interest is rare then the identification of separate cohorts will be necessary. In causal research, cohort studies usually test the hypothesis that disease incidence differs in people with different characteristics (exposures) at baseline; that is, there is an association between exposure and outcome.

The cohort study begins by establishing baseline data, usually from a cross-sectional study, or less commonly by the extraction of baseline data from sources such as the census (for legal and ethical reasons relating to data confidentiality such cohorts are rare and will become even rarer), or a routine information system such as a birth register.

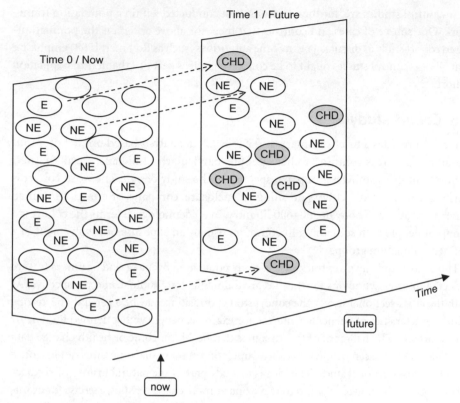

Fig. 9.7 Population concept of a cohort study.

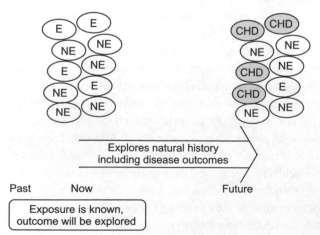

Fig. 9.8 Natural history of disease and cohort studies.

The cohort can either be followed up directly with repeated surveys of the same population or the baseline data can be linked to health records, so providing information on outcomes of interest, usually disease related but potentially also on risk factors. The new cases of disease identified are incident cases and can be enrolled into a case-control study. Controls can also be identified from within the cohort, and this is best done as each case occurs. This is known as a nested case-control study.

Where medical records permit accurate assessment of both risk factors and disease outcomes, only possible when data are collected systematically (and preferably computerized), cohort studies may be possible without any prospective work. The label retrospective cohort study is then applied. Essentially, the cohort is identified from past records of exposure status and this is the vital step. Usually, the outcome data are also obtained from records but this information can be supplemented with direct questioning of those subjects who are alive, and can be traced. Once identified the subjects can be followed up over time (prospectively) so using both currently available and future data on outcome. Figures 9.9 and 9.10 illustrate the concept in the context of populations

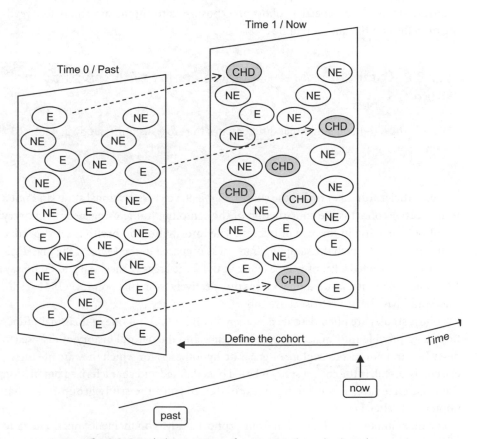

Fig. 9.9 Population concept of a retrospective cohort study.

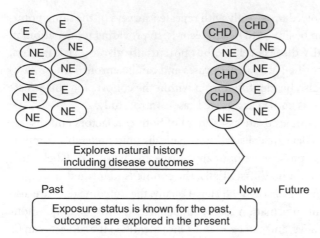

Fig. 9.10 Natural history of disease and retrospective cohort studies.

and the natural history of disease. The difference between this design and the prospective cohort is minimal; a retrospective cohort is assembled from historical records on exposure status, the prospective cohort on exposure status in the present. Before reading on reflect on the question in Box 9.8.

Box 9.8 **Comparing a retrospective cohort with the study in Table 9.3**

What is the essential feature that differentiates the cross-sectional study in Table 9.3 from a cohort study?

The essential feature that makes the study in Table 9.3 a cross-sectional study and not a retrospective cohort is the construction of the sampling frame using a contemporary list of people living in the area of interest. The information on health is retrospective from the point at which the sampling frame was prepared in the 1990s. If the investigators had constructed a list of people living in the same areas (zones A, B and C) in, say, 1940, and looked at consultation patterns prospectively from that point, say 1941–1946, this would have been a retrospective cohort.

Cohort studies are often described as analytic (Table 9.2) but one of their main functions is to provide information on the incidence and the natural history of disease (to describe) and not just to explore or generate hypotheses, for which they are of course, extremely useful. If the cohort study is based on a defined and characterized population the incidence rates can often be extrapolated beyond the study group to similar populations elsewhere.

The most important information from a cohort study is on incidence rates. The ratio of the incidence rates in the exposed and non-exposed groups derived from the cohort study is the relative risk, the primary basis for measuring the strength of an association, one of the keys to causal thinking in epidemiology. The calculation and interpretation of incidence rates was discussed in Chapter 7 and the relative risk was discussed in Chapter 8.

9.7 **Trials**

Tables 9.1 and 9.2 provide a brief summary and description based on dichotomous classifications. Trials are studies where an intervention designed to improve health has been applied to a population, and the outcome assessed at follow-up. Such studies may help us to understand disease causes, assess the effectiveness of interventions to influence the natural history of disease, and the costs and benefits of interventions. Trials are experiments, and may be described by various terms including intervention studies, clinical trials, and community trials. The term 'trial' is usually reserved for experiments that are not done in the laboratory setting, and are on human or whole animal studies. The trial has, essentially, the same design as a cohort study with one vital difference, that the exposure status of the study population has been deliberately changed by the investigator to see how this alters the incidence of disease or other features of the natural history (Figs 9.11 and 9.12).

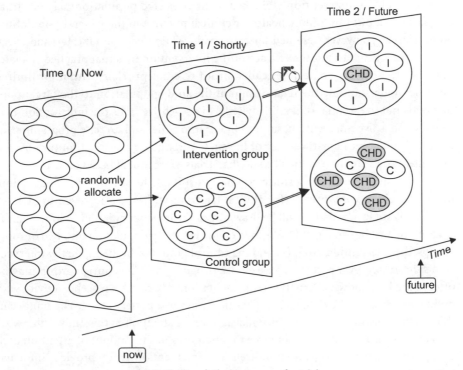

Fig. 9.11 Population concept of a trial.

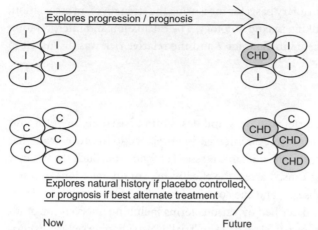

Now   Future

Fig. 9.12 Natural history of disease and trials.

Clinical and public health trials are difficult and important endeavours, which usually have a practical question to answer: whether a particular intervention is sufficiently effective to be introduced into clinical or public health practice. Such trials need to be based on a study population with proper understanding of how it relates to the (target) population which will be offered the intervention should it be shown to be successful. An intervention which works in a selected population may not fulfil its goals when put into public health or clinical practice in the general population. Some trials are, however, designed solely to produce knowledge about cause and effect, the intention being to test the efficacy of the intervention in actual practice at a later date. For these trials, sometimes called proof of concept trials, with their limited purpose, understanding the relationship of the study population to the target population is not so essential (but still advised). In preventive trials the intervention may be either an active intervention, say enrolment into a diet and exercise programme, or the manipulation of a natural way of life such as reducing the consumption of salt. Preventive trials are more difficult to do than trials of treatment based on drugs.

The first step is to define a study population suitable for answering the question, i.e. people either with disease (for clinical trials) or without (for prevention trials). Ideally, this study population will be drawn from the target population as shown in the ovals in the first box in Fig. 9.11. We then divide the study population into two or more groups, the intervention group(s) and the control group(s). In the figure the intervention symbolized by a cyclist, is an exercise programme. The control group may be offered the best known alternative (e.g. meditation classes) or a placebo activity with no known effect on the outcome (e.g. participation in a pottery class). The important thing is that the two groups gain an equal amount of attention in the study. Otherwise, the changes seen might be attributable to differences in the amount of attention each group receives, not the intervention itself. The intervention group provides information on prognosis, the control group on the natural history.

In the ideal trial, the study and control populations are at the same stage of the natural history of disease (Fig. 9.12), and are similar in the characteristics that affect disease outcomes, differing only in exposure to the intervention. To maximize the chances that the intervention and control groups are the same at baseline, and hence avoid confounding, the trial design should ensure that individuals in the study are assigned randomly to the groups. This process solves the problem of finding the right control group. This then is a randomized, controlled trial. Where there is no 'best known alternative' an intervention which is 'psychologically' of similar impact to the study intervention, but has no influence on the diseases process is used (a placebo, from the Latin word to please). This is a placebo-controlled randomized trial. To prevent bias, the subject, the field investigator, and the subjects' health carer, might not be told whether the subject receives the 'active' intervention or the control intervention (they are so-called 'blind'). This is a triple-blind, randomized, placebo-controlled trial (if the subject and the health carer do not know, this is 'double blind'). We now follow up the study populations and count the events of interest; in the example, the number of cases of coronary heart disease. Analysis is by comparing incidence rates of outcome (Chapters 7 and 8) or other outcome measures that are beyond the scope of this book.

9.8 **Overlap in the conceptual basis of the case-series, cross-sectional, case-control, cohort, and trial designs**

The cross-sectional study can be repeated using the same sampling methods to evaluate changes in time. The subjects in the second study will be different from those studied in the first, although there may be, by the laws of chance, some overlap. This is simply a repeat cross-sectional study. If, however, the same sample is studied for a second time (i.e. it is followed up), the original cross-sectional study now becomes a cohort study. The cohort study can also be turned into a trial. The key difference between a cohort design and a trial is that the investigator observes the study subjects in the former but imposes an intervention in the latter. If, during a cohort study, possibly in a subgroup, the investigator imposes an intervention, a trial begins. The cohort study also gives birth to case-control studies.

When people with a particular disease are compared with others without that disease, the study is a case-control study. Ideally, the case-control study should be of new, or incident, cases. Cases that are newly discovered in a cohort study are ideal. Failing that, cases could be from a cross-sectional study (though these are probably going to be prevalent ones) or from a case-series.

Cases in a case-series, particularly a population based one, may be the starting point of a case-control study or a trial. Case-series may provide the data on outcomes for a cohort study or trial. A cross-sectional study of people in a case-series is also possible.

These similarities and interrelations, overlooked in classifications which emphasize the distinctions in study design, unify a series of study designs. The important thing is to understand the principles behind, and the defining features of, a particular study design.

Not every epidemiological study fits neatly into one of the basic five designs in Box 9.1. However, such atypical studies are usually variants and amalgams of the basic designs, which can be grasped with an understanding of the key features and purposes of the five designs discussed. Table 9.4 develops this point by listing a range of epidemiological studies with their general aims and then indicating the usual design options. Investigators usually have a choice. In general, the simpler, cheaper approaches are adopted first. Experience indicates that the order of difficulty and expense of these studies is: case-series, cross-sectional, case-control, cohort, and trials. As we move along this sequence there are additional nuances; for example, the ethical and recruitment problems raised by trials add complexity to the challenge of follow-up, which is otherwise shared with cohort studies. The case-control adds the complexity of a control group to the one of establishing an unbiased case-series. The cross-sectional study adds the complexity of recruitment, consent, and a community base in comparison to a case-series. Before reading on do the exercise in Box 9.9.

Box 9.9 **Strengths and weaknesses of the study designs**

Based on the principles of study design and your knowledge of the purposes of epidemiology, consider the relative strengths and weakness of clinical and population case-series, cross-sectional, case-control and cohort studies, and trials. Put these in a table. You may find the following key words and phrases helpful in your reflection: ease, timing, maintenance and continuity, costs, ethics, data utilization, main contributions, observer and selection bias, analytic outputs.

Some of the strengths and weaknesses of each study design are given in Table 9.5. This is not a complete list. Full discussion of each point is beyond the scope of this book, and will be found in books concentrating on methods. The important point is that, contrary to a widely expressed view, each study has strengths and weaknesses and no one study design is superior. The 'hierarchy of evidence' whereby the trial is said to produce definitive evidence, and other designs weaker evidence, is a narrow idea that only applies to evaluation, particularly of drugs. Other designs are stronger for measuring the burden of disease and in understanding causality. As the history of epidemiology has demonstrated repeatedly, causal understanding comes from all types of study, and above all through deep reflection on disease patterns, however generated (see Chapter 5, e.g. Table 5.9). The landmark studies that have revolutionized medicine and public health, could be discarded by those who apply the checklist-based routines of 'evidence based medicine'. Understanding the concepts behind each study, however, is essential in choosing, interpreting, and evaluating reports of studies in the context of the research questions being addressed.

Table 9.4 Types, aim, and design of some epidemiological studies

Type of study	Main aims	Possible design(s)
Disease counts and description	Establish size of case-load; define characteristics of disease; generate hypotheses based on factors in common (similarity of cases); test hypotheses by seeing whether predicted associations occur	Case-series, preferably part of a clinical or population register
Incidence rates of disease or death, in relation to risk factors	(a) Establish disease rates; assess variation over time, place, and characteristics of cases; generate or test hypotheses (b) As above plus study natural history of disease; seek associations between risk factors and disease	(a) Population case-series with cases related to population usually defined by a census (b) Cohort studies with populations defined by exposure
International comparisons	Explore similarities and differences in disease rates, establish the relative importance of environmental anc genetic factors in disease, generate or test hypotheses	(a) Population case series, related to population census (b) Multicentre cross-sectional study (c) Multicentre cohort study
Prevalence of disease or risk factors	Quantify disease and risk factor burden; seek associations between disease and risk factors; generate or test hypotheses	(a) Cross-sectional study (b) Disease or at-risk registers related to a population census
Comparison of people with and without disease	Generate or test hypotheses by comparing similarities and dissimilarities between cases and controls	Case-control
Twin studies	Compare similarities and dissimilarities between people of similar genetic environment to give insight on the relative contribution of genetic and environmental factors in disease	Registers of twins studied by cohort design (often retrospective cohort)
Migrant studies	Follow effect of environmental change, to assess relative importance of genetic and environmental factors. Measure burden of disease in immigrant populations	Analysis of population case-series by country of birth, and cross-sectional or cohort studies of migrants in their adopted homeland compared with non-migrants in the land of origin
Evaluations	To assess effectiveness of interventions in decreasing disease, improving health or reducing risk factors	(a) Trial (b) Repeat cross-sectional study (c) Observations of change over time in population case-series data (d) Case-control studies

Table 9.5 Some of the strengths and weaknesses of each study design

Theme	Clinical case series	Population case-series	Cross-sectional	Case-control	Cohort	Trial
1. Ease	Easy to compile by clinicians or through clinicians	Difficult, as needs large number of data contributors and complex systems to ensure quality, comparable data	Difficulty depends on the study. Studies of natural living populations are hard compared with those at schools or other institutions	Usually difficult because of need for appropriate control group and problem of recall bias	Difficult because of added complexity of follow-up	Difficulty exceeds the cohort because of technical and ethical challenges of imposing an intervention
2. Timing	May be available very quickly especially if health administration systems record diagnosis	Needs much planning time Merging of data from clinical or administrative databases, if possible, can speed up the process greatly	Usually finished within months or a few years	Usually finished within months or a few years except those on incident cases of rare diseases	Usually long-term (decades) though sometimes (e.g. studies of birth outcomes) they can be quick	Usually deliberately designed to give an answer within a few years or a decade, i.e. usually shorter than cohort studies
3. Maintenance and continuity	Possible as along as clinical commitment remains	Demands continuing effort on part of clinicians and administrators	Study is usually stopped	Study is usually stopped	Long-term continuity is essential and problematic, particularly as observations are on free-living people	Similar to cohort studies but when trials are in patients with diseases, the commitment to the trial may be high
4. Costs	Costs are low in compiling the series because data are at hand	Costs are high but usually hidden in the administration of the health service	Costs depend on study but lower than cohort or trial of same size	Costs are usually comparable with cross-sectional studies and, as study size is small, the overall costs may be low	Costs are high both because numbers studied are large and because costs of retaining staff and systems to collect data over many years are high	Costs are high for the same reason as the cohort study and there are additional costs of the intervention, obtaining ethical approval, and trial management
5. Ethics	Ethical issues such as confidentiality are not	Data collection and storage systems must meet ever-	Standard ethical issues, and problem of obtaining	Standard ethical issues as in clinical case-series	Confidentiality issues are acute, particularly	The ethics of trials are complex and evolving

	usually difficult if investigator is the clinician	stricter legal and ethical standards	access to sampling frame	but also those of cross-sectional studies for community controls	as adverse outcomes may affect occupation and insurance premiums. Potential intrusion of repeated contact and measurement	and hinge on the issue of doing no harm and informed consent
6. Data utilization	Data are likely to be used for clinical and research purposes	Data are usually under-utilized	Usually under-utilized, as more information is collected than needed	As analysis is straight-forward, data are usually fully analysed	Data tend to be underutilized	Data concerning the central question are utilized
7. Main contribution	Contributes to clinical knowledge, health needs, disease burden and may spark causal hypotheses	Contributes to burden of disease, and sparking causal and testing hypotheses	Major contribution to burden of disease, substantial contribution to analysis of associations and may confirm or spark hypotheses	Major contribution to clinical knowledge, and sparking causal hypotheses. Control group may supply burden of need data	Major contribution to both burden of disease (incidence) and causal analysis	Main contribution is to understanding of effectiveness of interventions, and indirectly to disease mechanisms
8. Observer bias	May be compiled by single or few observers, minimizing observer bias	Multiplicity of contributors, so vast problem of observer bias	Small studies may be done by one observer, but for most studies inter-observer bias is a problem	Small studies may be done by one observer; large studies usually need a few	Usually requires multiple observers, though exceptionally, studies may be small	Usually requires multiple observers
9. Selection bias	Major problem	Minor problem as unselected cases but sometimes the diagnosis is inadequately confirmed	Selection bias arising from non-response is almost inevitable	Studies of prevalent cases have selection bias, those of incident cases minimize this. All studies have recall bias	Selection bias due to non-response at baseline is augmented by loss to follow-up	Selection biases are particularly severe because non-participation may be high and because intervention may only be suitable for some of the target population
10. Analytic output	Case numbers, percentages, proportional morbidity/mortality ratio	Main output is disease rates	Main output is prevalence though other measures including the odds ratio are possible (not the relative risk)	Proportions exposed and odds ratios	Incidence rate and the relative incidence, i.e. relative risk	Incidence, survival and numbers needed to treat or prevent

9.9 **Ecological studies: design or analysis?**

Ecology is the study of living organisms in relation to their environment. As we discussed in Chapter 1 epidemiology is, in many respects, an ecological discipline and in a general sense all or most epidemiological studies are ecological. The phrase 'ecological study', however, has come to mean (from Last), 'A study in which the units of analysis are populations or groups of people, rather than individuals.' The unit of analysis in epidemiology is always the group. Usually, though, data analysis is on aggregate measures made on individuals. Last gives as an example a study of the association between median income and cancer mortality rates in states and countries (p. 57, 4th edn). In such a study the cancer mortality rates are likely to derive from individual data from a population case-series held in a database (registry) of deaths, and median income from a census or other cross-sectional studies. In this example, the investigators have chosen to analyse their data by place (rather than, say, age, sex, or social class). This choice is not an inherent design feature but a mode of analysis. This type of analysis is also sometimes called correlational, demographic, or descriptive. For example, MacMahon and Trichochopolous inform us that ecological studies are descriptive studies based on routinely collected information. In this book these studies are described as population case-series, because the label ecological is not necessary and is potentially misleading. If the label is to be used, then it should be reserved for studies where the variables measure a feature of the place and not of individuals. How, then, must we conceptualize the ecological study?

There are variables which are truly not based on individual data and that are useful in epidemiology. Such variables were discussed in Chapter 2 (Section 2.5 in particular) and in Section 9.3. Sometimes such variables are merely a substitute for individualized data, which may not exist. For example, information on the duties (taxes) collected by governments on products such as alcohol and tobacco exist over long periods of time. Such data may be a partial substitute for information on consumption patterns in individuals and populations. Such data also provide additional information, for example, on government policy on the population's use of such products, the state of the economy, and the legal status of these products. Other variables that relate to a place may have no equivalent individual level counterpart (see also Chapter 2): gross national product, air quality measures, lead in water, the weather, expenditure on roads, the type of political structure, or the density of population. The variables might reasonably be described as ecological, particularly those relating to the natural environment. Such variables can be studied on their own with descriptions of time trends, variation between places, and differences by the characteristics of the populations in these places. Variables can be correlated with each other, for example, the relationship between expenditure on road traffic and particulate air pollution. Assuming such a study helps to study living organisms in relation to their environment, it could be said

Table 9.6 Design by mode of analysis

	Aggregate data on individuals	By aggregate data on places (ecological)
Ecological	–	✔
Case-series		
– clinical	✔	(✔)
– population	✔	✔
Cross-sectional	✔	(✔)
Case-control	✔	(✔)
Cohort	✔	(✔)
Trial	✔	(✔)

to be an ecological study, albeit a simple one and if it sheds light on the population pattern of disease it is also epidemiology.

There are other circumstances in which exposure data relating to a place and not to individuals (say hardness of water) are correlated with health data collected on individuals but summarized by place (say CHD rates). In this circumstance the boundaries are blurred. Here the study could simply be described as a population case-series study. Conceptually, the ecological component is an issue of data analysis and not study design. Cross-sectional, case-control, and cohort studies and trials (and not just population case-series) could also be analysed in relation to such 'ecological' variables and such units of analysis. This thinking leads us to modify our Box 9.1 as in Table 9.6. In Table 9.6 ecological studies are considered to be those using aggregate data on places. By this definition, the ecological design does not use aggregate information on individuals, simply because all of epidemiology does that. Studies on individuals of any design, however, can be analysed geographically using data on places. In practice, such analyses take place on population case-series and large cross-sectional studies such as the census. For other studies, the numbers of people enrolled and the geographical spread is usually too small. This is reflected by placing brackets around the tick in Table 9.6.

9.10 Size of the study

In planning a study the size of the study population is a crucial matter. Studies that are larger than they need to be are inefficient and wasteful not only of money but also scarce epidemiological expertise. Studies that are too small may provide misleading answers, or at least, imprecise ones.

Estimation of a desired study size is a complex issue, and one that is core to most statistics courses (and beyond this book). The principles, however, can be stated succinctly as follows:

- The sample size will be dictated by the research questions and stated study hypotheses.
- The study hypotheses need to be specified in a way that can be quantified; e.g. that the predicted incidence of a disease is 2 per cent per year, and that exposure to a risk factor (say smoking) doubles the incidence.
- The precision of the answer required needs to be stated; e.g. a study wishing to establish the incidence rate of a disease as 10/10 000 per year with no more than 10 per cent error, will be larger than one accepting an error of 40 per cent around the estimate.
- In studies where the hypothesis is based on a difference between groups, the size of the minimum difference that it is important to detect should be stated (alternatively, state the size of the difference expected).
- The sample size should be large enough to keep low the chances of two types of statistical error. Type 1 error is the error of rejecting a null hypothesis when it is true. In the context of most epidemiological studies a null hypothesis is one stating that there is no difference between comparison groups. In making this error one is claiming a difference when there is none and apparent differences have occurred by chance. In most research we wish the probability of making such an error to be lower than 5 per cent.
- Type 2 error is in failing to reject a null hypothesis when it is false. In epidemiology, this usually means declaring there is no difference between comparison groups when there is. Most studies aim to have less than 20 per cent probability of such an error. The power of a study is the probability that a type 2 error will not occur (so most studies aim for a power of 80 per cent or more).

With this type of information the stage is set to calculate sample size. Each study design, however, imposes its own specific requirements, and the reader will find guidance in books on statistical and epidemiological methods.

9.11 **Data analysis and interpretation**

The principles outlined in all the earlier chapters will be required to interpret data properly, particularly taking into account error, bias, and frameworks for analysis of associations. There is a multitude of choice in data analysis – the reader will need to consult one of many suitable textbooks – but the principles behind the basic measurements are in Chapters 7 and 8. The first step is to examine numbers of cases and percentages, and age and sex specific prevalence or incidence data (Chapter 7), to check for errors, obvious biases and patterns. Then choices of summary measures need to be made. The ideas behind, and strengths and limitations of, many of the key measures were discussed in Chapter 8. Every study design presents choices, but the principal outputs for each study design are given in Table 9.5 (analytic output). For calculating measures of association the 2×2 table (Chapter 8, Table 8.6) provides the standard way to present data. Table 5.9 shows how different study designs contribute towards judgements of cause and effect. Chapter 10 introduces the art of critical appraisal—a skill vital to data interpretation.

9.12 **Conclusion**

Study design is best thought of as a system of interlinked and mutually supporting methods. As the various designs have similar purposes, are rooted in population concepts of health and disease, and are conceptually overlapping, they are also subject to similar errors, biases, and problems of sampling, and similar challenges in data collection, analysis, and interpretation. In practice epidemiologists may use a mix of designs to solve a problem, and it may be difficult to name the design of the study. Most studies can be distinguished by their focus on either disease or exposure, the relationship of the observation to calendar time and the natural history of disease, and whether there is an imposed intervention.

Epidemiological designs are based on the theories discussed in earlier chapters, particularly that differential exposure to the causes of disease leads to differential population patterns of disease. Only one design—the cohort study—tests this theory directly. The trial tests it indirectly by seeing whether drugs or preventive procedures that interfere with the putative causes will prevent or control diseases thus leading to more favourable outcomes. Trials that deliberately exposed people to the causes of disease would be unethical. The other designs (case-series, case-control, and cross-sectional) test the theory indirectly and retrospectively. Studies of various designs, or more strictly, the data from such studies, helps to develop and refine causal theories of disease. The process of designing studies and interpreting data, and the unanswered questions arising, drive advances in methods and techniques.

This chapter only touches on the vast experience and writings on study design and methods; hopefully sufficient to allow the reader to understand more advanced writings and to link earlier concepts to methods. To implement a study requires a knowledge of scientific writing, preparation of proforma, sampling methods, statistics, computing, and data interpretation (and other skills, all beyond the scope of this book). The final chapter considers the art of reading and interpreting an epidemiological study, as discussed in the context of epidemiological theory, ethics, and practice. This skill, known as critical appraisal, is essential, and is best applied on a sound foundation of understanding of epidemiological concepts.

Summary

Epidemiological studies have apparently distinct designs but are unified by their common goal to understand the frequency and causes of disease, by their strategy of seeking associations between exposures (potential causes) and outcomes (disease), by their utilization of the survey method, and by their basis in defined populations. This explains why they complement each other, for example, in assessing the weight of evidence for cause and effect, and why small changes can change the design.

The population case-series and the cross-sectional survey lie at the core of the epidemiological method. A case-series is a coherent set of cases of a disease (or similar problem). A population case-series is a set of such cases arising in a defined population and time. Cases can be analysed as rates over time, between places, and by population characteristics to generate understanding of the burden of disease and to generate associations. If such cases are compared with non-cases we have a case-control study (see below). In a population studied at a specific time and place (a cross-section), measurements can be made of disease, the factors which may cause disease, or both simultaneously. This is a cross-sectional survey and its primary output is prevalence data, though associations between risk factors and disease can be generated and tested. Such a survey might be used to identify all cases of a particular disease in a population. If the characteristics of this group of cases are compared with those of a population without the disease, we have, again, a case-control study (of prevalent cases). If the population in a cross-sectional survey is followed up to measure health outcomes, this study design is a cohort study. Cohort studies produce data on disease incidence and on associations between risk factors and disease outcomes. Cases discovered in the course of follow-up in a cohort study may be compared with non-cases and, once again, give rise to a 'nested' case-control study. If the population of a cohort study is, at baseline, divided into two groups, and the investigators impose a health intervention upon one of the groups, the design is that of a trial. Trials produce data on incidence in treated populations in comparison with those untreated. They are used, primarily, to test rather then generate hypotheses, and their prime output is information on effectiveness of health interventions.

Studies based on aggregated data, usually based on geographically defined units of population, are commonly referred to as ecological studies. They represent a mode of analysis, rather than a design. All five epidemiological designs could, in theory, be analysed using 'ecologically' aggregated data. In practice, only population case-series and very large cross-sectional studies such as the census lend themselves to such a form of analysis, simply because other designs usually have insufficient numbers.

In all epidemiological studies interpretation and application of data are easier when the relationship between the population observed and the target population is understood. For example, case-series studies need a population to construct rates; the cross-sectional study needs a case or population register to construct a sampling frame; the case-control study should, ideally, be on a defined, representative population of incident cases; the cohort study should inform about risk factor–disease outcome relations in other populations; and the results of trials are only useful if they apply outside the study population.

All designs contribute, though unequally, to measuring disease burden for health policy and planning, and to testing causal hypotheses. The distinction between designs which serve one function or the other is not clear cut.

Theoretical, ethical, contextual, practical, and critical foundations for future epidemiology

Objectives

On completion of this chapter you should understand that:

- theory, method, and application are interrelated, therefore, evolution in the one leads to change in the others;
- epidemiology serves the community in a number of ways, but predominantly through its role as one of the underpinning sciences of public health and medicine;
- ongoing vigorous debate on the future of epidemiology probably heralds a paradigm shift;
- epidemiology is both broadening and specializing;
- the context in which epidemiology is learned and practised is important in determining its nature;
- epidemiological codes of ethics and good conduct need to encompass both science and the medical and public health applications;
- critical appraisal of research is an essential skill for epidemiologists and requires attention to fundamental issues including the social and geographical context of research;
- epidemiologists need to study their subject's history, classical studies, contemporary research, and debates that will shape the future.

10.1 The interrelationship of theory, methods, and application: a question of values

Epidemiology has entered the twenty-first century with both its exponents and critics questioning its foundations, record, and future. Epidemiology has been accused of being atheoretical; divorced from its source of problems, theories, and applications (public health); the source of spurious, confusing, and misleading findings; and over-dependent on the 'black box' risk factor approach. Even more seriously, there are questions about the relevance of epidemiology to resolving some major problems, such as the growing consumption of illegal drugs, the rising prevalence of smoking in developing countries, and the omnipresent problem of health inequalities. To participate in the resolution of such problems epidemiologists need to go beyond techniques.

In 1978 Alwyn Smith criticized the atheoretical, empirical, methodological orientation of modern epidemiology and called for an integration of social, political, and biological frameworks of health and disease into epidemiology. In his 1985 review of the evolution of epidemiology in the USA Melvyn Susser paid tribute to the methodological advances which had led to epidemiology reaching maturity as an academic discipline, but he echoed some of Smith's concerns, and emphasized that epidemiology originated as an applied public health discipline. Nancy Krieger (1992) concluded, based partly on an examination of textbooks, that attention has been diverted from theory and concepts of epidemiology to methods and technique. These and other influential observations, hopefully, will lead to a closer integration of theory, method, and application.

The philosophy and theory underpinning epidemiology, as in most other disciplines, is seldom made explicit and yet underpins all its work, is a driver of change, and guides the paradigms within which it works. A full exposition of the theoretical and philosophical basis of epidemiology is not within easy grasp, and is beyond this textbook, but a dialogue needs to be opened up. The following is a simple account that summarizes much that has been covered earlier.

Philosophically, epidemiology takes a positivist stance. The positivists' position is that problems can be solved and questions can be answered through the collection of data which are usually, but not always, quantitative. This stance has served epidemiology well. There are limitations in the quantitative approach, which is excellent for description, but insufficient for generating understanding. This book has repeatedly emphasized that great advances may follow inspiration and insights that are not based on quantitative data. A future epidemiology is likely to involve closer ties between qualitative and quantitative approaches.

The basic theory from which the aetiological contribution of epidemiology derives, is that systematic variations in the pattern of health and disease exist in populations and these are a product of differences in either the prevalence of, or susceptibility to, the causal factors. The fundamental epidemiological question is why these differences in prevalence and susceptibility occur, and the challenge is to link explanations to the observed phenomena and to predict one from the other. Ultimately, such predictions could generate the 'laws' of health and disease in populations. Epidemiological theory attributes the causes to an interaction within the causal triad of host, agent, and environment. This triad works particularly well for toxic and infectious diseases, but to make it more widely applicable it needs to be developed in more detail. Development will be derived from the expanding fields described by the labels of genetic, social, life-course, and chronic disease epidemiology. This way of causal thinking was discussed in Chapters 1, 2, 3, and 5. Before reading on do the exercise in Box 10.1.

> ## Box 10.1
>
> List five or six broad and fundamental influences on health and disease, i.e. those influences that change the population patterns of disease.

10.2 **Fundamental influences on health**

The influences on health and disease include natural changes in the environment; environmental change arising from human invention, discovery, and manipulation; changes in the interaction between humans, microbes, and animals usually for cultural reasons; changes in human circumstances, cultures, and behaviours; and the genetic evolution of microbes, animals, and humans. These complex and interacting influences, exerting their effect over long spans of time (for human genetic effects, likely to be measured in hundreds or thousands of years) are the underlying causes of population patterns in disease. Their initial impact may be on individuals and families or small groups. Over time, due to their varying circumstances, populations begin to differ from each other, leading to the population patterns in disease and health that epidemiologists describe (symbolized in the triad of time, place, and person). Epidemiological methods are designed to quantify variations in diseases and in their causes, to seek and quantify associations between them, and to generate and test resultant hypotheses, which are usually couched in more specific terms than above, but are embedded in the above concepts. Figure 10.1 provides a simplified diagrammatic representation of the above concepts.

Variations in disease frequency give rise to hypotheses which might help to explain the patterns observed, and give insight into the natural history and causes of disease. Classical epidemiological study designs (such as case-control and cohort) can be used to test such insights (Chapter 9) and, if supported, epidemiological criteria can be applied to assess the likelihood of associations representing cause and effect. Epidemiological models of cause (such as the triangle of causation) can help to conceptualize interventions for disease control (Chapter 5). Knowledge of cause and effect is essential to developing rational scientific interventions to prevent, control, and treat disease. To ensure these interventions work they need to be evaluated. Epidemiological study designs are also used for evaluating screening and diagnostic tests, in evaluating preventive and other procedures, in assessing the efficacy of drugs and other interventions in curative medicine, and in studies of prognosis. While all the study designs may contribute to evaluation, the most powerful one is the trial.

As many important advances derive from practical problems, epidemiological theory, research, and practice should intertwine. Morris, in his classic book, *Uses of Epidemiology* published in 1957, portrayed epidemiology as a discipline with multiple applications as reflected in his chapter headings: trends in disease, community diagnosis, working of health services, individual chances, completing the clinical picture, identification of

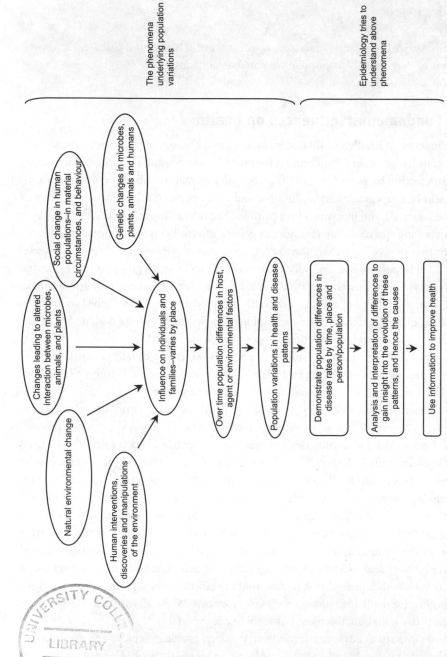

The phenomena underlying population variations

Epidemiology tries to understand above phenomena

Social change in human populations—in material circumstances, and behaviour

Genetic changes in microbes, plants, animals and humans

Changes leading to altered interaction between microbes, animals, and plants

Natural environmental change

Human interventions, discoveries and manipulations of the environment

Influence on individuals and families—varies by place

Over time population differences in host, agent or environmental factors

Population variations in health and disease patterns

Demonstrate population differences in disease rates by time, place and person/population

Analysis and interpretation of differences to gain insight into the evolution of these patterns, and hence the causes

Use information to improve health

Fig. 10.1 The basis of population differences in health and disease pattern: towards a theory.

syndromes, causal search, etc. In most contemporary textbooks, by comparison, the vision of epidemiology is narrower, and probably narrowing. Textbooks placing an emphasis on method, technique, and analysis wrongly imply that epidemiology is primarily about measuring disease in populations, and not primarily about how diseases develop, propagate, and are prevented in populations. Measuring disease is, however, merely the means to the end. One vital question under current debate is whether epidemiology is primarily an applied discipline or primarily a science where methods, technique, and theory dominate over practice and applications. Whatever the outcome the fact is that epidemiology has an impact on health and health care.

In measuring the frequency (incidence and prevalence) of disease in defined populations (Chapter 7), epidemiological studies almost invariably uncover morbidity, unmet healthcare need, and show the 'iceberg of disease' thus leading to new services (Chapter 6). Comparisons of disease patterns over time, between geographical areas, and by the characteristics of people within populations (e.g. by sex and age) also permit an understanding of how disease patterns are likely to change (Chapters 3 and 9). Disease trends, combined with information on demographic change and risk factor patterns, can be used to predict the future, and develop health targets. For example, epidemiological observations in the UK in the 1980s and 1990s on the trend in measles cases, with the prediction of an epidemic, gave priority to a national measles campaign targeted at school children; predictions of the HIV and AIDS epidemic in the mid-1980s gave priority to these problems; and the observations of variations in disease experience by socio-economic status have placed inequalities in health as one of the top ranking international and national priorities.

The traditional values of epidemiology are that it is concerned with the nature of health and disease in populations; that there is population group variation in disease that is worthy of scientific study; that it is important to medical and public health policy and practice; and that is it vital to prevent, control, and treat disease. To illustrate how theory, method, and application are interdependent I have chosen two topics of personal interest: setting priorities in health care and assessing the impact on health of local polluting industries.

10.3 Setting priorities in health and health care

> Setting priorities is an issue for any organisation. The process should be sensible; it should be founded on science; it should be based on experience and research.
>
> Virginia Bottomley (1993)

Priority setting within health and health care is a complex mix of science and politics. Epidemiological data on disease frequency, patterns, causes, risk factors, and effectiveness can stimulate and feed the political debate at the heart of priority setting. Epidemiological criteria for priority setting (e.g. frequency and severity of disease) need to be merged with clinical, economic, and political ones to make sense of past priorities and to help determine new ones. 'Our Healthier Nation', the national health strategy for England and Wales and similar national policy initiatives (including Healthy People 2000, the USA strategy for health (see US Department of Health and Human Services 1990)), are generally founded on epidemiology.

Priority setting cannot, however, be done by scientific data alone. Judgements need to be made within a decision-making framework. Some of the characteristics of diseases, conditions, and problems which tend to receive high priority in practice are listed in Table 10.1, which is based on judgements by the author shaped by successive groups of postgraduate public health students. In conjunction with other clinical sciences, epidemiology has a key role in studying the outcome of disease in terms of chronicity, severity, and case-fatality and in setting out the prospects for prevention, control, and treatment. With both laboratory and clinical sciences, epidemiology helps to define the relative importance of genetic, lifestyle, and external environmental factors in the causation of disease. The role of epidemiology is in providing background scientific information (part (a) of Table 10.1) that permits characterization of the importance of health problems.

The epidemiological principle, which has innate limitations, particularly in the context of the care of an individual patient, is that the most important problems are those that cause the greatest loss of life and illness, and are most amenable to prevention or effective treatment. The degree of loss can be expressed as the loss of life (mortality)

Table 10.1 Some characteristics of problems given high priority

---

A. Scientific factors

The problem is
—common
—increasingly common
—is commoner than expected compared with other similar populations
—severe in its effects
—long-lasting
—communicable
—epidemic
—externally, or iatrogenically, acquired
—one of the young
—treatable

B. Social, economic and political factors

The problem is
—of high public and political interest
—economically important
—lobbied for by pressure groups or powerful individuals
—low in stigma
—socially acceptable
—of interest to health professions

---

* Problems which do not have these characteristics, or have opposite characteristics, are given low priority.
This table is similar to the one published by the author in Bhopal (1998a), Health Needs Assessment in ethnic minority groups—with permission (see Permissions).

Table 10.2 The number of deaths, standardized mortality ratio (SMR) and potential years of life lost (PYLL) for selected causes of death, Newcastle upon Tyne, England, 1993

Cause of death	Number of deaths	Death rate per 100,00 population	PYLL	SMR
Cancer	943	335	6243	125
Ischaemic heart disease	884	314	3550	112
Cerebrovascular disease	348	124	1073	104
Accidents	72	26	1261	126
Suicide	26	9	870	94
All causes	3482	1236	19264	116

I acknowledge the work of Dr Mike Lavender in helping me think through the text that describes this table and for providing this table.

and the loss of life free of illness (morbidity) (as discussed in Chapter 8). Table 10.2 provides illustrative data on the number of deaths, the death rate, potential years of life lost (PYLL), and the standardized mortality ratios (SMR) for five health problems in an English health authority. In terms of providing diagnostic, advisory, and caring services, the data in Table 10.2, combined with basic clinical knowledge about the mode of presentation and severity of disease, show that cancers, ischaemic heart disease, and cerebrovascular disease occupy high priority. These three problems would be high priorities on the basis of the frequency data alone, but their major contributions to PYLL and the high SMR for cancer and ischaemic heart disease add to their priority status. Accidents and suicide cause relatively few deaths but the PYLL data enhance their priority status. Accidents also show a high SMR. The debate started by these data needs to be refined with information on the efficacy of treatment and preventive strategies (as discussed below in regard to risk factors), by adding the burden of disability and calculating disability adjusted life years (DALYs), and by including economic factors, for example, by using quality adjusted life years (QALYs) (Chapter 8).

Epidemiology also assesses the presence and impact of risk factors that influence mortality and morbidity. These data can be combined to estimate the risk of disease in a population that is attributable to one or more risk factors (Chapter 8). In conjunction with evaluation research these data, in turn, can be incorporated into health policy. For example, researchers have shown major variations in coronary heart disease (CHD) over time, between places, and within subgroups of populations, and have defined a number of important risk factors amenable to change (of which smoking, hypertension, and high levels of cholesterol are the best studied). Cross-sectional studies have defined the prevalence of risk factors in populations across the world, cohort and case-control studies have linked risk factors to disease outcome, and population-based trials have assessed the efficacy of preventive strategies. Health economics has been influential in helping to define the most cost-effective interventions that address the major issues highlighted by epidemiology. The sum of this knowledge contributes to judging the priority to be given to CHD prevention, in relation to the prevention of other disease, and in relation to 'curative' and palliative interventions.

Epidemiology provides information to use in the process of priority setting, which is largely a political one. (Some of the important political factors are given in Table 10.1 part (b).) The scientific factors and social/economic/political factors are not independent. Clearly, problems which are common and severe are more likely to interest health professionals and to be of economic and political interest. Problems which are of interest to pressure groups and politicians are more likely to be studied scientifically, and more data will become available to define the burden of disease and the scope for prevention or cure, thus raising its priority. The influence of politics and society on science, and vice versa, is an ethical matter (see Section 10.10).

Few topics fall more clearly into the domain of application than priority setting. The role of epidemiology, though vast, has seldom (if ever) been made explicit. Epidemiological theories and methods combine with other disciplines to help form difficult judgements. When the causation of a disease is known, it is easy to overlook the role of epidemiology, both in macro and micro decision making, but historical examples make it clear. In the case of cholera, the size of the problem gave it priority (macro) but which action should take priority: cleansing the streets of filth to reduce miasma or securing water supplies uncontaminated by sewage (micro)? In the case of pellagra (disease X) should we prioritize quarantine measures, assuming it is an infection, or supplement the diet, assuming it is a nutritional deficiency (micro)? For coronary heart disease do we prioritize cholesterol reduction or supplement the diet with folic acid to reduce endothelial dysfunction (micro)? New variant CJD (Creutzfeldt-Jakob disease) in humans, arising from BSE in cattle, is a priority on epidemiological grounds because it is increasingly common, externally acquired, severe, and potentially can result in an explosive epidemic (macro consideration). Theories on causation, and predictions of the size of the epidemic, are central to prioritizing this problem. These examples illustrate interdependence of theory and method in applied epidemiology.

In conclusion, this topic illustrates how epidemiological understanding of causation is complementary to descriptive data on the burden of disease and in aggregation helps us to develop a sense of priority, and guide public health , health policy, and medical care services. The needs of policy and practice have provided the stimulus for modes of analysis (PYLL, attributable risk, etc.) that are not essential to causal epidemiology, yet add additional insights. The application of epidemiological knowledge spurs new questions and advancement of both method and theory; for example, the description of inequalities in health is now giving way to understanding their causes and mechanisms.

10.4 Impact on health of local polluting industries: Teesside study of environment and health

Heavy industry is vital but there is a price to pay: pollution. People are increasingly reluctant to pay this price, and industries are facing complaints, adverse publicity, litigation, and public inquiries. Research on the impact of industrial pollution on the health of nearby populations is usually done in the midst of heavy media publicity and sometimes pending litigation. In our study of the impact of petrochemical and steel industries on the health of people in Teesside (Chapter 4, Box 4.6), my colleagues and I started with the testimony of general practitioners and with an analysis of mortality statistics. General practitioners feared, as had successive medical officers of health for the last hundred years, that the pollution caused premature death, cancer, asthma, and other chest problems. Routine statistics showed appallingly high mortality in the geographical areas, particularly Grangetown, close to industry. This type of problem typifies applied public health's dependence on epidemiological theory and method.

The first step was for us to devise the theoretical framework within which the problem was to be resolved. Ours was a positivist approach, that is, to seek the solution in epidemiological, empirical, objectively collected data. The second step was to propose hypotheses and a study design (see next paragraph). The third was to agree on how the data was to be interpreted. We agreed that if a disease or health problem was causally related to living close to industry, then there would be a gradient with distance, those closest having the highest rates, and those furthest the lowest. Proximity of residence to industry, then, was the key proxy measure for exposure to industrial pollution. These decisions are based on important values, assumptions, and theories of health and disease. For example, there is the value that empirical data are more reliable than the testimony of local people; and that an epidemiological approach would be more pertinent than a toxicological one where we focused on measuring the air quality, or chemicals in blood or other human tissues, rather than health status. The underlying theory of health and disease was that long-term exposure to low levels of industrial air pollution does harm, rather than good. These and many other similar important factors are seldom made explicit but play a vital role in guiding the research and its interpretation. (Indeed, they were not made explicit at all before, during, or after publication of the Teesside study, but after much reflection and in retrospect, their importance even at the time is clear.)

We had a number of hypotheses of which the key one was that the risk of mortality and disease, particularly for respiratory health, would be higher than expected in populations living close to industry. We defined four populations in geographical areas at varying distances from the main industrial complexes. We agreed that an association would be worthy of serious consideration as causal if there was a gradient with distance within the three areas in Teesside (called A, B, C) and if the three areas together had a higher rate than a fourth area some 20 miles distant in the City of Sunderland (called S). Our framework of causal thinking was based on the criteria (guidelines) discussed in Chapter 5.

We found that the death rates for lung cancer in women in area A were exceptionally high and in line with the pattern predicted in our prior hypothesis. For virtually every other cause of death and cancer, while health was poor, there was no such pattern; there was no evidence in favour of our prior hypothesis for birth weight, sex ratios at birth and perinatal mortality in infants; for self-reported health; and for general practice consultation patterns.

We applied our causal framework to analyse these associations. We concluded that there was evidence that local industrial pollution had a causal role in the high rates of lung cancer in women, but that for a wide range of other health concerns alternative explanations were necessary. While there was no room for complacency some reassurance was possible. We put particular emphasis on socio-economic deprivation and environmental degradation as causes of the general poor health in Teesside. We recommended a focus on poverty, new research on lung cancer in women and new studies of air quality around industry focusing on the public's concern. Our work provided data to resolve a public health problem that had been exercising medical officers of health since the turn of the century.

This work exemplifies how outwardly atheoretical, pragmatic, public health-orientated projects may be founded on important epidemiological theories and concepts. Those readers who do not share these theories and concepts, and who are neither familiar with nor confident about the methods, will not be comfortable with the results. In projects such as the Teesside one, the public may give more credence to individual case histories of illness, and general observations on the quality of the environment, than to epidemiological data. Environmental scientists may remain unconvinced by the epidemiological findings unless the specific sources and nature of exposures can be directly linked to disease mechanisms. The crucial step, interpretation, is also dependent on the theories and concepts that guide thinking. As epidemiologists need to communicate with both the public and other disciplines, it is important they understand how their theories and concepts compare with those of others. Indeed, epidemiologists should know and make explicit the paradigms that their work falls into.

10.5 **Paradigms: the evolution of epidemiology**

In this essay, 'normal science' means research firmly based upon one or more past scientific achievements, achievements that some particular scientific community acknowledges for a time as supplying the foundation for its further practice.

Thomas Kuhn *The Structure of Scientific Revolutions*

In 1996 Susser and Susser called for a paradigm shift in epidemiology. They identified four paradigm shifts (following Kuhn) in epidemiology in the last three hundred years or so (Table 10.3) and advocated a new paradigm of multilevel eco-epidemiology, which ranges from molecule to macro environment. Understanding the significance of their call requires some knowledge of Kuhn's concept of scientific paradigms. Paradigms are 'shared ideas which account for relative fullness of their [i.e. scientists'] communications and their relative unanimity of judgement'. Thomas Kuhn's view is that sciences mostly work, at any one time, within a single paradigm driven by exemplars of successful work. Sciences which are maturing or changing do not have a dominant paradigm.

The idea of scientific paradigms is complex, with many nuances (Table 10.4). Failure of the paradigm in solving current problems and explaining important observations

Table 10.3 Four paradigms in epidemiology identified by the Sussers

Exploratory description of disease (e.g. Graunt's analysis of the London Bills of Mortality in 1662, and Ramazzini and occupational exposures, 1700). In this period there was a change to sickness being seen as a result of disease entities not as humoral imbalance

Miasma theory of disease: the idea that disease arose from foul emanations from pollution (eighteenth century)

Germ theory of disease (nineteenth century)

Multiple causes as captured in the black box metaphor (twentieth century)

Table 10.4 Four components of a paradigm, or a disciplinary matrix as identified by Kuhn

Symbolic generalizations, e.g. the laws of physics as given in mathematical formulae

Beliefs in particular models, e.g. heat as kinetic energy

Values, e.g. the key goal of science being accurate predictions

Exemplars, i.e. classic examples of problems and their solutions, upon which Kuhn places special emphasis

inspires a search for a new paradigm which rapidly replaces the old one, which is then forgotten. This, he argues, is the foundation of scientific revolutions.

To call for a new paradigm is, therefore, a severe provocation for it declares the current paradigm inadequate. Vigorous debate and resistance to change are identified by Kuhn as precursors to change. Current resistance to a broader role for academic epidemiology (e.g. in achieving tobacco control or reducing health inequalities) might be explained as an intuition among epidemiologists that some of the dominant problems being identified lie outside the solution of current methods. Kuhn's view strikes a chord:

> one of the things a scientific community acquires with a paradigm is a criterion for choosing problems that, while the paradigm is taken for granted, can be assumed to have solutions. To a great extent these are the only problems that the community will admit as scientific or encourage its members to undertake.

This current debate in favour of new paradigms is fuelled by a combination of new patterns of disease (Section 10.6), challenging new applications, a perception that the current risk factor-disease outcome-based approach has not yielded the anticipated advances, and the availability of new techniques of data acquisition and analysis.

10.6 **Epidemiology: forces for change**

Diseases wax and wane. This has a profound effect on medical practice. Diseases that doctors saw a hundred years ago would baffle today's doctors, diseases we now see would baffle a doctor practising medicine a hundred years ago; and what we see now is likely to be very different from what our successors will see 50–100 years from now. Some of these changes are simply new diagnostic labels but there are also remarkably rapid changes in the pattern of disease, usually for reasons that are poorly understood.

The twenty-first century will rely on technology and science to resolve problems and these technologies are likely to speed up change. Before reading on do the exercise in Box 10.2.

Box 10.2 **Waning of diseases**

Reflect on the diseases that contemporary doctors either do not, or extremely rarely, see.

Now, reflect on diseases that may not be seen by doctors in a hundred years' time.

Examples of diseases never or rarely seen in contemporary medical practice in industrialized countries include smallpox (extinct), scurvy, beriberi, rickets, and erroneous diagnoses such as those previously attributed to masturbation, race, hysteria, and so on.

Many other massive changes, some anticipated (e.g. those due to climate change) but most not, will occur. Diseases that physicians in a hundred years' time may not see include mesothelioma (a cancer resulting from asbestos), tuberculosis, polio, measles, and Guinea worm infestation. With luck, even conditions such as stroke and heart disease, at least in the currently industrialized countries, may be rare. AIDS may be conquered by then. Epidemiology, and epidemiologists, need to follow and adapt to these changes. One adaptation that has already occurred is specialization.

10.7 **Scope of epidemiology and specialization**

The scope of epidemiology has broadened with the discovery or invention of new applications and methods. This, and the changing pattern of diseases, has encouraged subdivisions of epidemiology, though sometimes these are artificial. There is, for example, infectious disease epidemiology and chronic disease epidemiology, healthcare epidemiology, public health epidemiology, social epidemiology, clinical epidemiology, and genetic epidemiology. This list could be longer, and new forms of epidemiology could be proposed or created. The question is whether such divisions confer benefits, and whether these benefits exceed the costs.

The benefits are those of all forms of specialization: narrowing the scope of work permits the researcher or practitioner to deepen the field, particularly by working closely with colleagues in the specialized field; concepts and methods can be refined to suit a specific application; and specific applications give rise to innovations, that are often transferable. The costs of specialization are: fragmentation of the discipline; a loss of breadth by the specialist individual or group; and a reduction in communication and cross-fertilization between people working in the sub-disciplines.

The fundamental concepts used in most subdivisions of epidemiology are similar, as are the main measures of health and disease and study designs. The value of broad subdivisions such as chronic disease epidemiology is not clear, for the subdivision captures a vast territory, beyond the scope of a specialist, and the similarities between infectious disease and chronic disease epidemiology far outweigh the differences. In contrast, clinical epidemiology, in the sense of epidemiology applied to patients in the clinical setting, retains a relevant distinction, and its specific needs have driven the development of new techniques of data analysis and interpretation (e.g. numbers needed to treat). (The term clinical epidemiology may be used, wrongly, to distinguish medically qualified epidemiologists from others.) Subspecialization is heavily influenced by the context in which epidemiology is practised as discussed next.

10.8 The context of epidemiological practice: academic and service, USA and UK

Academic epidemiology in the USA is anchored in schools of public health which are mostly independent of medical schools. In recent decades, partly driven by the imperative to do and teach research, fewer people with a service public health background have been appointed to these schools, the posts being filled with laboratory scientists, epidemiologists, demographers, statisticians, or social scientists. The presence of clinically qualified staff (physicians and nurses) is also diminishing. In such schools of public health the vision of public health problems has become more scientific; issues of theory, measurement, and method receive close attention, so academic and service public health goals have diverged. In contrast, British academic epidemiology and public health is mostly associated with medical schools and public health service is within the NHS. These circumstances promote comparatively close links between public health and medicine and academia and service, and generate a focus on applied work.

The US School of Public Health environment is large enough to offer a career path within this system for professional researchers. There, the epidemiologists see themselves, by and large, as professional epidemiologists. There are sufficient of them to form a professionalized, self-contained group and set up and sustain organizations such as the Society for Epidemiological Research and the American College of Epidemiology. These are in addition to multidisciplinary societies such as the American Public Health Association. Many epidemiologists work in specialist departments of epidemiology. In contrast, many epidemiologists in the UK perceive themselves first as statisticians, physicians, public health specialists, or social scientists. They mostly work in multidisciplinary departments where they are usually a minority. Epidemiologists participate in multidisciplinary societies (Society for Social Medicine) or international epidemiological ones (IEA). There are no national epidemiology societies in the UK. These circumstances embed British epidemiologists within multidisciplinary and applied settings and allow US epidemiologists the option of specializing and standing apart from applied public health.

The fragmentation of American public health has been the subject of prolonged debate. An Institute of Medicine report stated that the 'nation has lost sight of its public health goals and has allowed the system of public health to fall into disarray'. A second report focused on the changing organization of health care, the changing role of government, the role of the community, and the need for partnership. The question for epidemiologists in such settings is: what is the role of epidemiology in such partnerships for public health?

The British system of academic public health is substantially founded on applied research relevant to health policy and planning, and medical and public health practice. Epidemiology is the backbone of the applied research effort. Rigorous training in the science of epidemiology is harder to achieve and most epidemiologists are trained through the public health disciplines. The question for epidemiologists working in such settings is: what is the role of epidemiology in the world of science, and how is theoretical and methodological work to be nurtured? These questions are developed below.

10.9 The practice of epidemiology in public health

There is general agreement that epidemiology is a key science that underpins public health and increasingly clinical practice too. Yet the gap between academic epidemiology and public health practice may be widening. Public health, according to the definition by Sir Donald Acheson, is 'The science and art of preventing disease, prolonging life and promoting health through the organised efforts of society'. Public health applies science in the social and political context, inevitably creating tensions between the scientific goal of gaining knowledge and the public health goal of improving health.

Epidemiology can be put into practice in many ways, including: understanding the relative impact of biology, environment, and health care on disease (e.g. the decline of tuberculosis); making the case for legislative change as was done following the London smog in 1953; setting up preventive programmes to tackle disease as done so vigorously in Finland to prevent CHD; predicting the future need for services using trends as in the field of AIDS; evaluating interventions; developing policy and clinical priorities; making clinical diagnosis in an individual patient; and providing the inspiration and methods for seeking new causal hypotheses as required for so many diseases (e.g. pancreatic cancer).

Epidemiological textbooks usually proclaim the applications of epidemiology as the foundation science of public health, but most focus on design and methods for causal research, rather than demonstrating clearly how epidemiology helps public health practice. The exemplars and classic studies used are mainly causal investigations yet much (maybe most) epidemiological effort in the public health field is on disease description and burden, prediction of trends, and evaluation of public health and clinical activity. (This book has attempted to achieve a balanced perspective.)

In a major review of epidemiology Susser picked two studies which established the reputation of epidemiology in the modern era: the Framingham cohort study and the case-control studies establishing smoking as a cause of lung cancer. Susser's choices, as opposed to other triumphs such as the poliomyelitis trial of 1954 (which he discusses in detail), illustrate the dilemma. While epidemiologists may spend much of their time working on applied public health work, they still respect causal contributions most, and this is reflected in their teaching. The reader needs to formulate an opinion on this vital issue. Acceptance of a role as an applied science imposes on epidemiology the need for a code of ethics and good conduct that serves both its scientific and public health purposes.

10.10 Ethical basis and proper conduct of epidemiology: the need for a code

To illustrate why applied sciences, including epidemiology, need an ethical code I have chosen to discuss three issues of interest to me: covert manipulation of scientists by the tobacco industry; the manipulation of authorship by researchers; and the purpose and direction of research on ethnicity and race (considered in some depth because of its exceptional importance in a millennium where all societies will surely become multi-ethnic ones).

10.10.1 Tobacco industry

The pervasive and covert influence of the tobacco industry on scientific research and publication has posed mighty ethical challenges for research institutions, researchers, and journal editors. The tobacco industry puts its commercial interests before those of society. Tobacco industry archives show how the industry has manipulated research into tobacco and health, for example, by fostering controversy about the effects of passive smoking on health; countering authoritative review articles through an international network of paid scientific 'consultants' whose activities included writing critical letters to academic journals; publishing 'review' articles; establishing a 'learned society' on indoor air quality; and performing research into non-tobacco causes of lung cancer (see Barnes and Bero 1998). The tobacco industry concealed or distorted evidence from its own research showing the addictive and harmful nature of smoking (see Hilts 1996). Epidemiologists working on topics such as tobacco need to be armed with an ethical code to protect them against such manipulation, and to guide them in making the right decisions in difficult circumstances, particularly when they are offered resources to pursue what are apparently good works.

10.10.2 Authorship

The authorship of scientific papers is increasingly important for the status of academic departments and for the reputations of researchers. There is a widespread view that only work that has passed the scrutiny of peers is reliable and trustworthy (a concept itself worthy of scrutiny). The main way of openly achieving and demonstrating peer scrutiny is through publication in peer-reviewed journals. Publication is a key factor in promotion, success in competing for an academic appointment (and sometimes in service appointments too), in winning research grants, and, in the UK, the finances coming into universities. Not surprisingly, the pressure to publish is great, tempting individuals to

> ## Box 10.3 The International Committee of Medical Journal Editors' criteria for authorship
>
> Authorship should be based only on a substantial contribution to:
> - conception and design, or analysis and interpretation of data; and
> - drafting the article or revising it critically for important intellectual content; and
> - final approval of the version to be published.
>
> International Committee of Medical Journal Editors (1997)

accept authorship on papers to which they have not contributed sufficiently, a practice called 'gift authorship'. Richard Horton, editor of the *Lancet*, recently said, 'The mantle of authorship has become a heavy robe of fake majesty that conceals those who seek credit unworthily, priority unjustly and reward improperly' (Horton 1998).

The criteria for authorship prepared by an international committee of medical journal editors are commonly flouted (Box 10.3). Scientists, including epidemiologists, recognize that allocation of authorship is complex and raises ethical issues central to scientific integrity. Epidemiologists need an ethical code, particularly as their work is often multidisciplinary and done in large teams, where misunderstandings about authorship are most likely to occur.

10.10.3 Ethnicity and race

Ethnicity and race are among the top five or so most important variables in epidemiology. Their utilization in science, however, has put many researchers in peril of being judged as racist. Knowledge of the history of racism in science and medicine provides the essential insight into how societies may abuse data on racial differences. Some two thousand years ago Hippocrates contrasted the feebleness of the Asiatic races to the hardiness of the Europeans (see Chadwick and Mann 1950). Hippocrates'concept of race was of human groups shaped by their ancestry in different environments especially climate. In the nineteenth century racial differences in anatomy, physiology, behaviour, and health status were avidly sought. The idea of races as distinct species, which was long and seriously debated, gave way to races as biological subspecies. Before reading on do the exercise in Box 10.4.

> ## Box 10.4 Ethnicity and race as artificial constructs
>
> Reflect on whether there is truth to the view that races and ethnic groups are socially constructed, artificial ways of categorizing human beings. Can you think of examples of times and places when the idea of race has been used to overtly political or social ends, particularly the suppression of some groups?

In the nineteenth century, differences among races were usually assumed to be biological, interpreted to show superiority of white races, and used to justify policies which subordinated 'coloured' groups. Racism results from the belief that some races are superior to others, which is used to devise and justify actions which create inequality among racial groups. Disraeli, then British Prime Minister said to the House of Commons (UK) in 1849, 'Race implies difference, difference implies superiority and superiority leads to predominance.'

Research focusing on problems more common in minority groups, combined with data presentation techniques designed to highlight differences in comparison with the majority population, so easily portrays the minorities as weaker. When research implies genetic factors rather than environmental ones as the cause of racial differences in health, racial minorities may be perceived as biologically weaker.

Science that indicated such weakness helped to justify slavery, social inequality, eugenics, immigration control, and racist practice of medicine. Race-pecific 'diseases' such as drapetomania (irrational and pathological desire of slaves to run away) were invented. John Down's theory of 'mongolism' (trisomy 21 or Down's syndrome) was that such infants were births from an inferior, Mongoloid, race. He interpreted this as indicating the unity of human races. The Tuskegee Syphilis Study in Alabama (discussed in Chapter 4 on bias) by the US Public Health Service, which lasted from 1932 to 1972, deceived and bribed 600 black subjects into cooperating with research which examined the progression of syphilis without treatment, even once penicillin (a cure) was available (see Jones 1993). In May 1997 President Clinton apologized on behalf of the USA to the survivors of this experiment. Tuskegee was not a unique racist research project. Osborne (Osborne and Feit 1992) concluded that much American health research on race and ethnicity contributes to the idea that some human groups are inferior. As Gladys Reynolds (1993) wrote 'We the scientific community ... bring everything we have been taught by our culture – our xenophobia, our homophobia, our racism, our sexism, our "classism", our tendency to "otherise"'.

Modern genetics undermined the biological concept of race and Nazi racism discredited eugenics. Races are now considered to be based on a few physical features (such as colour and facial features) of small direct importance to health, which serve important social rather than biological purposes. Nonetheless, the idea of the biological basis of health differences by race and ethnicity remains strong. This is the defining feature of the twentieth century race concept, supported by many contemporary dictionaries and encyclopedias, and permeating biomedical thinking. The view that race is a social, not biological, reality is, however, emergent. The concept of ethnicity is that human beings identify themselves as belonging to a group because they differ culturally in fundamental ways including language, food, religion, lifestyle and, of course, their geographical origins. In epidemiological practice, race and ethnicity are virtually used as synonyms for similar underlying concepts.

The division of people on the basis of race and ethnicity raises questions about human values, for the consequences of such divisions have been great. Studies of ethnic and racial variations in disease pose a challenge to the maintenance of high ethical standards in epidemiology. The concepts of race and ethnicity are commonly applied in epidemiology to the study of the health of immigrant and ethnic minority groups in the hope of advancing causal understanding of disease. Contemporary race, ethnicity, and health research is mostly 'black box' epidemiology, concentrating on so-called ethnic health issues, and generating a multiplicity of interesting hypotheses. As Kiple and King (1981) discuss, the idea of a package of specific 'racial' or 'ethnic' diseases that deserve special attention and research has unfortunate echoes in history. 'Negro' susceptibility to particular diseases, such as leprosy, tetanus, pneumonia, scurvy, and sore eyes, was instrumental in 'branding blacks as an exotic breed', and the differences were explained by hypotheses on causation that can now be seen as nonsense.

Racial prejudice is fuelled by research portraying ethnic minorities as different, usually inferior to the majority. Infectious diseases, population growth, and culture are common foci for publicity. Following the release of statistics on the ethnicity of single mothers, the *Sunday Express*, an important UK newspaper, ran the headline (13 August 1996) 'The ethnic time bomb'. Toni Morrison (1993) wrote in her book *Beloved* 'A whip of fear broke through the heart chambers as soon as you saw a Negro's face in a paper' (for this signalled singularly bad news). Researchers cannot be responsible for media reporting, but epidemiologists must be aware of the attractions of their work to the media and of potential impact of their work on race relations.

Race and ethnicity are epidemiological variables that show, dramatically and unequivocally, the importance of historical, political, and social awareness among epidemiologists.

10.11 **Ethical guidelines**

Ethical guidelines for epidemiological research have included broad statements about the duties of epidemiologists to be honest and impartial, not to distort the truth, and to uphold the public interest rather than narrow sectional interests. Other guidelines have given more specific guidance, including that epidemiologists should not accept contractual obligations contingent on reaching particular conclusions from research proposals; or accept grants or contracts in which the funder retains the right to edit or suppress results. In 1998, the International Epidemiology Association's European Group published a code of practice for epidemiologists. This states, that among other principles, epidemiologists should:

- seek the truth in good faith without doing harm or jeopardizing personal integrity;
- judge their own work and ideas and those of colleagues in an impartial manner;
- disclose conflicts of interest to ethical review committees;
- publicly acknowledge all research sponsorship;

◆ publish all research with scientific merit;

◆ refuse requests to withhold findings, change, or tone down the content of reports, or delay publication unreasonably;

◆ ensure sponsors agree in writing that results will be published regardless of outcome and agree to the independence of the investigators;

◆ declare sources of funding and possible conflicts of interests in publications.

The reader is encouraged to study these guidelines in more detail (the World Wide Web address is given in the References). To seek the truth and judge with impartiality (first and second points above) requires, above all, a sound understanding of critical appraisal.

10.12 Critical appraisal in epidemiology: separating fact from error and fallacy

> Scepticism is the scalpel which frees accessible truth from the dead tissue of unfounded belief and wishful thinking.
>
> Petr Skrabenek and James McCormick in
> *Follies and Fallacies in Medicine*, p. 144.

Medicine and public health are not sciences; they use sciences to seek solutions from agreed knowledge. Sciences seek to acquire new knowledge. In an era emphasizing information and research evidence as the foundation of medicine and public health, the scalpel of critical appraisal is likely to be as important to the twenty-first century doctor as the surgical scalpel was to the nineteenth century doctor. Critical appraisal is important because much of what we know as the truth is wrong, sometimes dangerously so (Box 10.5).

Box 10.5 Reflection on medical and public health activities shown to be wrong

Reflect on some medical and public health activities which were widely practised but are now known to be wrong, some dangerously so. Your reflection should include both historical activities, say, before the turn of the twentieth century and more recent ones. Now, reflect on some current policies and practices that may meet the same fate.

Historical examples of erroneous medical activities abound and include cautery, bloodletting, purging, vomiting, enemas, and surgery for psychiatric disorders. Many public health actions were equally wrong; for example, fumigation of towns and persecution of ethnic minority groups to control epidemics of cholera, typhus, and yellow fever. At the time, however, these actions must have made sense to those who put them into practice. Erroneous actions are a characteristic of modern times too. Examples of follies of the twentieth century include surgery for the floating kidney; ECT (electro-convulsive therapy) for a wide range of psychological and psychiatric disorders for which it did not work; prolonged (six weeks or longer) enforced bed rest after a heart attack when we now know that patients need to be mobilized within hours or days; and treatment of heart rhythm disorders during a heart attack with the drug lignocaine. These actions were, in retrospect, dangerous.

Only with the 'retrospectoscope' can we identify follies and fallacies. At this moment life and death decisions are being made by applying uncertain knowledge about the causes, prevention, diagnosis, and management of disease. For example, is hospital birth safer than home birth for a healthy mother? Is screening for cervical and breast cancer saving lives or causing unnecessary costs and anxiety? Are drugs for moder-ate/mild high blood pressure, obesity, depression, and anxiety effective and safe? Why are so many antibiotics prescribed for non-bacterial illnesses? Does health education about drugs and safer sex prevent or augment problems? We often don't have clear-cut answers about the effectiveness or cost effectiveness of the activities we undertake. Before reading on do the exercise in Box 10.6.

Box 10.6 **Reasons for the lack of clear answers**

Reflect on and list reasons why, historically, medical and public health practice has not sought, or has not achieved, clear research-based answers to important questions.

The reasons include the following:
- the tendency and preference to base practice on personal experience;
- the tendency to act on good, common-sense ideas, often based on general scientific principles, in the absence of research evidence;
- the tendency to follow the fashions and ideas of distinguished colleagues;
- the difficulty of doing research that gives clear-cut answers;
- the difficulty of extracting the correct interpretation of data;
- error in research.

Error commonly accompanies human endeavour, and science is not exceptional, as the regular notification of errors in every journal shows. (Several thousand are recorded annually in the *Index Medicus* and the prestigious journal the *Lancet* has a column called Department of Error.) The popular image of the scientific process is that of steady accumulation of knowledge which is sound. The fault with science, if any, is usually said to lie in the abuse of knowledge, rather than in its accumulation and interpretation. The scientific paper, the carrier of scientific knowledge, has the author-ity of its authors, the elaborate peer review system, and the editorial processes of the publishing journal, and is expected to be accurate. Accuracy is a characteristic cherished and demanded by scientists. Both lay and expert readers may easily overlook errors in published work, precisely because they are unexpected. They can then be perpetuated by quotation in secondary sources. The editorial and peer review processes are not, however, proof against error. The publication and continued citation of fraudulent research provides the most extreme example of the limitations of current means of detecting error. Fraud, however, represents an important but small proportion of errors in the scientific literature. Several studies of the use of statistics in medical journals have shown that error is a massive problem. Most errors are subtle and are made unwittingly by researchers who wish and try to avoid them.

Critical appraisal is the use of the 'scalpel of scepticism' to extract truth from error in research. In evaluating research, particularly epidemiological research, researchers need to consider both technical excellence and its value in historical, political, social, and geographical context. These are heavy obligations on epidemiologists. This book has provided the background concepts to guide the reader in critical appraisal. In preparation for application of these concepts the reader will need to consult other books and papers. Petr Skrabanek and James McCormick's book *Follies and Fallacies in Medicine* (I acknowledge my debt to them here) is a gold mine of examples, and the brief exposition in Sections 10.12.1 to 10.12.10 is heavily based on their discussion of fallacies.

10.12.1 The fallacy of association being causal

Humankind needs explanations, and this need leads us to confuse association, which is easily demonstrated, with causation, which is problematic. This matter has been discussed throughout this book. The axiom, 'association is not causation, but it may be', is a safeguard, as is remembering that an association between factor A and disease B may be a result of: coincidence or chance; confounding (A and B share a common cause D); B causes A (consequence); A causes B (cause). This can be easily remembered as the four Cs.

10.12.2 The weight of evidence fallacy

The idea that pooling together weak evidence can turn it into better evidence is tempting but wrong. It is wrong to discard discordant evidence, even if it is scanty. The Popperian view of science is that progress is made by rejecting hypotheses and the example of the hypothesis 'All swans are white' is memorable. More is learned about this hypothesis by observing a single black swan than 1000 white ones.

10.12.3 The fallacy of repeated citation

Is spinach a good source of iron as claimed by the cartoon of Popeye the sailor man? The answer, according to Skrabanek and McCormick, is no. In the original paper reporting these data, the decimal point on the iron content was misplaced giving a 10-fold overestimate. (As I have not checked the original citation, this is an example of repeated citation.)

10.12.4 **The fallacy of authority**

Simply because an article or book is published does not make it right. Equally, the fact that it is not published because it is rejected by peer review does not make it wrong.

10.12.5 **The fallacy of simple explanation**

Scientists and the public alike have a preference for simple explanations (usually referred to in science as elegant or parsimonious hypotheses). The emphasis in epidemiology on searching for single risk factors as causes, as opposed to ways of summarizing and studying the complex interaction of multiple risk factors, is a reflection of this preference. A quotation from H.L. Hencken summarizes Skrabanek and McCormick's view on this matter: 'for every complex problem there is a solution that is simple, direct and wrong'.

10.12.6 **The fallacy of risk**

Skrabanek and McCormick discuss a WHO study showing that women who had used oral contraceptives for 2.5 years had a relative risk of 1.5 for cervical cancer, that is, 50 per cent more than those who did not. Is this association reflecting a causal relationship, they asked? Second, does it matter and is it something for women to worry about? In terms of life expectancy women aged 20–24 reduced, on average, their lifespan by 11 days. The principle here is: presented with a relative risk, ask yourself, what does it matter in terms of absolute risk?

10.12.7 **The fallacy of inappropriate extrapolation**

Just because something is unhealthy in excess (salt, milk, zinc, alcohol, weight, serum cholesterol, radiation, or water) does not mean it is unhealthy in moderation. Beware of investigators who extrapolate beyond their data, warn Skrabanek and McCormick.

10.12.8 **The fallacy of significance tests**

Any difference between two groups, no matter how small, can be shown to be 'statistically significant' if the sample size is large enough, but the important question is whether the difference is clinically important. Skrabanek and McCormick ask us to beware of statistically significant differences in big studies and remember that the validity of the probability that a particular set of results has occurred by chance, shown by the significance tests (and illustrated by the p-value), depends on a prior hypothesis. They also remind us that statistically significant results are more likely to be published and that there may be unpublished studies showing the opposite.

10.12.9 **The fallacy of obfuscation**

Beware of the use of complex language to obfuscate. The use of words such as 'essential', 'multifactorial', or 'functional', when describing diseases really means we don't know the causes. Such words hide ignorance yet give authority to the user.

10.12.10 The fallacy of covert bias

Use of language, particularly adjectives, may reflect the bias of the investigator. One writer may see a difference as important, another as insignificant. The reader needs to avoid being misled by the bias of the writer.

10.12.11 The nature of critical appraisal

Despite its name critical appraisal is not just about criticism and has a kinship to a book, film, or theatre review which aims to assess how good the work is in relation to expectations and what has gone before. *Citizen Kane* is an acclaimed film, but one wouldn't judge it in relation to the state of knowledge or technology of today. Similarly, in appraising a scientific paper, give credit for ideas. Do not criticize a cross-sectional study because it is not a trial! Give a balanced view. Second, scientific papers have a structure and purpose. You can only do critical appraisal when you know what this is.

The next step is for the reader to attempt critical appraisal. To make this a meaningful activity engaging in the world of science the reader is advised to work on contemporary papers and prepare the appraisal as a letter to the editor and, if good enough, submit it for publication. The educational benefits of preparing a concise, critical evaluation of a scientific paper are considerable. Researchers reviewing a field should routinely search for, summarize, and cite relevant correspondence and other comments. An original scientific paper is simply incomplete without the accompanying published comment. On-line journals now offer the ideal of electronic linkage of corrections, retractions, and correspondence to original articles. Ideally, inter-library loan requests for a paper should be for the paper together with its related commentary, whether correspondence or editorial. The next section outlines some questions of particular relevance in epidemiological appraisal.

10.13 Some questions relevant to the appraisal of epidemiological research

Austin Bradford Hill posed four simple questions to guide the reading of scientific papers: Why did the authors start? What did they do? What did they find? What does it mean? These four questions are an excellent starting point. Additional general questions include these:

◆ What is the importance of the research this paper describes?

◆ Have the authors made explicit the concepts guiding their work and defined their terms?

◆ What are the objectives, hypotheses, and research questions under investigation?

◆ Were the methods appropriate to meeting the objectives, testing the hypotheses, and answering the research questions?

◆ Is the sample of the right size to meet the study objectives?

◆ What biases are inherent in these methods and what steps have been taken to minimize these?

◆ Do the results help to resolve the problem addressed?

◆ Do you agree with the discussion and conclusions?

◆ What is the next step in terms of policy, practice, and research?

Such general questions can be combined with those below to produce a critical appraisal specific to epidemiological research.

◆ Is an epidemiological approach appropriate to the problem under study? What alternative methods would also help to resolve the problem?

◆ What is the study design and is it suitable for the problem addressed?

◆ Are the dates on which the sampling frame was compiled given?

◆ Is the date or time period over which data were collected given?

◆ For conditions which have a cyclical pattern, has the timing of measurements been stated? For example, for blood pressure the timing needed may be time of day, time of week, month, and season.

◆ Have the precise geographical boundaries of the study been given? If this is not a geographically defined population, can the sampled population be related to a place?

◆ Have the populations been defined in terms of their social and economic standing, and geographical and cultural origins?

◆ Have terms/labels used to describe populations or sub-populations been defined and justified?

◆ Is the study sample representative of a larger population and, hence, are the results likely to be more widely generalizable?

◆ Are the sampling and measurement methods equivalent in the groups to be compared?

◆ Are compared populations or subgroups similar on key variables?

◆ If not, are the differences sufficiently small to permit adjustment using a weighting technique such as age standardization, or other statistical techniques such as logistic regression (see Glossary)?

◆ Do the analyses provide information on both absolute and relative risks?

◆ If odds ratios are given and used as an estimate of relative risk, are the required assumptions met?

◆ If the study is one exploring causality is the causal model given? Are the data interpreted within a causal framework? If so, is this made explicit?

The subject of critical appraisal is a large one, and the interested reader will be able to find guidance on how to critically appraise studies both in different fields and with different designs. We now turn to the need to reflect on both the past and the future, as a means of continuing education in epidemiology.

10.14 Building on an epidemiological education: role of historical landmarks

One path to a solid epidemiological education is to study the classics, or in Kuhn's terminology, exemplars. Exemplars provide inspiration as well as instruction. I have chosen three examples to illustrate the value of historical studies to contemporary work.

Lind investigated scurvy and reported his findings in 1753 (see Lind 1753). He wrote 'Scurvy alone, during the last war, proved a more destructive enemy, and cut off more valuable lives, than the united efforts of the French and Spanish wars'. He also noted that scurvy 'raged with great violence in some journeys, not at all in others'. The first observation identified the immense size of the problem, the second told him that scurvy was preventable. He generated many causal hypotheses including the role of sea climate and particularly the moist air. He chose to investigate diet and conducted his famous experiment on the ship *Salisbury* in 1747 where he 'ordered' 12 patients, divided in pairs, to take cider, elixir vitriol, vinegar, sea water, an electuary (consisting of garlic, mustard seed, radishes, balsam of Peru, gum myrrh), and oranges and lemons. He found that 'the most sudden and visible good effects were perceived from the use of the oranges and lemons'. Sadly, many lives were to be lost before his remedy was accepted and adopted decades later. A deficiency of vitamin C was later shown to be the cause of scurvy. Vitamin C was the first vitamin to be synthesized in 1932, nearly two hundred years later. This story illustrates the importance of reflecting on the differing patterns of disease, here, scurvy in some journeys and not in others, and then generating a number of plausible hypotheses and testing the most likely ones. It shows that putting research into practice is a long-term endeavour. Finally, this story shows that precise mechanistic understanding, though valuable, is not crucial to put epidemiology into public health practice.

Smallpox is one of history's most important diseases. The story of how Edward Jenner, a country practitioner in Gloucester, investigated the role of vaccination with cowpox virus is well known but where did he get the idea? What was the observation that inspired him to take the cowpox virus from the hands of Sarah Nelmes and insert it into the arm of 'a lad of the name of Phipps' on 14 May 1796? The observation on which he reflected was this: that milkmaids have clear complexions and are generally free of pockmarks (a disease pattern) and that it is hard to inoculate them using smallpox virus, an observation that we would disparagingly call an old wives' tale. Jenner investigated this tale and the local practice of exposing people to cowpox as a means of protecting against smallpox. He inferred that milkmaids' exposure to the cowpox protected them from smallpox. If so, he thought, why not inoculate with cowpox, rather than with smallpox, a practice that was widespread but risky. His bold gamble was to vaccinate Phipps, and then expose him to inoculation with the smallpox virus six weeks later. Phipps did not react to the smallpox inoculation. Jenner was convinced he had demonstrated a new technique for the prevention of smallpox and, perhaps surprisingly, his contemporaries agreed (see Jenner). Jenner correctly forecast the elimination of the disease. Indeed the World Health Organization declared smallpox to be eradicated in 1980. I believe this is history's supreme medical advance. Smallpox is the only disease to be completely eradicated through deliberate public health endeavour. This story illustrates the need to listen to the public with an open mind, and to test a hypothesis with experiment. Finally, it shows that those making a discovery need to be champions of its dissemination and implementation.

The classic investigation of cholera by John Snow also illustrates important principles. The pandemics in the nineteenth century sweeping from the East into Europe were causing terror, as thousands died. The description by Roy Porter gives a feel for the terror that an outbreak involving hundreds or thousands of people might cause.

> Internal disturbances, nausea and dizziness led to violent vomiting and diarrhea, with stools turning to a gray liquid (often described as 'rice water') until nothing emerged but water and fragments of intestinal membrane. Extreme muscular cramps followed, with an insatiable desire for water, followed by a 'sinking stage' during which the pulse dropped and lethargy set in. Dehydrated and nearing death, the patient displayed the classic cholera physiognomy: puckered blue lips in a cadaverous face. There was no agreement about its cause; many treatments were tried; nothing worked.
>
> Roy Porter (1997) *The Greatest Benefit to Mankind*, p. 403.

At the time the miasma theory was favoured. Miasma was atmospheric pollution arising from decaying organic matter. John Snow investigated this disease for 20 years, culminating in his study of what he described as 'the most terrible outbreak of cholera which ever occurred in this kingdom', the epidemic of cholera in Broad Street, Soho, London (see Snow). On reaching the scene he immediately suspected some contamination of the water in the Broad Street pump, a conclusion he supported by his observations that the dead lived or worked near the pump; a nearby workhouse and brewery had their own water supply and little cholera; and people living far away but drinking Broad Street pump water were afflicted. The homes of people dying from cholera were clustered around the pump. Water, not miasma in the air, he concluded, is the source of the morbid matter that causes cholera. He published in 1849 and 1855, and gave evidence to many learned committees including one in the House of Commons. He was unable to convince those in power and died in 1858 before his ideas were accepted. John Snow's book cost him two hundred pounds to publish and he sold 56 copies in three years, making 3 pounds, 12 shillings. The lessons here are numerous. How much emphasis can we place on either peer review or indicators of popularity such as the science citation index, in assessing the importance of research? It is worth reflecting on the fact that John Snow was, primarily, an anaesthetist for whom epidemiology was a passion. All doctors, perhaps all health professionals, should see themselves as potential contributors to epidemiology. Another lesson is that confronting an established theory (miasma here) is a formidable challenge.

Based on these early achievements, epidemiology and public health advanced rapidly with triumphant insights into the causes and control of diseases including puerperal fever, pellagra, typhus, beriberi, congenital rubella, adenocarcinoma of the vagina, lung cancer, coronary heart disease, and, more recently, AIDS and sudden infant death syndrome. These landmarks showed how society could conquer disease by organized research and action.

These are the examples that provide the inspiration and, rightly, take pride of place in our textbooks. Kuhn identified textbooks as vehicles for perpetuating scientific paradigms and as necessary for rapid progress by the novice, including through the study of exemplars (classics). The further reading lists at the end of the book offer choices on reading exemplars, and on the wide range of epidemiological textbooks.

10.15 **Building on an epidemiological education: a reflection on the future of epidemiology**

To predict and plan for the future is fraught with difficulty, but requires reading the latest journals, attending seminars and conferences and a great deal of reflection. Some trends are evident.

In industrialized countries the challenges for epidemiology will, increasingly, lie in the prevention and control of the diseases of older people. Paradoxically, the solutions to these problems of old age may lie in improving maternal, fetal, and infant health. According to the fetal origins hypothesis, the environmental conditions that the fetus is subjected to programme metabolic adaptation, and lay the foundations for disease of middle and later life. Relative poverty in early life, and wealth in later life, may be the basis of maladaptation, triggering diseases such as coronary heart disease and diabetes (the adaptation–dysadaptation hypothesis).

In many developing countries the traditional public health problems of poverty (inadequate sanitation, inadequate nutrition, and the communicable disease) are combining with those of the post-industrial era (cancer, heart disease, stroke, and road traffic accidents) to create a public health nightmare. Disentangling the interacting effects of changing circumstances of poverty and wealth in the causation of disease (health in populations in economic transition) is a vast challenge for epidemiology.

Economic and health inequalities will hold centre stage in public health as they have done for two hundred years. Modern communications exposes the injustice of gross waste in some countries, and horrendous poverty in others. The traditional 'solution' based on the moral regeneration of the poor through schooling on sobriety, frugality, and industry is insufficient. Poverty is now seen as a potent and direct cause of ill-health, and vice versa. Epidemiology has made a vast contribution both in describing such inequalities, and in helping to understand them, given the limitations of studying a matter of such complexity. The future holds an ethical and a technical challenge. The ethical one is whether epidemiology should be an advocate for eradication of health inequalities (i.e. participate in the policy debate) or a dispassionate observer (i.e. seek the neutral stance associated with sciences). The technical challenge is whether epidemiology can provide insights on the mechanisms by which wealth and health interact, and whether it can design and implement efficient and solid trials of interventions. This work falls into the growing realm of social epidemiology. The other end of the spectrum is the biology and, particularly, genetics of disease.

The human genome mapping project will re-ignite the question of the relative importance of genetic and environmental factors as the underlying causes of disease. In assessing disease causation and prevention, even though the environment–gene interaction is all-important, the categorization of disease into 'genetic' or 'environmental' is often the first step. A few important principles will help to guide epidemiologists in the coming tidal wave of genetic research.

Within populations the genetic pool changes slowly and genetic variations between populations are small; in contrast, the environment changes rapidly, and differs greatly from place to place. The frequency of occurrence of most common diseases shows massive geographical and time period variation. For instance, heart disease rates in Japan are a fraction of those in Europe. Even more strikingly, rates of many diseases, including heart disease, have been shown to vary as much as threefold between neighbouring areas in cities; areas distinguished by little more than their affluence. Variations in the incidence of cancer are also particularly striking. Geographical variations between populations appearing over short periods of time are not genetic. Changes in the incidence of disease over brief time spans, say between single generations, point to the dominance of environmental causes.

The incidence of many diseases has changed dramatically in recent decades. In the UK, for example, stroke, gastric cancer, chronic bronchitis and, most striking of all, infections including tuberculosis, have been in decline. At the same time, however, asthma, AIDS, skin cancers, and hip fractures are among problems that are increasing. The epidemiological pattern of coronary heart disease (CHD) exemplifies the oscillating nature of disease. While rare at the beginning of this century, CHD reached a peak in many industrialized countries in the 1960s, 1970s, or 1980s. However, the cause of this great epidemic has never been fully understood and now that it is in rapid decline the reasons are again unclear. Diseases fluctuate in frequency and severity, and we are left in wonder and ignorance at the pace of change in the pattern of disease. The speed of change, however, unequivocally implicates the environment rather than genetics, as the primary factor in the causative process. Studies have underlined the role of genetic inheritance in many multifactorial disorders although their interpretation is often difficult. Great advances in genetics will follow the mapping of the human genome. The genetic contribution to disease causation will be clarified and there will be a revolution in diagnostic and therapeutic medical techniques. However, the genetic revolution will not match the revolution in public health which, based on environmental change, has within a few generations added decades to the average human lifespan. Genetic factors provide the stage in the great drama of disease causation, but the environment is the leading player.

Epidemiology will need to embrace and benefit from the advances in molecular biology. While it is difficult to predict all the demands that the advances in genetics will make to epidemiology, two are clear. Firstly, advances in genetics will undoubtedly have an impact on the diagnosis and management of disease in the future, and ultimately on population disease patterns. Secondly, epidemiologists will need to be trained in genetics to a much greater depth than at present.

Molecular science will deepen understanding of the interaction between the environment, lifestyle, and the gene, for example, demonstrating why some people have high serum cholesterol and how this causes atherosclerotic diseases. Yet, the public health dividend will come from altering the pattern of risk factors in the whole population. Reducing serum cholesterol from the currently pathological level of 6 mmol per litre and more in some populations, to a physiologically normal value of 4 mmol per litre or even less, without mass medication, requires an understanding of how people and societies change. It is not simply biochemistry that determines an individual and population's serum cholesterol level, but what and how food is grown, processed, purchased, cooked, and eaten. These factors are determined by more than personal taste. Trade agreements, agricultural policy, marketing, and economic subsidy are crucial determinants of costs, availability and consumption.

One of the future challenges for epidemiology will be to set priorities, and to avoid being deflected from its crucial purpose, which is understanding the causes and consequences of diseases in populations, and acquiring and presenting the evidence advocating the appropriate actions to improve health. In addition to maintaining the solid middle ground of today's epidemiology, we will need to make much clearer and better observations on how diseases are generated through the interactions that people make when living in groups, in other words, the population determinants of disease. Epidemiologists would do well to work with social scientists who have a more sound understanding of how societies work and can be changed to promote health. Epidemiology could also potentially make a much greater contribution to clinical research. Clinicians fully trained in epidemiology are best placed for this work.

There has been a massive increase in knowledge of methods, which has not been matched with development of theoretical frameworks. Development of theory and concepts is a pressing need. An even closer collaboration between epidemiologists and researchers in other fields will be a stimulus to such advances. Epidemiology as a discipline will grow in the next 10–20 years and will become a vital area of knowledge for all clinical and public health researchers. Epidemiology will help them to envision the causes of ill-health and diseases and the health needs of their populations and hence to develop coherent policies, laws, and healthcare systems to generate health from the pattern of disease.

Summary

The philosophy and theory underpinning epidemiology is seldom made explicit, and yet underpins all work, drives change, and guides the paradigms within which it works.

Epidemiology takes a positivist stance. The basic theory, from which the aetiological contribution is derived, is that systematic variations in the pattern of health and disease exist in populations and these are a product of differences in the prevalence of, or susceptibility to, the causal factors. Epidemiological methods are designed to quantify variations in disease patterns and their causes, to establish associations, and to test resultant hypotheses on causes. Diseases arise from complex interactions of causal forces. This knowledge is applied to prevent, control, and treat disease. Theory, method, and application are interdependent.

A vigorous ongoing debate on the future of epidemiology, and the paradigms within which it works, is fuelled by a combination of the changing pattern of disease; new challenging applications; a perception that the current risk factor-disease outcome-based approach has not yielded the anticipated advances; and availability of new techniques of data acquisition and analysis. Major changes are anticipated. Already, epidemiology is both broadening and specializing. We can predict the rise of genetic epidemiology and, at the opposite spectrum, of social epidemiology.

While epidemiology is applied in several health domains, it is a prime force in public health, whether influencing policy, making strategic and planning decisions, or in disease prevention and control. It is the underpinning (but not sole) science of public health. It also has a big role in clinical medicine. This imposes on epidemiology the need for a code of ethics and good conduct that serves both its scientific and its applied purposes.

Errors in study design and data collection and interpretation may impair human health. Critical evaluation of research is, therefore, a crucial skill, and essential in the ethical conduct of epidemiology. In evaluating research, epidemiologists need to attend both to technical excellence, and to its value in the historical, political, social, and geographical context. Epidemiology is rooted in the populations it studies, and in place and time, and in that context it contributes to the guardianship of health.

These obligations require epidemiologists to have an understanding of the wide determinants of health and disease. This can only be achieved by broad studies of the history and achievement of the key disciplines contributing to epidemiology, combined with a keen interest in contemporary debates and future trends.

References and further reading

To be effective in the science and craft of epidemiology readers of this book will need to reflect on a broad range of issues—conceptual, technical and social. An excellent starting point is a dictionary. You will probably need at least a general dictionary, an epidemiological dictionary and a medical and biological dictionary. I have drawn repeatedly upon many dictionaries but particularly:

- **Last, J.M.** (2001) *A dictionary of epidemiology* (4th edn). Oxford University Press, New York.
- *The Oxford dictionary of current English*. Oxford University Press, Oxford. ISBN 0 19 281 91 94
- *Pocket Medical Dictionary* (14th edn, 1987). Roper, N. (Ed). Churchill Livingstone, Edinburgh.

Your next need is to be aware of the range of material in, and approach of, the many excellent textbooks on epidemiology and related topics. Twenty-five textbooks were formally reviewed by me in preparation for writing this book and this may be of use to the reader:

Bhopal, R.S. (1997) Which book? A comparative review of 25 introductory epidemiology textbooks. *J Epidemiol Community Health*, **51**, 612–622.

Compilations of classic papers are particularly valuable and an excellent example is:

Buck, C., Llopis, A., Najera, E., and Terris, M. (1988) *The challenge of epidemiology. Issues and selected readings*. Pan American Health Organization, Washington DC.

The references listed below indicate the sources I have drawn upon and bring to attention others of potential interest. Many of the references are relevant to much of the book though only a few are cited in more than one chapter.

The references are, with a few exceptions, not linked directly to the text, which means readers will need to browse the list for each chapter to find the references relevant to the text. The drawbacks are balanced by the more fluid writing style this approach permits, and by the encouragement it gives the reader to scan the reference lists.

Excellent reading lists are available in many books, including Last's *Dictionary of epidemiology* (with some websites) and Rothman and Greenland's book *Modern epidemiology* (see Chapter 5 reference list).

Happy reading!

Chapter 1
References drawn upon or referred to in text

Alderson, P. (1998) The importance of theories in health care. *BMJ*, **317**, 1007–10.

Bhopal, R.S. (1999) Paradigms in epidemiology textbooks: In the footsteps of Thomas Kuhn. *American Journal of Public Health*, **89**, 1162–5.

Chadwick, J. and Mann, W.N. (1950) *The medical works of Hippocrates*. Blackwell Scientific Publications, Oxford.

Department of Health (1998) *Our healthier nation*. London.

Fraser, D.W., Tsai, T.R., Orenstein, W., Parkin, W.E., Beecham, H.J., Sharrar, R.G., Harris, J., Mallison, G.F., Martin, S.M., McDade, J.E., Shepard, C.C., and Brachman, P.S. (1977) Legionnaires' disease: description of an epidemic of pneumonia. *New England Journal of Medicine*, **297**, 1189–97.

Goldberger, J. (1964) *Goldberger on pellagra*. A collection of Goldberger's papers on pellagra (ed. with an introduction by M. Terris). Louisiana State University Press, Baton Rouge.

Krieger, N. (1994) Epidemiology and the web of causation: has anyone seen the spider? *Social Science and Medicine*, **39**, 887–903.

Kuhn, T.S. (1996) *The structure of scientific revolutions* (3rd edn). The University of Chicago Press, Chicago.

Kuller, L.H. (1999) Invited commentary: circular epidemiology. *American Journal of Epidemiology*, **150**, 897–902.

Last, J.M. (2001) *A dictionary of epidemiology* (4th edn). Oxford University Press, New York.

Marmot, M.G., Adelstein, A.M., and Bulusu, L. (1984) *Immigrant mortality in England and Wales 1970–78*. HMSO, London.

Morris, J.N. (1964) *Uses of epidemiology* (2nd edn). The Williams and Wilkins Company, Baltimore.

Popper, K.R. (1989) *Conjectures and refutations: the growth of scientific knowledge* (5th edn). Routledge, London.

Roe, D. (1973) *A plague of corn: the social history of pellagra*. Cornell University Press, Ithaca.

Senior, P.A. and Bhopal, R.S. (1994) Ethnicity as a variable in epidemiological research. *British Medical Journal*, **309**, 327–30.

Shy, C.H. (1997) The failure of academic epidemiology: witness for the prosecution. *American Journal of Epidemiology*, **145**, 479–84.

Skrabanek, P. (1994) The emptiness of the black box. *Epidemiology*, **5**, 553–5.

Susser, M. (1985) Epidemiology in the United States after World War II: the evolution of technique. *Epidemiologic Reviews*, **7**, 147–77.

Susser, M. and Susser, E. (1996*a*) Choosing a future of epidemiology: I eras and paradigms. *American Journal of Public Health*, **86**, 668–73.

Susser, M. and Susser, E. (1996*b*) Choosing a future for epidemiology: II From black box to Chinese boxes and eco-epidemiology. *American Journal of Public Health*, **86**, 674–7.

Taubes, G. (1995) Epidemiology faces its limits. *Science*, **269**, 164–9.

Other references of interest

Bhopal, R.S. (1997) Which book? A comparative review of 25 introductory epidemiology textbooks. *Journal of Epidemiology and Community Health*, **51**, 612–22.

Goldberger, J. (1914) Considerations on pellagra. *Public Health Reports*, **29**, 1683–6. (Reprinted in Buck *et al.*, 99–102.)

Goldberger, J., Wheeler, G., and Sydenstricker, E. (1920) A study of the relation of family income and other economic factors to pellagra incidence in seven cotton-mill villages of South Carolina in 1916. *Public Health Reports*, **46**, 2673–714. (Reprinted in Buck *et al.*, 584–609.)

Goldberger, J., Waring, C., and Tanner, W.F. (1923) Pellagra prevention by diet among institutional inmates. *Public Health Reports*, **38**, 2361–8. (Reprinted in Buck *et al.*, 726–730.)

Savitz, D.A. (1994) In defence of black box epidemiology. *Epidemiology*, **5**, 550–2.

Walker, A.M. (1997) Kangaroo Court: invited commentary on Shy's The failure of academic epidemiology: witness for the prosecution. *American Journal of Epidemiology*, **145**, 485–6.

Chapter 2

References drawn upon or referred to in text

Christakis, N. and Lamont, E. (2000) Extent and determinants of error in doctors' prognoses in terminally ill patients: prospective cohort study. *British Medical Journal*, **320**, 469–74.

Diamond, J. (1998) *Guns, germs and steel—A short history of everybody for the last 13,000 years*. Vintage, London.

Durkheim, E. (1951) *Suicide: a study in sociology* (trans. J.A. Spalding and G. Simpson) (ed. with an introduction by G. Simpson). Free Press, Illinois. (First published 1897.)

Herbst, A., Ulfelder, H., and Poskanzer, D. (1971) Adenocarcinoma of the vagina: Association of maternal stilbestrol therapy with tumour appearance in young women. *New England Journal of Medicine*, **284**, 878–81.

Kahn, R., Wise, P., Kennedy, B., and Kawachi, I. (2000) State income inequality, household income, and maternal mental and physical health; cross-sectional national survey. *British Medical Journal*, **321**, 1311–15.

Kinlen, L.J., Dickson, M., and Stiller, C.A. (1995) Childhood leukaemia and non-Hodgkin's lymphoma near large rural construction sites, with a comparison with Sellafield nuclear site. *British Medical Journal*, **310**, 763–8.

Lind, J. (1753) *A Treatise of the Scurvy in three parts, containing an inquiry into the nature, causes, and cure of the scurvy*. Excerpted from James Lind, *A Treatise of the Scurvy in Three Parts, Containing an enquiry into the nature, causes and cure of that disease, together with a critical and chronological view of what has been published on the subject*. Sands, Murray and Cochran, Edinburgh, and re-printed in, Buck, C., Llopis, A., Najera, E., and Terris, M. (1988) *The challenge of epidemiology. Issues and selected readings*. pp. 20–23. Pan American Health Organization, Washington DC.

Roe, D. (1973) *A plague of corn: the social history of pellagra*. Cornell University Press, Ithaca.

Rose, G. (1985) Sick individuals and sick populations. *International Journal of Epidemiology*, **14**, 32–8.

Rose, G. (1994) *The strategy of preventive medicine*. Oxford University Press, New York.

US Department of Health and Human Services—Public Health Service (1990) *Healthy People 2000. National health promotion and disease prevention objectives*. Department of Health and Human Services, Washington, DC.

Wilkinson, R. (1997) Health inequalities: relative or absolute material standards? *British Medical Journal*, **314**, 591–5.

Other references of interest

Bland, J. (1990) The population mean predicts the number of deviant individuals. *British Medical Journal*, **301**, 1031–4.

Kogevinas, M. (1998) The loss of the population approach puts epidemiology at risk. *Journal of Epidemiology and Community Health*, **52**, 615–16.

Rose, G. (1987) Environmental factors and disease: the man made environment. *British Medical Journal*, **294**, 963–5.

Rose, G. and Day, S. (1990) The population mean predicts the number of deviant individuals. *British Medical Journal*, **301**, 1031–4.

Walberg, P., McKee, M., Shkolnikov, V., Chenet, L., and Leon, D.A. (1998) Economic change, crime and mortality crisis in Russia: regional analysis. *British Medical Journal*, **317**, 312–18.

Weitoft, G., Haglund, B., and Rosen, M. (2000) Mortality among lone mothers in Sweden: a population study. *Lancet*, **355**, 1215–19.

Chapter 3
References drawn upon or referred to in text

Bhopal, R.S. (1991) A framework for investigating geographical variation in diseases, based on a study of Legionnaires' disease. *Journal of Public Health Medicine*, **13**, 281–9.

Bhopal, R.S., Fallon, R.J., Buist, E.C., Black, R.J., and Urquart, J.D. (1991) Proximity of the home to a cooling tower and the risk of non-outbreak Legionnaires' disease. *British Medical Journal*, **302**, 378–83.

Bhopal, R.S., Diggle, P., and Rowlingson, B. (1992) Pinpointing clusters of apparently sporadic Legionnaires' disease. *British Medical Journal*, **304**, 1022–7.

Fraser, D.W., Tsai, T.R., Orenstein, W., Parkin, W.E., Beecham, H.J., Sharrar, R.G., Harris, J., Mallison, G.F., Martin, S.M., McDade, J.E., Shepard, C.C., and Brachman, P.S. (1977) Legionnaires' disease: description of an epidemic of pneumonia. *New England Journal of Medicine*, **297**, 1189–97.

Gregg, N.M. (1941) Congenital cataract following German measles in the mother. *Transactions of the Ophthalmological Society of Australia*, 3, 35–46. Reprinted in Buck, C., Llopis, A., Najera, E., and Terris, M. (1988) *The challenge of epidemiology. Issues and selected readings.* pp. 426–434. Pan American Health Organization, Washington DC.

Openshaw, S. and Blake, M. (1995) Geodemographic segmentation systems for screening health data. *Journal of Epidemiology and Community Health*, **49**(suppl 2), S34–8.

World Health Organisation (1992) ICD-10: International statistical classification of diseases and related health problems. World Health Organisation, Geneva.

Other references of interest

Olsen, S.F., Martuzzi, M., and Elliott, P. (1996) Cluster analysis and disease mapping—why, when, and how? A step by step guide. *British Medical Journal*, **313**, 863–6.

Chapter 4

References drawn upon or referred to in text

Bhopal, R. (1997) Is research into ethnicity and health racist, unsound, or important science? *British Medical Journal*, **314**, 1751–6.

Bhopal, R.S., Phillimore, P., Moffatt, S., and Foy, C. (1994) Is living near a coking works harmful to health? *Journal of Epidemiology and Community Health*, **48**, 237–47.

Bhopal, R.S., Moffatt, S., Pless-Mulloli, T., Phillimore, P.R., Foy, C., Dunn, C.E., and Tate, J. (1998) Does living near a constellation of petrochemical, steel, and other industries impair health? *Occupational and Environmental Medicine*, **55**, 812–22.

Bhopal, R.S., Tate, J.A., Foy, C., Moffatt, S., and Phillimore, P.R. (1999) Residential proximity to industry and adverse birth outcomes. *Lancet*, **354**, 920.

Gould, S.J. (1984) *The mismeasure of man*. Pelican, London.

Greenland, S. (1980) The effect of misclassification in the presence of covariates. *American Journal of Epidemiology*, **112**, 564–9.

Health Education Authority (1994) *Health and lifestyles: Black and minority ethnic groups in England*. HEA, London.

Jones, J.H. (1993) *Bad blood. The Tuskegee Syphilis Experiment* (2nd edn). Free Press, New York.

Key, T.J., Fraser, G.E., Thorogood, M., Appleby, P.N., Beral, V., Reeves, G., Burr, M.L., Chang-Claude, J., Frentzel-Beyme, R., Kuzma, J.W., Mann, J., and McPherson, K. (1999) Mortality in vegetarians and nonvegetarians: detailed findings from a collaborative analysis of 5 prospective studies. American Journal of Clinical Nutrition, **70**(suppl 3), 516S–24S.

Kuhn, T.S. (1996) *The structure of scientific revolutions* (3rd edn). The University of Chicago Press, Chicago.

Lillie-Blanton, M., Anthony, J.C., and Schuster, C.R. (1993) Probing the meaning of racial/ethnic group comparisons in crack smoking. *Journal of the American Medical Association*, **269**, 993–7.

Moffatt, S., Phillimore, P., Hudson, E., and Downey, D. (2000) 'Impact? What impact?' Epidemiological research findings in the public domain: a case study from North-East England. *Social Science and Medicine*, **51**, 1755–69.

Popper, K.R. (1989) *Conjectures and refutations: the growth of scientific knowledge* (5th edn). Routledge, London.

Rose, G. (1985) Sick individuals and sick populations. *International Journal of Epidemiology,* **14**, 32–8.

Other references of interest

Brusin, S. (1999) The communicable disease surveillance system in the Kosovar refugee camps in the former Yugoslav Republic of Macedonia April–August 1999. *Journal of Epidemiology and Community Health,* **54**, 52–7.

Ecob, R. and Williams, R. (1991) Sampling Asian minorities to assess health and welfare. *Journal of Epidemiology and Community Health,* **45**, 93–101.

Moffatt, S., Mulloli, T.P., Bhopal, R., Foy, C., and Phillimore, P. (2000) An exploration of awareness bias in two environmental epidemiology studies. *Epidemiology,* **11**, 199–208.

Chapter 5

References drawn upon or referred to in text

Beiser, C. (1997) Recent advances: HIV infection–II. *British Medical Journal,* **314**, 579.

Bhopal, R.S. (1992) Smoking and suicide. *Lancet,* **304**, 1095.

Bhopal, R.S., Phillimore, P., Moffatt, S., and Foy, C. (1994) Is living near a coking works harmful to health? *Journal of Epidemiology and Community Health,* **48**, 237–47.

Bradford Hill, A. (1965) The environment and disease: association or causation? *Occupational Medicine,* 295–300.

Chadwick, J. and Mann, W.N. (1950) *The medical works of Hippocrates.* Blackwell Scientific, Oxford.

Charemza, W.W. and Deadman, D.F. (1997) New directions in econometric practice: general to specific modelling, cointegration, and vector autoregression (2nd edn). Elgar, Cheltenham.

Cottingham, J. (1996) *Western philosophy—an anthology.* Blackwell, Oxford.

Doll, R. and Bradford Hill, A. (1956) Lung cancer and other causes of death in relation to smoking. *British Medical Journal,* **2**, 1071–81.

Evans, A. (1978) Causation and disease: a chronological journey. *American Journal of Epidemiology,* **108**, 249–58.

Gould, S.J. (1984) *The mismeasure of man.* Pelican, London.

Herbst, A., Ulfelder, H., and Poskanzer, D. (1971) Adenocarcinoma of the vagina: Association of maternal stilbestrol therapy with tumour appearance in young women. *New England Journal of Medicine,* **284**, 878–81. (Reprinted in Buck *et al.* p. 446–50.)

Hicks, J. (1979) Causality in economics, Blackwell, Oxford, 1–18.

Krieger, N. (1994) Epidemiology and the web of causation: has anyone seen the spider? *Social Science and Medicine,* **39**, 887–903.

Kuhn, T.S. (1996) *The structure of scientific revolutions* (3rd edn). The University of Chicago Press, Chicago.

Mausner, J.S. and Kramer, S. (1985) *Epidemiology* (2nd edn). W.B. Saunders, Philadelphia.

Rothman, K.J. (1986) *Modern epidemiology* (1st edn). Little, Brown, Boston.

Rothman, K.J. and Greenland, S. (1998) *Modern epidemiology.* Lippincott-Raven, Philadelphia.

Semmelweis, I. (1983) *The etiology, concept and prophylaxis of childbed fever.* (Translated by K. Codell Carter). University of Wisconsin, Madison. Excerpted and reprinted in Buck, C., Llopis, A., Najera, E., and Terris, M. (1988) *The challenge of epidemiology. Issues and selected readings.* pp. 46–59. Pan American Health Organization, Washington DC.

Skrabanek, P. (1994) The emptiness of the black box. *Epidemiology*, **5**, 553–5.

Smith, G.D., Phillips, A.N., and Neaton, J.D. (1992) Smoking as 'independent' risk factor for suicide: illustration of an artifact from observational epidemiology? *Lancet*, **340**, 709–12.

Susser, M. (1977) *Causal thinking in the health sciences* (2nd edn). Oxford University Press, New York.

Tesh, S.N. (1988) *Hidden arguments.* Rutgers University Press, New Brunswick.

Other references of interest

Doll, R. (1998) Uncovering the effects of smoking: historical perspective. *Statistical Methods in Medical Research*, **7**, 87–117.

Elwood, J.M. (1992) *Causal relationships in medicine* (2nd edn). Oxford University Press, New York.

Kaufman, J.S. and Cooper, R.S. (1999) Seeking causal explanations in social epidemiology. *American Journal of Epidemiology*, **150**, 113–20.

McPherson, K. (1998) Wider 'causal thinking in the health sciences'. *Journal of Epidemiology and Community Health*, **52**, 612–13.

Renton, A. (1994) Epidemiology and causation: a realist view. *Journal of Epidemiology and Community Health*, **48**, 79–85.

Rigas, J., Feretis, C., and Papavassiliou, E.D. (1999) John Lykoudis: an unappreciated discoverer of the cause and treatment of peptic ulcer disease. *Lancet*, **354**, 1634–5.

Rothman, K.J. (1988) *Causal inference.* Epidemiology Resources Inc., Chestnut Hill, Massachusetts.

Vineis, P. (1997) Proof in observational medicine. *Journal of Epidemiology and Community Health*, **51**, 9–13.

Weed, D. (1997) On the use of causal criteria. *International Journal of Epidemiology*, **26**, 1137–41.

Chapter 6
References drawn upon or referred to in text

Fowkes, F. (1986) Diagnostic vigilance. *Lancet*, **i**, 493–4.

Holland, W. and Stewart, S. (1990) *Screening in health care.* Nuffield Provincial Hospitals Trust, London.

Jones, J.H. (1993) *Bad blood. The Tuskegee Syphilis Experiment* (2nd edn). Free Press, New York.

Last, J. (1963) The iceberg 'completing the clinical picture' in general practice. *Lancet*, **ii**, 28–31.

Last, J.M. (2001) *A dictionary of epidemiology* (4th edn). Oxford University Press, New York.

Raffle, A.E. (2000) Honesty about new screening programmes is best policy. *British Medical Journal*, **320**, 872.

Rothman, K.J. and Greenland, S. (1998) *Modern epidemiology.* Lippincott-Raven, Philadelphia.

Wilson, J.M.G. and Jungner, G. (1968) *Principles and practice of screening for disease.* World Health Organization, Geneva.

Chapter 7
References drawn upon or referred to in text

Bodansky, H.J., Airey, C.M., Chell, S.M., Unwin, N., and Williams, D.R.R. (1997) The incidence of lower limb amputation in Leeds, UK: setting a baseline for St Vincent. International Diabetes Federation Meeting. *Diabetologia*, A1850.

Elandt-Johnson, R. (1975) Definition of rates: Some remarks on their use and misuse. *American Journal of Epidemiology*, **102**, 267–71.

International Working Group for Disease Monitoring and Forecasting (1995*a*) Capture-recapture and multiple-record systems estimation I: History and theoretical development. *American Journal of Epidemiology*, **142**, 1047–58.

International Working Group for Disease Monitoring and Forecasting (1995*b*) Capture-recapture and multiple-record systems estimation II: Applications in human diseases. *American Journal of Epidemiology*, **142**, 1059–68.

Last, J.M. (2001) *A dictionary of epidemiology* (4th edn). Oxford University Press, New York.

Pickles, W.N. (1939) *Epidemiology in country practice*. Wright, Bristol.

Rothman, K.J. and Greenland, S. (1998) *Modern epidemiology*. Lippincott-Raven, Philadelphia.

Unwin, N., Alberti, K.G.M.M., Bhopal, R., Harland, J., Watson, W., and White, M. (1998) Comparison of the current WHO and the new ADA criteria for the diagnosis of diabetes in three ethnic groups in the UK. *Diabetic Medicine*, **15**, 554–7.

Other references of interest

Berlin, A., Bhopal, R.S., Spencer, J.A., and van Zwanenberg, T.D. (1993) Creating a death register for general practice. *British Journal of General Practice*, **43**, 70–2.

Calman, K. (1996) Cancer: science and society and the communication of risk. *British Medical Journal*, **313**, 799–802.

Calman, K. and Royston, G. (1997) Risk language and dialects. *British Medical Journal*, **315**, 939–42.

Choi, B., de Guia, N., and Walsh, P. (1998) Look before you leap stratify before you standardize. *American Journal of Epidemiology*, **149**, 1087–96.

Department of Health (1997) *Communicating about risks to public health: Pointers to good practice*, pp. 1–35. Department of Health, London.

Gottlieb, S. (1999) Updates for US heart disease death rates. *British Medical Journal*, **318**, 79.

Maudsley, G. and Williams, E. (1996) 'Inaccuracy' in death certification—where are we now? *Journal of Public Health Medicine*, **18**, 59–66.

Sonderegger-Iseli, K., Burger, S., Muntwyler, J., and Salomon, F. (2000) Diagnostic errors in three medical eras: a necropsy study. *Lancet*, **355**, 2027–32.

World Health Organisation (1992) *ICD-10: International statistical classification of diseases and related health problems*. World Health Organisation, Geneva.

Chapter 8
References drawn upon or referred to in text

Charlton, J.V.R. (1986) Some international comparisons of mortality amenable to medical intervention. *British Medical Journal*, **292**, 295–301.

Cornfield, J. (1951) A method of estimating comparative rates from clinical data. Applications to cancer of the lung, breast and cervix. *Journal of the National Cancer Institute*, **11**, 1269–1275.

Cornfield, J. and Haenszel, W. (1960) Some aspects of retrospective studies. *Journal of Chronic Disease*, **11**, 523–34.

Doll, R. and Hill, A.B. (1950) Smoking and carcinoma of the lung: preliminary report. *British Medical Journal*, Vol 2, (**September**), 739–748.

Doll, R. and Bradford Hill, A. (1956) Lung cancer and other causes of death in relation to smoking. *British Medical Journal*, **2**, 1071–81.

Herbst, A., Ulfelder, H., and Poskanzer, D. (1971) Adenocarcinoma of the vagina: Association of maternal stilbestrol therapy with tumour appearance in young women. *New England Journal of Medicine*, **284**, 878–81.

Lee, W. (1998) The meaning and use of the cumulative rate of potential life lost. *International Journal of Epidemiology*, **27**, 1053–6.

Mackenbach, J.P., Bouvier-Colle, M.H., and Jougla, E. (1990) 'Avoidable' mortality and health services: a review of aggregate data studies. *Journal of Epidemiological and Community Health*, **44**, 106–11.

Mackintosh, J., Bhopal, R.S., Unwin, N., and Ahmad, N. (1998) *Step-by-step guide to epidemiological health needs assessment for ethnic minority groups*. Department of Epidemiology and Public Health, University of Newcastle upon Tyne, Newcastle upon Tyne. (Available on www.minority health. gov.uk/docs/step_by_step.doc)

Marmot, M.G., Adelstein, A.M., and Bulusu, L. (1984) *Immigrant mortality in England and Wales 1970–78*. HMSO, London.

Mausner, J.S. and Kramer, S. (1985) *Epidemiology* (2nd edn). W.B. Saunders, Philadelphia.

Murray, C.J.L. and Lopez, A.D. (1997) Mortality by cause for eight regions of the world: Global burden of disease study. *Lancet*, **349**, 1269–76.

Pless-Mulloli T., Phillimore, P., Moffatt, S., Bhopal, R., Foy, C., Dunn, C., and Tate, J. (1998) Lung cancer, proximity to industry, and poverty in northeast England. *Environ Health Perspect*, **106**, 189–96.

Roman, E., Beral, V., Inskip, H., McDowall, M., and Adelstein, A.A. (1984) Comparison of standardised proportional mortality ratios. *Statistics in Medicine*, **3**, 7–14.

Other references of interest

Arnesen, T. and Nord, E. (1999) The value of DALY life: problems with ethics and validity of disability adjusted life years. *British Medical Journal*, **319**, 1423–6.

Bartlett, C.J. and Coles, E.C. (1998) Psychological health and well-being: why and how should public health specialists measure it? Part 1: rationale and methods of the investigation, and review of psychiatric epidemiology. *Journal of Public Health Medicine*, **20**, 281–94.

Bland, J. and Altman, D. (2000) The odds ratio. *British Medical Journal*, **320**, 1468.

Cook, R. and Sackett, D. (1995) The number needed to treat: a clinically useful measurement of treatment effect. *British Medical Journal*, **310**, 452–6.

Julious, S., Nicholl, J., and George, S. (2000) Why do we continue to use standardized mortality ratios for small area comparisons? *Journal of Public Health Medicine*, **23**, 39–46.

Rockhill, B., Newman, B., and Weinberg, C. (1998) Use and misuse of population attributable fractions. *American Journal of Public Health*, **88**, 15–19.

Schwartz, L., Woloshin, S., and Welch, H. (1999) Misunderstandings about the effects of race and sex on physicians; referrals for cardiac catherization. *New England Journal of Medicine*, **341**, 279–85.

Silcocks, P.B.S., Jenner, D.A., and Reza, R. (2000) Life expectancy as a summary of mortality in a population: statistical considerations and suitability for use by health authorities. *Journal of Epidemiology and Community Health*, **55**, 38–43.

Vandenbroucke, J. (1989) Statistical modelling: the old standardisation problem in disguise? *Journal of Epidemiology and Community Health*, **43**, 207–8.

Wyatt, J. (1999) Same information, different decisions: format counts. *British Medical Journal*, **318**, 1501–2.

Chapter 9

References drawn upon or referred to in text

Barbenel, J., Jordan, M., Nicol, S., and Clark, M.O. (1977) Incidence of pressure-sores in the Greater Glasgow Health Board area. *Lancet*, **2**, 548–50.

Bhopal, R.S., Moffatt, S., and Pless-Mulloli, T. *et al.* (1998) Does living near a constellation of petrochemical, steel, and other industries impair health? *Occupational and Environmental Medicine*, **55**, 812–22.

Bhopal, R.S., Unwin, N., White, M., Yallop, J., Walker, L., and Alberti, K.G.M.M. *et al.* (1999) Heterogeneity of coronary heart disease risk factors in Indian, Pakistani, Bangladeshi and European origin populations: cross sectional study. *British Medical Journal*, **319**, 215–20.

Harland, J., Unwin, N., Bhopal, R.S., White, M., Watson, B., Laker, M., and Alberti, K.G.M.M. (1997) Low levels of cardiovascular risk factors and coronary heart disease in a UK Chinese population. *Journal of Epidemiology and Community Health*, **51**, 636–42.

Herbst, A., Ulfelder, H., and Poskanzer, D. (1971) Adenocarcinoma of the vagina: Association of maternal stilbestrol therapy with tumour appearance in young women. *New England Journal of Medicine*, **284**, 878–81.

McMahon, B. and Trichopoulos, D. (1996) *Epidemiology* (2nd edn). Little, Brown, Boston.

Pearce, N. (2000) The ecological fallacy strikes back. *Journal of Epidemiology and Community Health*, **54**, 326–7.

Rothman, K.J. and Greenland, S. (1998) *Modern epidemiology*. Lippincott-Raven, Philadelphia.

Other references of interest

Coker, W.J., Bhatt, B.M., Blatchley, N.F., and Graham, J.T. (1999) Clinical findings for the first 1000 Gulf war veterans in the Ministry of Defence's medical assessment programme. *British Medical Journal*, **318**, 290–4.

Concato, J., Shah, N., and Horwitz, R.I. (2000) Randomized, controlled trials, observational studies, and the hierarchy of research designs. *New England Journal of Medicine*, **342**, 1887–92.

Cornfield, J. and Haenszel, W. (1960) Some aspects of retrospective studies. *Journal of Chronic Disease*, **11**, 523–34.

Dawber, T., Kannel, W., and Lyell, L. (1963) An approach to longitudinal studies in a community: The Framingham Study. *Annals New York Academy of Sciences*, **107**, 539–56. (Reprinted in Buck *et al.*, 1988).

Diez-Roux, A. (1998) Bringing context back into epidemiology: variables and fallacies in multilevel analysis. *American Journal of Public Health*, **88**, 1–13.

Uusitalo, U., Feskens, E., Tuomilehto, J., Dowse, G., Haw, U., and Fareed, D. *et al.* (1996) Fall in total cholesterol concentration over five years in association with changes in fatty acid composition of cooking oil in Mauritius: cross sectional survey. *British Medical Journal*, **313**, 1044–6.

Chapter 10

References drawn upon or referred to in text

Action on Smoking and Health UK. Philip Morris Scandal documents show how Philip Morris and its lawyers, Covington and Burling invented and orchestrated controversy around passive smoking by infiltrating highly respected science and policy institution and by buying up scientists. Available from: URL: http://www.ash.org.uk/

Alper, J.S. and Natowicz, M.R. (1992) The allure of genetic explanations. *British Medical Journal*, **305**, 666.

Barnes, D.E. and Bero, L.A. (1998) Why review articles on the health effects of passive smoking reach different conclusions. *Journal of the American Medical Association*, **279**, 1566–70.

Bhopal, R. (1997) Is research into ethnicity and health racist, unsound, or important science? *British Medical Journal*, **314**, 1751–6.

Bhopal, R.S. (1998*a*) Setting priorities for health care in ethnic minority groups. In *Health needs assessment in ethnic minority groups* (ed. S. Rawaf and V. Bahl). Royal College of Physicians, London.

Bhopal, R.S. (1998*b*) The context and role of the American School of Public Health: Implications for the UK. *Journal of Public Health Medicine*, **20**, 144–8.

Bhopal, R.S. (1999) Paradigms in epidemiology textbooks: in the footsteps of Thomas Kuhn. *American Journal of Public Health*, **89**, 1162–5.

Bhopal, R.S. (2000) Race and ethnicity as epidemiological variables. In *Ethnicity and health* (ed. H. Macbeth), pp. 21–40. Taylor and Francis, London.

Bhopal, R.S. (2001) Generating health from the pattern of disease. *Proceedings of the Royal College of Physicians of Edinburgh*, **31**, 293–298.

Bhopal, R.S. and Tonks, A. (1994) The role of letters in reviewing research. *British Medical Journal*, **308**, 1582–3.

Bhopal, R.S., Rankin, J., McColl, E., Thomas, L., Kaner, E., Stacy, R., Pearson, P., Vernon, B., and Rodgers, H. (1997) The vexed question of authorship: views of researchers in a British medical faculty. *British Medical Journal*, **314**, 1009–12.

Bottomley, V. (1993) Priority setting in the NHS. Ch 3 in *Rationing in Action*, p. 25. British Medical Journal, London.

Chadwick, J. and Mann, W.N. (1950) *The medical works of Hippocrates*. Blackwell Scientific, Oxford.

Committee for the Study of the Future of Public Health (Institute of Medicine) (1988) *The future of public health*. National Academy Press, Washington, DC.

Committee of Inquiry (1988) *Public health in England*. HMSO, London.

Down, J.L.H. (1995) Observations on an ethnic classification of idiots (reprinted from *Journal of Mental Science*, 1867). *Mental Retardation*, **3**, 54–6.

Edwards, R. and Bhopal, R. (1999) The covert influence of the tobacco industry on research and publication: a call to arms. *Journal of Epidemiology and Community Health*, **53**, 261–2.

Gamble, V. (1993) A legacy of distrust: African Americans and medical research. *American Journal of Preventive Medicine*, **9**, 35–7.

Herbst, A., Ulfelder, H., and Poskanzer, D. (1971) Adenocarcinoma of the vagina: Association of maternal stilbestrol therapy with tumour appearance in young women. *New England Journal of Medicine*, **284**, 878–81.

Hilts, P.J. (1996) Smokescreen: the truth behind the tobacco industry cover-up. Addison-Wesley, Massachusetts.

Horton, R. (1998) The unmasked carnival of science. *Lancet*, **351**, 688–9.

International Committee of Medical Journal Editors (1997) Uniform requirements for manuscripts submitted to biomedical journals. *Journal of the American Medical Association*, **277**, 927–34.

Jenner, E. (1798) An inquiry in to the causes and effects of the variolae vaccine. Excerpt in *The challenge of Epidemiology. Issues and selected readings* (ed. C. Buck, A. Llopis, E. Najera and M. Terris), pp. 31–2. Pan American Health Organization, Washington DC. (1988)

Jones, J.H. (1993) *Bad blood. The Tuskegee Syphilis Experiment* (2nd edn). Free Press, New York.

Kiple, K.F. and King, V.H. (1981) *Another dimension to the black diaspora.* Cambridge University Press, London.

Krieger, N. (1992) The making of public health data: paradigms, politics, and policy. *Journal of Public Health Policy*, **65**, 412–27.

Krieger, N.D., Rowley, D.L., and Herman, A. (1993) Racism, sexism and social class: implications for studies of health, disease, and wellbeing. *American Journal of Preventive Medicine*, **9**, 82–122.

Kuhn, T.S. (1996) *The Structure of Scientific Revolutions* (3rd edn). The University of Chicago Press. Chicago.

Last, J.M. (1990) Guidelines on ethics for epidemiologists. *International Journal of Epidemiology*, **19**, 226–9.

Lilienfeld, D.E. and Stolley, P.D. (1994) *Foundations of epidemiology* (3rd edn). Oxford University Press, New York.

Lillie-Blanton, M., Anthony, J.C., and Schuster, C.R. (1993) Probing the meaning of racial/ethnic group comparisons in crack smoking. *Journal of the American Medical Association*, **269**, 993–7.

Lind, J. (1753) *A Treatise of the Scurvy in three parts, containing an inquiry into the nature, causes, and cure of the scurvy.* Excerpted from James Lind, *A Treatise of the Scurvy in Three Parts, Containing an enquiry into the nature, causes and cure of that disease, together with a critical and chronological view of what has been published on the subject.* Sands Murray and Cochran, Edinburgh, and re-printed in, Buck, C., Llopis, A., Najera, E. and Terris, M. (1988) *The challenge of epidemiology. Issues and selected readings.* pp 20–23. Pan American Health Organization, Washington DC.

MacMahon, B., Pugh, T.F., and Ipsen, J. (1960) *Epidemiological methods.* J & A Churchill, London.

Marmot, M.G., Adelstein, A.M., and Bulusu, L. (1984) *Immigrant mortality in England and Wales 1970–78.* HMSO, London.

Mausner, J.S. and Kramer, S. (1985) *Epidemiology* (2nd edn). W. B. Saunders Company, Philadelphia.

Morris, J.N. (1964) *Uses of epidemiology* (2nd edn). The Williams and Wilkins Company, Baltimore.

Morrison, T. (1993) *Beloved.* Chatto and Windus, London.

Osborne, N.G. and Feit, M.D. (1992) The use of race in medical research. *Journal of the American Medical Association*, **267**, 275–9.

Pearce, N. (1996) Traditional epidemiology, modern epidemiology, and public health. *American Journal of Public Health*, **86**, 678–83.

Porta, M. and Alvarez-Dardet, C. (1998) Epidemiology: bridges over (and across) roaring levels. *Journal of Epidemiology and Community Health*, **52**, 605.

Porter, R. (1997) *The greatest benefit to mankind: A medical history of humanity from antiquity to the present.* Harper Collins, London.

Reynolds, G. (1993) Foreword. *Annals of Epidemiology*, **3**, 119.

Rothman, K., Adami, H., and Trichopoulos, D. (1998) Should the mission of epidemiology include the eradication of poverty? *Lancet*, **352**, 810–13.

Semmelweis, I. (1983) *The etiology, concept and prophylaxis of childbed fever.* (Translated by K. Codell Carter). University of Wisconsin, Madison. Excerpted and reprinted in Buck, C., Llopis, A., Najera, E., and Terris, M. (1988) *The challenge of epidemiology. Issues and selected readings.* pp. 46–59. Pan American Health Organization, Washington DC.

Skrabanek, P. and McCormick, J. (1992) *Follies and fallacies in medicine* (2nd edn). Tarragon Press, Chippenham, UK.

Smith, A. (1978) The epidemiological basis of community medicine. In *Recent advances in community medicine* (ed. A.E. Bennett). Longman, Edinburgh.

Snow, J. (1949) *The Cholera near Golden Square* (extracted from *Snow on Cholera*, Cambridge, Hybrid University Press.) Reprinted in, Buck, C., Llopis, A., Najera, E. and Terris, M. (1988)

The challenge of epidemiology. Issues and selected readings. pp. 415–418. Pan American Health Organization, Washington DC.

Stoto, M., Abel, C., and Dievler, A. *Healthy communities: New partnerships for the future of public health (Institute of Medicine).* National Academy Press, Washington DC.

Susser, M. (1985) Epidemiology in the United States after World War II: the evolution of technique. *Epidemiologic Reviews,* **7,** 147–177.

Susser, M. (1998) Does risk factor epidemiology put epidemiology at risk? Peering into the future. *Journal of Epidemiology and Community Health,* **52,** 608–11.

US Department of Health and Human Services—Public Health Service (1990) *Healthy People 2000.* National health promotion and disease prevention objectives. Department of Health and Human Services, Washington, DC.

Winkelstein, W. (1996) Editorial: Eras, paradigms, and the future of epidemiology. *American Journal of Public Health,* **86,** 621–2.

Other references of interest

Ashton, J. (ed.) (1994) *The epidemiological imagination. A reader.* Open University Press, Philadelphia.

Barkan, E. (1992) *The retreat of scientific racism.* Cambridge University Press, London.

Beauchamp, T.L. Cook, R.R. Fayerweather, W.E., Raabe, G.K., Thar, W.E., Cowles, S.R., *et al.* (1991) Ethical guidelines for epidemiologists. *Journal of Clinical Epidemiology,* **44,** 151S–169S.

Bhopal, R.S. and Thomson, R.A. (1991) Form to help learn and teach about the assessment of medical audit papers. *British Medical Journal,* **303,** 1520–2.

Blettner, M., Sauerbrei, W., Schlehofer, B., and Scheuchenpflug, T. (1999) Traditional reviews, meta-analyses and pooled analyses in epidemiology. *International Journal of Epidemiology,* **28,** 1–9.

Blettner, M., Heuer, C., and Reeder, R.C. (2000) Critical reading of epidemiological papers. *European Journal of Public Health,* **11,** 97–101.

Bobrow, M. and Grimbaldeston, A. (2000) Medical genetics, the human genome project and public health. *Journal of Epidemiology and Community Health,* **54,** 645–9.

Bonneux, L., Barendregt, J., and Van der Maas, P. (1998) The expiry date of man: a synthesis of evolutionary biology and public health. *Journal of Epidemiology and Community Health,* **52,** 619–23.

Brown, P. (1992) Popular epidemiology and toxic waste contamination: Lay and professional ways of knowing. *Journal of Health and Social Behaviour,* **33,** 267–81.

Colditz, G. (1997) Epidemiology—future directions. *International Journal of Epidemiology,* **26,** 693–7.

Cooper, R. (1984) A note on the biological concept of race and its application in epidemiological research. *American Heart Journal,* **108,** 715–23.

Day, R.A. (1994) *How to write and publish a scientific paper* (4th edn). Oryx, Phoenix.

Greenland, S. (ed.) (1987) *Evolution of epidemiologic ideas: Annotated readings on concepts and methods.* Epidemiology Resources Inc, Massachusetts.

Huth, E.J. (1990) *How to write and publish papers in the medical sciences* (2nd edn). Williams and Wilkins, Baltimore.

Saracci, R. (1997) The World Health Organization needs to reconsider its definition of health. *British Medical Journal,* **314,** 1409–10.

Stepan, N. (1982) *The idea of race in science.* MacMillan Press, London.

Terris, M. (1978) Epidemiology as a basic science in the education of health professionals. *International Journal of Epidemiology*, 7, 294–6.

Weed, D.L. and McKeown, R.E. (1998) Epidemiology and virtue ethics. *International Journal of Epidemiology*, 27, 343–9.

Wright, J., Williams, R., and Wilkinson, J. (1998) Development and importance of health needs assessment. *British Medical Journal*, 316, 1310–14.

Index

page numbers in **bold** refer to figures and tables

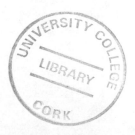